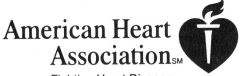

American Heart
Association℠

*Fighting Heart Disease
and Stroke*

Monograph Series

PULMONARY
EDEMA

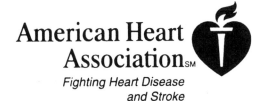

American Heart Association℠

Fighting Heart Disease and Stroke

Monograph Series

PULMONARY EDEMA

Edited by

E. Kenneth Weir, MD

*Professor of Medicine,
VA Medical Center and
University of Minnesota
Minneapolis, MN*

and

John T. Reeves, MD

*Professor Emeritus,
Pediatrics and Medicine,
University of Colorado
Denver, CO*

Futura Publishing
Company, Inc.
Armonk, NY

Copyright © 1998
Futura Publishing Company, Inc.

Published by
Futura Publishing Company
135 Bedford Road
Armonk, New York 10504

Library of Congress Cataloging-in-Publication Data

Pulmonary edema / edited by E. Kenneth Weir and John T. Reeves.
     p.   cm. — (American Heart Association monograph series)
    Includes bibliographical references and index.
    ISBN 0-87993-689-4
    1. Pulmonary edema.   I. Weir, E. Kenneth.   II. Reeves, John T.
III. Series.
    [DNLM: 1. Pulmonary Edema—physiopathology.   2. Extravascu-
lar Lung Water.   3. Water-Electrolyte Balance.   WF 600 P98343028
1998]
    RC776.P8P842   1998
    616.2'4—dc21
    DNLM/DLC
    for Library of Congress   97-34820
                                           CIP

LC #: 97-34820
ISBN #: 0-87993-6894

Foreword

It's been nearly 20 years since I edited the first multiauthor research book on pulmonary edema.[1] Since then, I have seen or participated in many advances in our understanding of the normal regulation of lung liquid and protein exchange, and of the pathophysiology of pulmonary edema. However, although we know a great deal and have improved the treatment of pulmonary edema, especially in association with acute lung injury, there is still much to be learned. For example, we have little insight into how the lung's microvascular endothelium "knows" how tightly to make the intercellular junctions normally. We have no explanation as to why the pulmonary microvascular barrier is not sensitive to histamine, whereas the nearby bronchial venular barrier (a systemic circulation) is.

As we approach the third millennium of the current era (January 1, 2001), I applaud the editors for bringing their concept for this book to fruition; namely, to bring together a summary of where research on lung liquid exchange stands and where new ideas and new technologies may lead us over the next decade.

When Ken Weir asked me to participate in the planning group, I almost refused. I was approaching retirement and was not sure I could contribute in a useful manner. That's a lie, of course—I was just lazy and didn't want to get involved. He assured me that I wouldn't have to write anything, such as a chapter on the history of pulmonary edema, which I had recently done anyway.[2] So, here I am writing a *Foreword* in spite of myself. I proposed a set of themes, which I hoped would help us avoid narrow authoritarianism, chauvinism, and sectarianism, some of the oldest and cheifest sins among scientists. I wanted the several themes to be open-ended, so as to promote broad participation. Dr. Weir and his coeditor accepted many of my suggestions, then they asked for specific topics and authors from several advisors. In this way they obtained a broad working list of most of those actively engaged in investigations related to lung liquid and protein exchange.

Interestingly, no one who contributed a chapter in my 1978 book participated in this one, with the exception of Professor Aubrey E. Taylor, who helped with the planning. I think that is a real advance; so often we see the same authors repeating themselves again and again in books—part of the authoritarianism I mentioned earlier—which seriously detracts from bringing out new thinking and new investigators with new directions if research. There, I wrote that last sentence without using the central word of molecular biology, "novel."

When research books are planned, the editors sometimes fail to include authors whose investigations appear at first glance not to be directly related to the central topic. This, of course, is a failure of the planning process. There are no such limitations in this book because the editors wisely sought broad input. Unfortunately, not every actively creative investigator is included, and for that I am sorry; some could not participate, one or two were overlooked, and space limitations forced the editors to make choices.

When I got into the pulmonary edema business in about 1962, granting agencies did not include pulmonary edema as a research category; neither did the *Index Medicus*. Few regarded pulmonary edema as anything more than an annoying, sometimes fatal, complication of heart failure.[2] Later, as the awake sheep chronic lung lymph fistula model became available, pulmonary edema rapidly accelerated.[3,4] In the 1970s and early 1980s, physiological and pathophysiological advances in lung liquid and protein exchange came fast and furious.[5-8] As with other areas of endeavor, research along whole animal physiological lines eventually reached a plateau.

Now, cellular and molecular physiology offer opportunities for another period of research growth. Eventually, the combination of whole animal physiology and biotechnology will raise our understanding of the edema process to new heights. Whether that expectation will come true concerned me greatly during the planning of the book; but I worried needlessly. Without direction from authority, the various authors made many of the combinations I had dreamed about.

Beginning with comparative physiology and a variety of animal models including the newborn, there are chapters related to liquid flow within the lung and its reabsorption from the alveoli, several chapters describing activity within microvascular endothelial cells, hydrostatic pressure effects (central to any discussion of pulmonary edema), the still vexing problem of increased leakiness of the alveolar-capillary barrier, and the possible interactions with particular barrier molecules (the barriers we so glibly describe are living, organized communities of cells and matrix), and finally, therapeutic approaches to the edema associated with lung injury (almost unknown 30 years ago).

Scientists are always seeking new territories for investigation. There is a general human law called the Pareto Principle. Applied to biological research, it states that 80% of advances are made by 20% of the scientists. Unfortunately, deciding who the 20% are ahead of time (a priori) has proven disastrous. A way around some of the disasters that have plagued biotechnology in the last decade would be to invoke the Comroe Principle (the long-held view of my mentor), that shows clearly that discovery cannot be planned.[9] The efficient way to foster research discovery, he believed, is to find active and productive biologists, give them a place to work and money to do research, leave them alone, and some of them (20%) will discover important things. That view goes against the grain of every government apologist. Remember how the war on cancer was won?

One of the beneficial effects of this book is that it will act as a stimulus for new young scientists to think about and then investigate lung liquid and protein exchange. What better testimonial does a book need!

NORMAN C. STAUB SR., MD
Professor of Physiology Emeritus
University of California, San Francisco
July 21, 1997

References

1. Staub NC (ed): Lung water solute exchange. In: *Lung Biology in Health and Disease.* vol 7. New York: M. Dekker; 1978.
2. Staub NC. Lung liquid and solute exchange. In: West JB (ed): *Respiratory Physiology: People and Ideas.* London: Oxford University Press; 1996;108–139.
3. Staub NC. The pathophysiology of pulmonary edema. *Hum Pathol* 1970;1:419–432.
4. Staub NC. Steady-state transvascular water filtration in unanesthetized sheep. *Circ Res* 1971;28/29(suppl 1):135–139.
5. Brigham KL, Woolverton WC, Blake LH, Staub NC. Increased sheep lung vascular permeability caused by Pseudomonas bacteremia. *J Clin Invest* 1974;54:792–804.
6. Erdmann AJ III, Brigham KL, Woolverton WC, Staub NC. Effect of increased vascular pressure on lung fluid balance. *Circ Res* 1975;37:271–284.
7. Bland R, Demling R, Selinger S, Staub NC. Effects of alveolar hypoxia on lung fluid and protein transport in unanesthetized sheep. *Circ Res* 1977;40:269–274.
8. Matthay MA, Landolt CC, Staub NC. Differential liquid and protein clearance from the alveoli of anesthetized sheep. *J Appl Physiol* 1982;53:96–104.
9. Dripps RD, Comroe JH Jr. Scientific basis for the support of biomedical science. *Science* 1976;192(4235):105–111.

Contributors

Steven Abman, MD   Department of Pediatrics, University of Colorado Health Science Center, Denver, CO

Jenny Allard, BS   Pulmonary Hypertension Center, University of Colorado Health Science Center, Denver, CO

Hans Bachofen, MD   Professor of Medicine, Division of Pneumology, Department of Medicine, University of Berne, Switzerland

Gordon R. Bernard, MD   Professor of Medicine and Director of Medical Intensive Care, Division of Allergy, Pulmonary, and Critical Care Medicine, Vanderbilt University School of Medicine, Nashville, TN

Yves Berthiaume, MD, MSc Associate Professor of Medicine, Centre for Research, Hôtel-Dieu de Montréal and Department of Medicine, Université de Montréal, Montréal, Québec, Canada

Peter B. Bitterman, MD   Professor of Medicine, Department of Medicine, Pulmonary and Critical Care Division, University of Minnesota Medical School, Minneapolis, MN

Rena Bizios, PhD   Professor, Department of Biomedical Engineering, Rensselaer Polytechnic Institute, Troy, NY

Ellen C. Breen, PhD   Assistant Research Biologist, Department of Medicine, University of California, San Diego, La Jolla, CA

Edward D. Crandall, PhD, MD   Hastings Professor of Medicine, Will Rogers Institute Pulmonary Research Center, Chief, Division of Pulmonary and Critical Care Medicine, Chairman, Department of Medicine, University of Southern California, Los Angeles, CA

Nicholas P. Curzen, PhD, MRCP   MRC Training Fellow in Critical Care/Cardiology, Unit of Critical Care, Royal Brompton Hospital, London, United Kingdom

Doloretta D. Dawicki, PhD   Assistant Professor of Medicine, Providence VA Medical Center, Brown University School of Medicine, Providence, RI

Claire M. Doerschuk, MD   Associate Professor, Department of Environmental Health, Harvard University School of Public Health, Boston, MA

Nicholas A. Doyle, MS   Graduate Student, Indiana University School of Medicine, Indianapolis, IN

Timothy W. Evans, BSc, MD, FRCP, PhD, EDICM   Professor of Intensive Care Medicine, Unit of Critical Care, Royal Brompton Hospital, London, United Kingdom

K. Falke, MD Professor, Klinik fur Anaesthesiologie und Operative Intensivmedizin, Universitatsklinikum Rudolf Virchow, Berlin, Germany

Candice D. Fike, MD   Associate Professor, Department of Pediatrics, Medical College of Wisconsin, Children's Hospital of Wisconsin, Milwaukee, WI

Joe G.N. Garcia, MD   Dr. Calvin H. English Professor of Medicine, Professor of Physiology and Biophysics, Indiana University School of Medicine, Indianapolis, IN

Mary E. Gerritsen, PhD   Principal Staff Scientist, Institute of Bone and Joint Disorders and Cancer, Bayer Corporation, West Haven CT

Lydia I. Gilbert-McClain, MD   Pulmonary Fellow, Indiana University School of Medicine, Indianapolis, IN

Simeon E. Goldblum, MD   Professor of Medicine, Division of Infectious Diseases, Department of Medicine, VA Maryland Health Care System, University of Maryland School of Medicine, Baltimore, MD

Casilda I. Hermo, MD   Center for Lung Research, Vanderbilt University Medical Center, Assistant Professor of Pediatric Cardiology, Meharry Medical College, Nashville, TN

Alan H. Jobe, MD, PhD   Professor of Pediatrics, Division of Pulmonary Biology, Children's Hospital Medical Center, Cincinnati, OH

Pavel L. Khimenko, MD, PhD　　Instructor, Department of Physiology, University of South Alabama College of Medicine, Mobile, AL

Hiroshi Kubo, MD, PhD　　Research Fellow, Physiology Program, Department of Environmental Health, Harvard University School of Public Health, Boston, MA

Gregory J. Kutkoski, BS　　Research Assistant, Physiology Program, Department of Environmental Health, Harvard University School of Public Health, Boston, MA

Stephen J. Lai-Fook, PhD　　Professor, Center for Biomedical Engineering, Wenner-Green Research Laboratory, University of Kentucky, Lexington, KY

Laura L. Likar, MD　　Pulmonary/Critical Care Post-Doctoral Fellow, Providence VA Medical Center, Brown University School of Medicine, Providence, RI

Richard L. Lubman, MD　　Assistant Professor of Medicine, Will Rogers Institute Pulmonary Research Center, Division of Pulmonary and Critical Care Medicine, University of Southern California, Los Angeles, CA

Hazel Lum, PhD　　Assistant Professor of Pharmacology, Department of Pharmacology, College of Medicine, University of Illinois at Chicago, Chicago, IL

Robert J. Mangialardi, MD　　Fellow in Pulmonary and Critical Care Medicine, Division of Allergy, Pulmonary, and Critical Care Medicine, Vanderbilt University School of Medicine, Nashville, TN

Odile Mathieu-Costello, PhD　　Professor, Department of Medicine, University of California, San Diego, La Jolla, CA

Barbara Meyrick, PhD　　Professor of Pathology and Medicine, Vanderbilt University Medical Center, Nashville, TN

Giuseppe Miserocchi, MD　　Professor of Physiology, Instituto di Fisiologia Umana, Università degli Studi, Milano, Italy

Timothy M. Moore, PhD　　American Heart Association Alabama Affiliate Research Fellow, Department of Pharmacology, University of South Alabama, Mobile, AL

Hideaki Motosugi, MD, PhD   Research Fellow, Indiana University School of Medicine, Indianapolis, IN

Alan B. Moy, MD   Assistant Professor of Medicine and Biomedical Engineering, University of Iowa, Iowa City, IA

John H. Newman, MD   Chief of Medical Service, Department of Veteran's Affairs Medical Center, Professor of Medicine, Vanderbilt University School of Medicine, Nashville, TN

Annie Lin Parker, MD   Assistant Professor of Medicine, Providence VA Medical Center, Brown University School of Medicine, Providence, RI

Vitaly Polunovsky, PhD   Assistant Research Professor of Medicine, Department of Medicine, Pulmonary and Critical Care Division, University of Minnesota Medical School, Minneapolis, MN

William M. Quinlan, BA   Research Assistant, Indiana University School of Medicine, Indianapolis, IN

J. Usha Raj, MD   Professor of Pediatrics, University of California Los Angeles School of Medicine, Department of Pediatrics, Harbor-UCLA Medical Center, Torrance, CA

R. Rossaint MD,   Professor, Chairman, Klinik für Anäesthesiologie, Universitatätsklinikum-Rheinisch—Westfäliche Technische Hochschule Aachen, Aachen, Germany

Sharon Rounds, MD   Professor of Medicine, Providence VA Medical Center, Brown University School of Medicine, Providence, RI

Jan E. Schnitzer, MD   Associate Professor of Pathology, Department of Pathology, Harvard Medical School, Beth Israel Hospital, Boston, MA

Eric A Schwartz, BS   Doctoral Degree Candidate, Department of Biomedical Engineering, Rensselaer Polytechnic Institute, Troy, NY

D. Michael Shasby, MD   Professor of Medicine, Division of Pulmonary, Critical Care, and Occupational Medicine, Department of Internal Medicine, University of Iowa College of Medicine, Iowa City, IA

Alan W. Smits, PhD   Associate Professor, Department of Biology, Quinnipiac College, Hamden, CT

Aubrey E. Taylor, PhD   Professor and Chairman, Department of Physiology, University of South Alabama College of Medicine, Mobile, AL

Norbert F. Voelkel, MD   Professor of Medicine, Pulmonary Sciences and Critical Care Medicine, University of Colorado Health Sciences Center, Denver, CO

E.R. Weibel, MD   Professor and Chairman, Department of Anatomy, University of Berne, Maurice E. Müller Foundation, Switzerland

John B. West, MD, PhD, DSc   Professor of Medicine and Physiology, Department of Medicine and Physiology, University of California, San Diego, La Jolla, CA

Contents

SECTION III
Increased Permeability and Pulmonary Edema

SECTION IV
Treatment of Pulmonary Edema

The Physiology of Lung Fluid Balance

Chapter 1

Fluid Balance in Vertebrate Lungs:
Are All Lungs "Dry"?

Allan W. Smits, PhD

Introduction

In the normal nondiseased state, mammalian lungs have been repeatedly described as being "dry" with respect to fluid balance; presumably, this refers to the small amount of fluid that is retained by the lung interstitium during its dynamic perfusion by the entire cardiac output. Implied with this dry status is that gas exchange, by a reduction in air-blood diffusion distances, is maximized. The bases for this dry status reside in mechanisms that closely balance transcapillary pressures, a comparatively high resistance to membrane fluid flux, and an effective pulmonary lymphatic system (see reviews by Staub[1] and Taylor and Rippe[2]).

While comparatively little research has been applied to lung fluid balance in nonmammalian vertebrates, sufficiently different patterns of transcapillary fluid dynamics have emerged to cause us to question whether the dry lung is a phenomenon representative of all air-breathing vertebrates. Net filtration fluxes in lungs of amphibians and reptiles appear so enormous that suggestions of a vertebrate "wet" lung are prevalent, albeit largely untested. This brief chapter reviews the evidence for and the probable basis for high pulmonary filtration rates in lower vertebrates, and addresses whether the filtration bias seen in these species supports the notion of a wet lung.

Evidence of High Transcapillary Filtration in Lungs

The first suggestion that fluid balance in lower vertebrate lungs might differ from those of mammals came in 1982 with a study by

From: Weir EK, Reeves JT (eds). *Pulmonary Edema.* Armonk, NY: Futura Publishing Company, Inc.; ©1998.

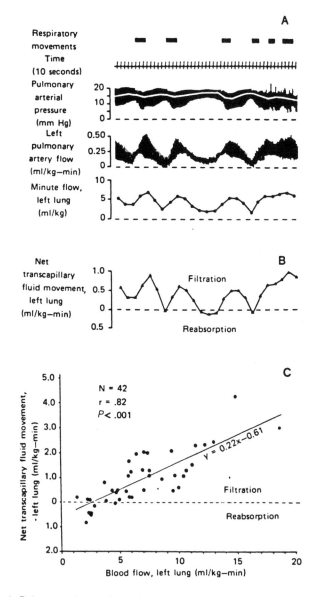

Figure 1. Pulmonary hemodynamics and respiratory movements (A) in a 1 kg aquatic turtle (*Chrysemys scripta*) during normal intermittent breathing, and concurrent changes in net transcapillary fluid flux in the lungs (B). Panel C represents a correlation plot of net transcapillary fluid flux and pulmonary blood flow from 42 measurements. From Reference 3.

Burggren.[3] Using the concentration of erythrocytes in blood samples drawn simultaneously from pulmonary arterial and venous sites as indicators of net transcapillary exchange, Burggren showed that conscious turtles (*Chrysemys scripta*) possessed enormous rates of pulmonary filtration (Figure 1). Large increases in pulmonary perfusion during breathing (a common reflex in diving lower vertebrates) resulted in as much as 20% to 30% of the fluid that enters the lung being filtered out of the pulmonary circulation (Figure 1, panels A and B). Sharp reductions in pulmonary blood flow during diving (apnea) reduced the rate of filtration to minimum levels, and occasionally initiated net pulmonary absorption (Figure 1, panel B). Mean pulmonary arterial pressure actually fell during the breathing events and associated lung hyperperfusion (Figure 1, panel A), indicating a dramatic fall in pulmonary vascular resistance. Thus, the net transcapillary filtration was best correlated with lung blood flow rather than lung blood pressure (Figure 1, panel C). The size and duration of this filtration bias led Burggren to suggest a wet lung syndrome in these and, potentially, in other lower vertebrates.

Supporting evidence for comparatively high net filtration in lower vertebrates came shortly thereafter from Smits et al,[4] who reported on lung fluid dynamics in a dramatically different species, the marine toad (*Bufo marinus*). Using a technique similar to that of Burggren, Smits et al not only showed a comparable degree of net filtration in this amphibian, but by manipulation of the lung hemodynamics by denervating baroreceptor afferents, they correlated lung fluid filtration best (among 11 cardiovascular variables measured) with pulmonary blood flow (as with the turtle). In response, Smits et al suggested that the flow-related changes in net pulmonary filtration might best be explained by

Table 1.

Pulmonary Filtration Rates of Vertebrate Species[a]

Species	ml·min^{-1}	ml·h^{-1}·kg^{-1}	Reference
Toad (*Bufo marinus*) conscious, at rest temp=20–22°C	0.21	43.8	Smits et al (1986)[4]
Toad (*Bufo marinus*) conscious, bilateral denerv. of pulmocut baroreceptors	2.24	466.2	Smits et al (1986)[4]

Table 1.   Continued

Species	ml·min^{-1}	ml·h^{-1}·kg^{-1}	Reference
Iguana lizard (*Sauromalus hispidus*) BM=0.55 kg, temp.=22–25°C; conscious, at rest	0.87	94.9	Smits and Burggren (Unpublished)
Varanid lizard (*Varanus exanthematicus*) BM=1.75 kg; temp.=22°C; conscious at rest	0.22	7.5	Smits and Burggren (Unpublished)
Pond turtle (*Chrysemys scripta*) BM=1.0 kg; temp.=22–23°C; conscious, volunt. diving	0–2.0[b]	0–120.0[b]	Burggren (1982)[3]
Dog BM=22 kg; temp.=37°C; anesthet., closed chest; spontan. breathing	0.043	0.12	Courtice (1951, 1963)[30,31]
Cat BM=22 kg; temp.=37°C; anesthet., closed chest; spontan. breathing	0.009	0.13	Courtice (1963)[31]
Rat BM=0.3 kg; temp.=37°C; anesthet.; closed chest; spontan. breathing	0.002	0.33	Schooley (1958)[32]
Rabbit BM=2.5 kg; temp.=37°C; anesthet., closed chest; spontan. breathing	0.005	0.12	Hughes et al (1956)[33]
Sheep BM=50 kg; temp.=37°C; anesthet., closed chest; spontan. Breathing	0.093	0.11	Boston et al (1965)[34]
Sheep BM=35 kg; temp.=37°C; conscious	0.13	0.18	Brigham et al (1974)[35]
Human BM=70kg	0.09–0.18	0.07–0.14	Blake (1978)[36]

[a]Values for mammalian species were calculated from Staub (1974).[1]
[b]Minimum and maximum values were during apnea (diving) and breathing.
BM = body mass.

increases in capillary recruitment. Smits and Burggren subsequently extended these measurements of pulmonary filtration to two other species of lower vertebrates (an iguanid lizard and varanid lizard), which supported the initial studies in absolute and mass-corrected amounts (Table 1), and illustrated the disparity between fluid flux in amphibian and reptile lungs and in those of mammals.[5]

Basis for High Filtration in Lower Vertebrates

Based on the current understanding of fluid dynamics of the microcirculation in vertebrate animals, it must be concluded that the high filtration bias observed above results from a gross imbalance of the transcapillary forces, that lower vertebrate lung capillaries are comparatively "leaky," or both.

No published accounts of all transcapillary pressures in lower vertebrate lungs exist. Further, the available literature on capillary hydraulic conductivity in lower vertebrates (which is extensive) is exclusively for nonlung capillaries (skeletal muscle, mesenteric). Therefore, the clear-cut evidence for either possibility (mismatch of transcapillary forces and/or "leaky" capillaries) is currently lacking, and can only be surmised by a number of inferences.

Loss of large volumes of circulating body fluids in amphibians and reptiles is not a new discovery, and is best documented in the early works by Conklin,[6] Danielli,[7] and Isayama[8] that suggest incredibly high rates of plasma turnover under a variety of hemodynamic conditions. More recent studies[9-11] confirm these high rates of plasma turnover—primarily those studies that demonstrate rapid onsets of hypovolemia in amphibians when the lymphatic system (including lymph hearts) is compromised. Hemorrhage studies, used as tools to test for shifts in body fluid compartments, have consistently shown an incredible mobility of extravascular fluid recruitment from a comparatively large extracellular fluid space in reptiles.[12-14] In turtles, an excess of 100% of the initial blood volume could be removed without a significant loss of cardiovascular integrity,[13] owing to an extremely rapid transcapillary absorption rate. Systemic fluid shifts in reptiles are also well documented in response to systemic arterial hypertension, as up to 20% of the blood volume is transiently lost from the circulation during mild exercise in two snake species.[15] The extent to which the lung capillaries contribute to this whole-body lability in blood volume is unclear. However, it is interesting that the capillary filtration coefficient (CFC) for skeletal muscle microcirculation, which is typically lower than that of lungs in mammals,[2] is nearly 10 times higher in the toad hindquarters than that measured in mammalian skeletal muscle.[16] If capillaries of lower vertebrate lungs are "leakier" than their skeletal muscle capillaries, the high rates of pulmonary transcapillary filtration documented above may indeed relate largely to the structure of the capillaries.

The other basis for comparatively high pulmonary filtration in lower vertebrates is a mismatch among the transcapillary pressures. The two dominant pressures that are most easily measured, and thus deserve immediate attention, are capillary hydrostatic and capillary oncotic pressures. Maloney and Castle[17] made direct measurements (servo-null micropipets) of intravascular pressures on both sides of the pulmonary capillary bed in the frog (*Rana catesbeiana*) at a variety of perfusion pressures (Figure 2). Using their data combined with the typical mean pulmonary arterial pressure of conscious frogs (20 to 25 mm Hg),[18] the mean arteriolar (approximately 10 mm Hg) and venular (approximately 8 mm Hg) pressures would closely match capillary pressures observed in mammal lungs.[19,20] This estimate of capillary pressure (8 to 10 mm Hg) agrees well with estimates of capillary pressure made by pulmonary arterial wedge (7 to 8 mm Hg; Smits AW, and West NH, unpublished data, July, 1985) and both arteriolar micropipet measurements (8 to 10 mm Hg) and double occlusion studies (10 to 12 mm

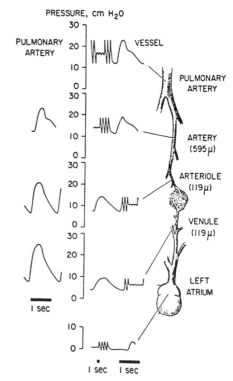

Figure 2. Dynamic intravascular pressures measured across the pulmonary vascular hierarchy of the bullfrog (*Rana catesbeiana*), using servo-null micropipets. Simultaneously measured pressures in the pulmonary artery are illustrated on the left side of the figure. From Reference 17.

Hg) performed by Smits (unpublished data, August, 1992). These data, which support the idea that pulmonary capillary pressures are not unusually high, must be viewed cautiously, especially in lower vertebrates. Due to the incompletely divided ventricle of most amphibians and reptiles, systemic and pulmonary circuits are perfused in parallel, leading to the possibility of elevated capillary pressures during increased cardiac output (see review by Johansen and Burggren).[21] An extensive autonomic innervation of the heart and pulmonary vasculature coordinates lung perfusion in concert with lung ventilation, resulting in highly variable pulmonary arterial pressures as well.[22–24] Thus, the available literature suggesting a similarity in pulmonary capillary pressures between mammals and other vertebrates, which was derived from anesthetized animals, is tenuous at best. The only datum that experimentally suggests a minor to nonexistent role of capillary hydrostatic pressure as a basis for high pulmonary filtration rates is that of Smits et al,[4] in which pulmonary arterial afferent nerves (baroreceptors) were severed to stimulate elevated lung perfusion and pulmonary arterial pressure. Immediately following baroreceptor denervation, high rates of pulmonary filtration were observed in the toad in response to peak elevations in lung blood pressure and flow (Figure 3).

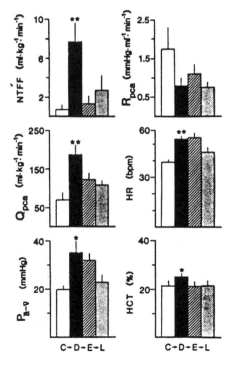

Figure 3. Mean changes (± 1 SE) in six cardiovascular variables measured in marine toads (*Bufo marinus*) during control, normotensive periods (C), 5 minutes following bilateral rLN denervation (D), and during early (E) and late (L) postdenervation 0.5 and 1.5 hour following denervation, respectively. Variables are pulmonary net transcapillary fluid flux (NTFF), pulmocutaneous arterial flow (Q_{pca}), mean driving pressure across the lung (P_{a-v}), pulmonary vascular resistance (R_{pca}), heart rate (HR), and pulmocutaneous arterial hematocrit (HCT). Levels of significance are indicated by *($P<0.05$) and **($P<0.01$). From Reference 4.

As time progressed, pulmonary arterial pressures returned toward normal levels, but both lung blood flow and high capillary filtration persisted. Because capillary filtration did not decrease proportionally with pulmonary arterial pressure, the authors proposed that pulmonary filtration is more flow-dependent than pressure-dependent in this amphibian lung.[4]

Although the evidence for the role of capillary hydrostatic pressure in lower vertebrate pulmonary fluid balance is less than resolved, there is a much clearer picture of how the plasma oncotic pressure opposes filtration. Following an extensive review of measured plasma oncotic pressure in vertebrates (Figure 4), it is obvious that all nonmammalian species (including birds) appear to have lower capacities for colloid-dependent capillary absorption. According to these data, lower vertebrates possess oncotic pressures that are approximately equal to the estimated capillary hydrostatic pressures (8 to 10 mm Hg). If, like

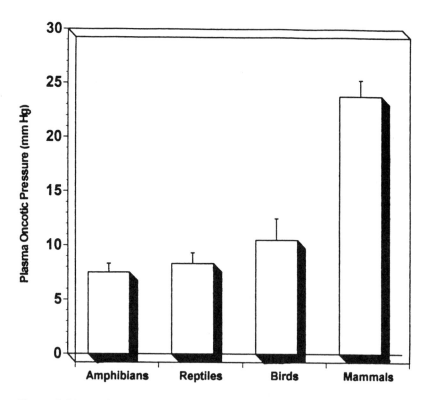

Figure 4. Mean plasma colloid osmotic pressures (±1 SE) recorded for four vertebrate classes. Literature-based information included species and samples (N, n) for mammals (56,58), birds (3,3), reptiles (8,8) and amphibians (5,12). From Reference 5.

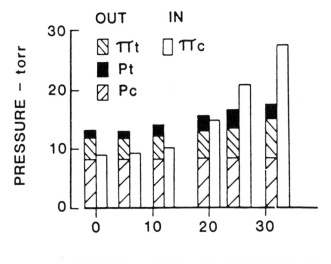

Figure 5. Summary of transcapillary forces in the integument of the toad (*Bufo marinus*) at various stages of dehydration. Note that the outward forces (favoring filtration) are not balanced by inward forces (favoring absorption) until body water loss exceeds 20% of the original body mass. From Reference 25.

mammals, lower vertebrates possess interstitial hydrostatic and oncotic pressures that favor transcapillary filtration, the likelihood for a mismatch of the pulmonary transcapillary forces is clear. Hillman et al[25] have documented strong evidence for a transcapillary pressure mismatch in the integument of the toad (*Bufo marinus*) and frog (*Rana catesbeiana*), where an estimation of all four capillary pressures revealed a clear filtration bias of 4 to 5 mm Hg (Figure 5). Because their value for capillary hydrostatic pressure was based on central venous pressure, the net transcapillary pressure gradient was probably underestimated by several mm Hg. If the lungs share similar transcapillary pressures with those of the integument, the inherently low plasma oncotic pressure, evident in all lower vertebrates, represents a likely basis for the comparatively high pulmonary filtration.

Evidence Against a Wet Lung

Given the extremely high rates of pulmonary filtration that have been documented in lower vertebrates, it is perhaps tempting to assume that "wet lungs," in the form of interstitial or alveolar fluid accumulation, result. After all, transcapillary filtration in turtle lungs alone, after applying mammalian rates of lymphatic return, would reduce the turtle's blood volume by 70% in 1 hour![5] Such a net flow of filtrate into lung tissue might be expected to 1) substantially increase the resting proportion of extravascular lung water, 2) result in certain edema when pulmonary hypertension occurs, and 3) lower the capacity for gas exchange due to greater diffusion distances. However, none of these expectations are borne out by the available literature.

First, the most sensitive expression of lung water, the ratio between extravascular lung water (ELW) and dry, blood-free lung mass (LM $_{dry}$) is surprisingly similar between mammals lungs (ELW/LM $_{dry}$ = 4.0 in sheep, 3.7 in dogs),[1] and lungs of toads (ELW/LM$_{dry}$ = 4.3),[26] despite major differences in lung design and function. Birds, which might also be suspect of possessing wet lungs due to their low plasma colloid osmotic pressures (see Figure 4), appear to have dramatically "drier" lungs than mammals, as demonstrated by Weidner in the domestic fowl (ELW/LM$_{dry}$ = 2.1).[27] Thus, based strictly on the extravascular pool of lung water, there is no obvious sign of filtration-based fluid accumulation in either lower vertebrates or birds.

Second, no qualitative or quantitative signs of edema were observed by Smits[26] in toad lungs when extremely high rates of pulmonary flow, pressure, and capillary filtration were experimentally induced. Bilateral sectioning of recurrent laryngeal nerves to eliminate baroreceptor input increased mean pulmonary arterial pressure by nearly 25 mm Hg, and pulmonary blood flow increased fourfold and resulted in a tenfold increase in net pulmonary filtration. However, extravascular fluid volumes of hypertensive toads were not significantly different from those of control (resting, normotensive) toads (Table 2).[26]

Table 2.

Fluid Volumes Measured in Left Lungs of
Control (normotensive) and Baroreceptor-Denervated
(early and late denervates) Toads

	Control	Early Denervates	Late Denervates
n	12	6	6
Total Lung Water	7.15±0.22	8.43±0.30	8.72±0.96
Extravascular Water	4.35±0.18	4.57±0.21	4.50±0.35
Blood Volume	3.23±0.23	4.51±0.23	4.95±1.05
Intravascular Water	2.81±0.21	3.87±0.15	4.23±0.88

Values are means±SE normalized to mL/g of blood-free dry lung mass.
Lungs of early denervates were measured 12 to 18 min after bilateral denervation of recurrent laryngeal nerves; lungs of late denervates were measured 45 min after denervation. From Reference 26.

The failure to induce pulmonary edema under these extreme cardiovascular states not only weakens support for a wet lung phenomenon, but simultaneously strongly suggests that mobilization of pulmonary filtrate through lymphatic routes is unusually effective in these animals. Indeed, our recent work delineating the pathways of fluid removal from reptile lungs strongly indicates that pulmonary surfactant, which is present in comparatively high amounts, assists the lymphatic pathway of lung fluid efflux.[28,29]

Finally, induction of a wet lung syndrome would be expected to decrease the effectiveness of gas exchange, owing to an increase in alveolar-blood diffusion distances. This was directly tested by measuring the lung diffusing capacity (D_L) of toads by use of isotopic CO and mass spectrometry before and following an induction of pulmonary hypertension. As seen in Figure 6, lung diffusing capacities were not signifi-

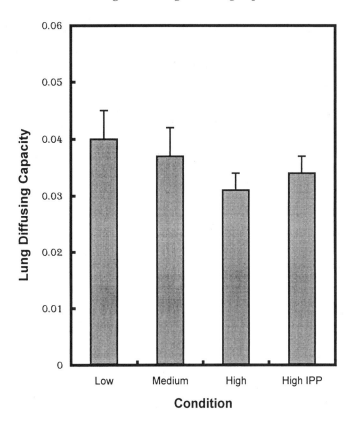

Figure 6. [13]CO-Lung diffusing capacities (mL [13]CO/min/kg) measured in toad lungs (*Bufo marinus*) perfused at low, intermediate, and high rates of perfusion, as well as at high flows with positive (>3 cm H2O) intrapulmonary pressures (High IPP). Means (±1 SE) were not significant across the treatment groups.

cantly diminished under high flow (hypertensive) conditions. Not even an elevation in intrapulmonary pressure, which might be expected to invoke a mechanical assist of lung lymphatics, significantly altered D_L.

Admittedly, data from fluid dynamics in toad lungs alone cannot be used to dismiss the possibility of wet lungs in all other lower vertebrates. However, given the similar capacities for blood volume lability and the similar design of their cardiovascular systems in amphibians and reptiles, as well as the lack of evidence to document wet lungs, our working hypothesis should remain that all vertebrate lungs are comparatively dry.

Summary

The contention that species of lower vertebrates possess unusually high rates of pulmonary fluid filtration is now well documented. The basis for such transcapillary flux appears grounded in both low resistance of the pulmonary capillary walls and gross imbalances of the transcapillary forces, particularly the comparatively low colloid osmotic pressure. The temptation to assume that the enormous flux of filtrate into the lung tissue results in excess fluid accumulation (wet lungs) cannot be supported by the literature, and in fact, no known study has documented wet lungs in healthy individuals of lower vertebrates. In contrast, comparisons of lung water compartments across vertebrates reveal no overt signs of extracellular fluid storage in lungs of lower vertebrates compared to mammals, and in fact, attempts to experimentally induce edema in toad lungs despite substantial hypertension and hyperperfusion have failed. We can only assume that the lymphatic efficacy of lower vertebrate lungs is sufficient to deal with this unsusally high rate of pulmonary fluid turnover, and further wonder what adaptive value, if any, resides with having such a high flux of fluid through the pulmonary circuit.

References

1. Staub NC. Pulmonary edema. *Physiol Rev* 1974;54:678–811.
2. Taylor AE, Rippe B. Pulmonary edema. In: Andreoli TE, Hoffman JF, Fanestil DD, Schultz SG (eds): *Physiology of Membrane Disorders*. New York: Plenum; 1986;1025–1039.
3. Burggren WW. Pulmonary blood plasma filtration in reptiles: A "wet" vertebrate lung. *Science* 1982;215:77–78.
4. Smits AW, West NH, Burggren WW. Pulmonary fluid balance following pulmocutaneous baroreceptor denervation in the toad. *J Appl Physiol* 1986;61:331–337.
5. Smits AW. Fluid balance in vertebrate lungs. In: Wood SC (ed): *Compara-*

tive Pulmonary Physiology: Current Concepts. New York: Marcel-Dekker (Lung Biology in Health and Disease series, Vol. 39); 1989;503–537.

6. Conklin RE. The formation and circulation of lymph in the frog: II. Blood volume and pressure. *Am J Physiol* 1930;95:91–97.

7. Danielli JF. Capillary permeability and oedema in the perfused frog. *J Physiol (Lond)* 1940;98:109–129.

8. Isayama S. Uber Geschwindigkeit des Flussigkeitsanstauches zwischen Blut und Gewebe. *Z Biol* 1924;82:101–106.

9. Zwemer RL, Foglia VG. Fatal loss of plasma volume after lymph heart destruction in toads. *Proc Soc Exp Biol Med* 1943;53:14–17.

10. Baustian M. *The contribution of the lymph hearts in compensation for acute hypovolemia stress in the toad Bufo marinus.* Portland State University; 1986. Thesis.

11. Baustian M. The contribution of lymphatic pathways during recovery from hemorrhage in the toad *Bufo marinus. Physiol Zool* 1988;61:555–563.

12. Lillywhite HB, Smith LH. Hemodynamic responses to hemorrhage in the snake, *Elaphe obsoleta obsoleta. J Exp Biol* 1981;94:275–283.

13. Smits AW, Kozubowski MM. Partitioning of body fluids and cardiovascular responses to circulatory hypovolaemia in the turtle, *Pseudemys scripta elegans. J Exp Biol* 1985;116:237–250.

14. Smits AW, Lillywhite HB. Maintenance of blood volume in snakes: Transcapillary shifts of extravascular fluids during acute hemorrhage. *J Comp Physiol [B]* 1985;155:305–310.

15. Lillywhite HB, Smits AW. Lability of blood volume in snakes and its relation to activity and hypertension. *J Exp Biol* 1984;110:267–274.

16. Smits AW, Ilowite R. Transcapillary fluid exchange in isolated toad hindlimbs. *FASEB J* 1989;3:A559.

17. Maloney JE, Castle BL. Dynamic intravascular pressures in the microvessels of the frog lung. *Respir Physiol* 1970;10:51–63.

18. Shelton G, Jones DR. A comparative study of central blood pressures in five amphibians. *J Exp Biol* 1968;49:631–643.

19. Michel RP, Hakim TS, Chang HK. Pulmonary arterial and venous pressures measured with small catheters in dogs. *J Appl Physiol* 1984;57:309–314.

20. Townsley MI, Korthuis RJ, Rippe B, Parker JC, Taylor AE. Validation of double occlusion method for $P_{c,i}$ in lung and skeletal muscle. *J Appl Physiol* 1986;61:127–132.

21. Johansen K, Burggren WW. Cardiovascular function in lower vertebrates. In: Bourne GH (ed): *Hearts and Heart-Like Organs, Vol. 1.* New York: Academic Press; 1980;61–117.

22. Burggren WW. The pulmonary circulation of the chelonian reptile: Morphology, haemodynamics and pharmacology. *J Comp Physiol [B]* 1977;116: 303–323.

23. Milsom WK, Langille BL, Jones DR. Vagal control of pulmonary vascular resistance in the turtle. *Can J Zool* 1977;55:359–367.

24. deSaint-Aubain ML, Wingstrand KG. A sphincter in the pulmonary artery of the frog *Rana temporaria* and its influence on blood flow in skin and lungs. *Acta Zool (Stockholm)* 1979;60:163–172.

25. Hillman SS, Zygmunt A, Baustian M. Transcapillary fluid forces during dehydration in two amphibians. *Physiol Zool* 1987;60:339–345.

26. Smits AW. Lack of edema in toad lungs after pulmonary hypertension. *Am J Physiol* 1994;266:R1338–1344.

27. Weidner WJ. Extravascular lung water content in the domestic fowl (Gallus domesticus). *Physiol Zool* 1978;51:267–271.

28. Smits AW, Orgeig S, Daniels CB. Pulmonary surfactant functions as an antiglue in the lungs of the lizard, *Pogona vitticeps*. *FASEB J* 1995;9(4):A861.
29. Orgeig S, Smits AW, Daniels CB, Herman JK. Surfactant regulates pulmonary fluid balance in reptiles. *Am J Physiol* 1997; In press.
30. Courtice FC. Extravascular protein and the lymphatics. *Aust N Z Assoc Adv Sci* 1951;28:115–119.
31. Courtice FC. Lymph flow in the lungs. *Br Med Bull* 1963;19:76–79.
32. Schooley J. Lymphocyte output and lymph flow of thoracic and right lymphatic duct in anesthetized rats. *Proc Soc Exp Biol Med* 1958;99:511–513.
33. Hughes RA, May AJ, Widdecombe JC. The output of lymphocytes from the lymphatic system of the rabbit. *J Physiol (Lond)* 1956;132:384–389.
34. Boston RW, Humphreys PW, Reynolds EOR, Strang LB. Lymph flow and clearance of fluid from the lungs of the foetal lamb. *Lancet* 1965;2:473–474.
35. Brigham KL, Woolverton WC, Staub NC. Reversible increase in pulmonary vascular permeability after *Pseudomonas aeruginosa* bacteremia in unanesthetized sheep. *Chest* 1974;65 (suppl):515–535.
36. Blake LH. Mathematical modeling of steady state fluid and protein exchange in the lung. In: Staub NC (ed): *Lung Water and Solute Exchange, Vol. 7.* New York: Marcel Dekker (Lung Biology In Health and Disease series); 1978;99–128.

Chapter 2

Structure-Function Relationships in the Pathogenesis of Pulmonary Edema

Hans Bachofen, MD and E.R. Weibel, MD

Introduction

Pulmonary edema is usually divided into two paradigmatic models according to the presumed particular pathogenetic mechanisms: (1) permeability pulmonary edema (PPE), which is characterized by high concentrations of plasma proteins in the edema fluid, and which is thought to be caused by direct injuries to the blood-gas barrier, ie, to the endothelial and epithelial cell layers of pulmonary capillaries with leakage of plasma and blood cells into the interstitial and alveolar spaces, and (2) hydrostatic (hemodynamic) pulmonary edema due to increases in pulmonary microvascular pressure, which results in transudation of fluid across the capillary walls into the interstitial spaces and eventually into the alveolar air spaces. It is commonly viewed as a passive filtration process with no, or minimal, injury to the cell barriers, which maintain in part a sieving property, as reflected by protein concentrations being lower in the edema fluid than in the capillary plasma.

This basic concept has served well in the management of many clinical conditions in that hemodynamic disorders and the sequelae of direct lung tissue damage require different treatments. However, there are many situations where the distinction between these two types of pulmonary edema is blurred, and more recent observations challenge

From: Weir EK, Reeves JT (eds). *Pulmonary Edema*. Armonk, NY: Futura Publishing Company, Inc.; ©1998.

Supported by Grants from the Swiss National Science Foundation.

the simplistic pathogenetic models. In fact, even in "pure" hemodynamic pulmonary edema, there is evidence of structural alterations, such as disruptions of the permeability barriers,[1–5] whereas in "pure" permeability edema, extra-alveolar lesions might be routes of protein leakage,[6] and disequilibria of forces regulating pulmonary fluid exchange may play an important role.[7–9]

Permeability Pulmonary Edema

The hallmark of PPE is a protein-rich edema fluid in both interstitial and alveolar spaces that cannot be explained by barrier lesions caused by excessive microvascular pressures. With regard to its definition, causes, and pathogenesis, it appears to be more complicated than hemodynamic pulmonary edema.[8,10] The complexity stems not only from the large variety of etiologies and pathogenetic mechanisms, but also from the imprecise use of the term *permeability*. In the clinic, "increased permeability" is used for increased diffusive and convective protein transport across the blood-gas barrier, and it even includes diffuse ruptures of microvessels as in severe pulmonary contusion.

With most etiologies of clinical importance it is thought that the essential route of protein loss is through injuries of both the capillary endothelium and alveolar epithelium, so that macromolecules can traverse the blood-gas barrier[8,11–14] (the basement membrane is highly permeable for liquids, macromolecules, and even for cells).[15] However, analyses of the fine structure of lung parenchyma are not always conclusive with regard to the structure-function relationship. In human lungs with PPE, frequent and large gaps can be seen predominantly in the alveolar epithelium[12,13]; the endothelial cell layer, on the other hand, appears to be continuous and rather well preserved. It has been supposed that this conspicuous discrepancy is due to the delay in obtaining human tissue specimens (these are usually not available before 24 hours after the onset of PPE). During this period, endothelial leaks may be covered, owing to the particular plasticity and high repair capacity of the endothelium.[16,17] This hypothesis is supported by experiments done on oleic acid-damaged dog lungs. Measurements of vascular permeability to macromolecules by positron emission tomography (PET) have been quantitatively compared with structural lesions of the alveolar-capillary barrier assessed by morphometry.[14] With regard to both location and to extent of protein escape, an excellent correlation was found between PET measurements and barrier damages. In particular, the prevalence of epithelial lesions and endothelial lesions was about equivalent in this very acute stage of lung injury. However, this example of PPE, which illustrates a rather convincing structure-function relationship, does not imply a uniform mechanism of PPE, and there is evidence that other noxious agents might open other routes for alveolar flooding with proteinaceous fluid. Quite recent experiments point to alternative routes of fluid and protein escape. In lungs perfused with hydrogen peroxide solutions, leakage of protein through extra-alveolar vessels, ie, through transendothelial gaps in small pulmonary arteries, could be demonstrated.[6] Progressive extravasation of the perfusate resulted in interstitial edema as reflected by increases in lung weight and the formation of perivascular cuffs. Signs of concomitant increase in microvascular permeability were absent. This particular pathogenetic model might be of clinical relevance in some types of PPE associated with extrapulmonary inflammation. In such cases, leaks in small arteries could be the primary site of fluid escape; the edema fluid first accumulates in the interstitial spaces, and eventually reaches the alveoli by retrograde flow,[18] where the inflammatory exudate may secondarily damage the delicate epithelial cell layer. Thus, the complexities of PPE are still with us in that a seemingly plausible structure-function relationship observed at a given time may not reflect the true cause-effect relationship.

Hydrostatic Pulmonary Edema

In contrast to permeability lung edema that results from primary barrier lesions, the pathogenesis of hydrostatic (hemodynamic) lung edema, in particular the exact sites of fluid and protein leakage into alveoli, has been even more controversial.[18–24] In the past, an attractive hypothesis was the reversible stretching of "pores" in endothelial and epithelial cell layers,[25–27] which might escape morphological observation. However, more recent studies have demonstrated that the formation and morphology of hydrostatic pulmonary edema are rather complex in that there is a marked inhomogeneity in fluid filtration into the interstitial spaces and of alveolar flooding, and that endothelial and epithelial breaks occur when microvascular pressure is abnormally increased.[2–5]

The preservation of edema fluid is essential for study of the structure-function relationship of lung edema, and in particular the accumulation and distribution of alveolar fluid. To this aim, special techniques must be used, since free alveolar fluid cannot be readily fixed. One way to preserve both tissue and fluid is to rapidly freeze the lungs and to process cryosamples using a low-temperature scanning electron microscopy system.[28] Alternatively, edematous lungs can be fixed by vascular perfusion, provided that the protein concentration of alveolar fluid is sufficiently high. The following discussion focuses on the latter model, ie, on excised rabbit lungs perfused with a 6% albumin solution in which edema was induced by increased microvascular pressures prior to fixation by vascular perfusion with glutaraldehyde and osmium tetroxide.[4] Certainly, this model gives interesting insight into the pathogenesis of lung edema, but it cannot be considered as *pars pro toto*: first, the model is not fully physiological in that among other flaws it has no bronchial circulation and a severed lymphatic system, and second, species differences in lung structure call for cautious extrapolation of all findings to other mammals.

Sites and Distribution of Edema Fluid

Chest radiographs of patients with beginning pulmonary edema usually show a rather inhomogeneous, patchy distribution of extravascular fluid accumulation with an apicobasal gradient. In rabbit lungs, a quite similar morphological pattern can be seen with inhomogeneities at three different levels. First, there is a clear-cut apicobasal gradient with much more interstitial and alveolar edema in the lower lobes than in the upper lobes.[4,29] Second, considerable differences in edema formation can occur between right and left lungs. Third, and most interestingly, at the same lung height, both interstitial and alveolar edema fluid is irregularly distributed between acini and even between groups of alveoli around the same alveolar duct, and the volume of interstitial edema fluid does not necessarily correlate with the amount of fluid in the adjacent alveoli (Figure 1).

The apical to basal increase in interstitial and alveolar edema might be explained by gravity, which increases the filtration pressure at the lung bases and favors intrabronchial drainage of edema fluid. However, the mechanism of this seemingly trivial finding appears to be more complex. As expected, the interstitial fluid in the apices of lungs increases with increasing filtration pressure.[29] In contrast, the apical air spaces remain virtually dry, regardless of capillary pressure changes within the range of 30 mm Hg. Most interesting is the observation that in lungs suspended in a top-down position, the alveolar fluid is distributed without gravity-dependent direction. All of these observations suggest that anatomic and/or functional heterogeneities influence the pattern of edema formation in addition to the mean local hydrostatic pressures.

As striking as the inhomogeneities of fluid distribution, are spatial variations in the albumin concentration of the edema fluid, as they are reflected by differences in the density of the fixed proteinaceous material (Figure 2). There are marked differences between neighboring alveoli, as well as between alveoli and adjacent interstitial spaces; appar-

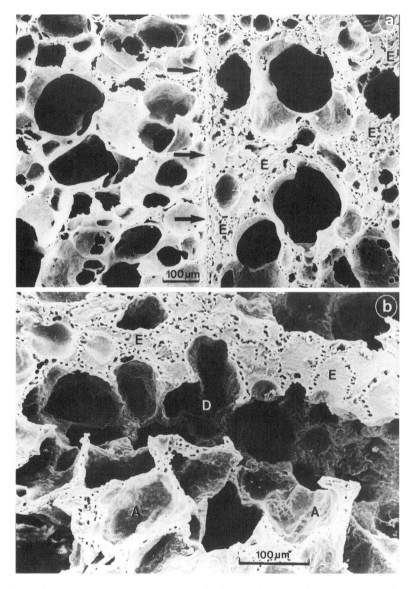

Figure 1. Scanning electron micrographs illustrating the inhomogeneous distribution of edema fluid. (a) Lobule with marked alveolar edema (right) adjacent to a fairly "dry" lobule (left). Arrows indicate the interlobular septum. (b) Differences in fluid accumulation within the same alveolar duct. D = alveolar duct; E = alveoli completely filled with edema fluid; A = air-filled alveoli.

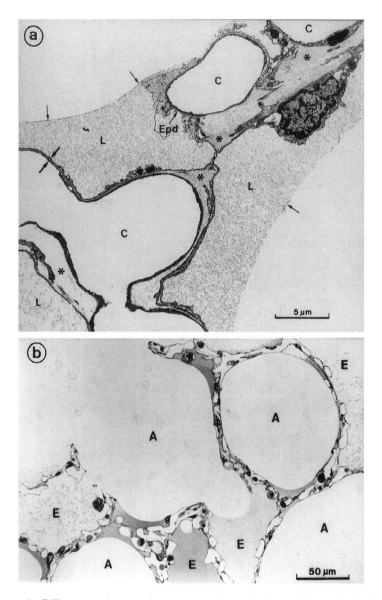

Figure 2. Differences in protein concentrations in interstitial and alveolar edema fluid. (a) Asterisks indicate interstitial edema pools with varying protein contents (electron micrograph). C = capillaries; L = alveolar edema; Epd = damaged epithelial cell. (b) Alveolar fluid pools with different protein content (light micrograph). A = alveolar air spaces; E = alveolar edema fluid.

ently, endothelial leaks are not necessarily matched by opposite epithelial leaks. Concentration gradients exist even within the interstitium along short distances. Furthermore, in some individual alveoli, there are sharply demarcated layers of different densities, sometimes separated by continuous films of surfactant, which point to different leakage sites with local differences in the sieving property.

These observations strongly suggest that there are substantial differences in fluid filtration and in the reflection coefficients for macromolecules. Apparently, a simple uniform membrane model of passive fluid and solute movement following pressure gradients is not valid for hydrostatic pulmonary edema. It is, rather, the result of complex alterations in structure and function of the important components of the blood-gas barrier, ie, of both the endothelial and epithelial cell layers; this is a consequence of, or in addition to, increased hydrostatic pressures.

Barrier Lesions

High-pressure pulmonary edema has been thought to arise from the imbalance of forces affecting the normal process of fluid exchange, as described by the Starling hypothesis, rather than from structural alterations of the barriers. This concept was supported by two clinical observations: the rapid termination of the outflow of edema fluid once the equilibrium of forces is reestablished, and the preservation of a selective permeability of the barrier, as indicated by the amount and type of proteins in the edema fluid.[26,30–32] Most important, previous ultrastructural findings obtained in edematous animal lungs and in lungs from patients with left-sided heart failure revealed rather intact endothelial and epithelial cell layers.[19,26,33]

The rabbit lung model appears to confirm the previous finding only in part, in that minimal injuries to the endothelium are minimal, indeed. At this point, a further peculiarity of this experimental model must be noted: the lungs have not been fixed under high-pressure conditions, but rather after the reestablishment of normal perfusion pressures. Hence the scarcity of endothelial lesions may be explained by the fact that the capillary distension was released before fixation. In the endothelial cell layer, the clefts probably occurred by the opening of the relatively weak intercellular junctions which, thus, prevented disruptions of the cells. The swift repair upon pressure release can be explained by the integrity of the cells, their high repair capacity, and the restitution of the original geometry of the microvessels.

There are, however, distinct and numerous lesions of the "tight" part of the barrier, ie, the epithelial cell layer. In lungs subjected to high microvascular pressures (approximately 30 mm Hg), different types of epithelial leaks occur on both the thin parts (consisting of a fused basement membrane between thin epithelial and endothelial cell layers only) and the thick parts of the blood-gas barrier; disruptions are even present at intercapillary parts of alveolar septa that were distended by interstitial edema fluid. Interestingly, the lesions on the thin barrier parts assume the pattern of vesicular fragmentation, ie, the disrupted cells or cytoplasmic fragments are resealed such that the edge of the break consists of a smoothly rounded membrane (Figure 3). These breaks must be distinguished from open cell junctions, which are barely detectable. On the thick parts, on the other hand, wide clefts and a scaling off of epithelial cell extensions from the basement membrane are more common.

The total area of epithelial breaks is considerable and can amount to 3% to 5% of the total surface area of the basement membrane; breaks are much more frequent in the lower regions of lungs filled with alveolar edema.[29] In contrast, the area of breaks of the endothelial cell layer related to the area of the capillary basement membrane is less than 1%.

On the other hand, if lung edema is induced by rather moderate capillary pressures (approximately 15 mm Hg) associated with a slow extravasation of fluid (approximately 0.5 mL/min), epithelial discontinuities are rather rare. In this situation, the most conspicuous alterations of the barrier are epithelial blebs of various size and appearance (Figure 4). Blebs can be small, resembling enlarged pinocytotic vesicles, they can be pockets formed by an extended cell layer segment detached from the basement membrane, and they can be large blisters surrounded by seemingly intact attenuated cell extensions. Three further features of epithelial blebs are noteworthy. First, they occur only at sites of abundant alveolar edema, whereas they are absent in dry alveolar regions. Second, they are filled with proteinaceous fluid, the protein concentrations of which are usually quite similar to that in the adjacent interstitial space, but which may be quite different from that in the surrounding alveolar edema fluid. Third, the frequency of such alterations is considerable. They can be observed in almost every fluid-filled alveolus; approximately 4% of the alveolar epithelial surface are transformed into blebs; and their volume accounts to approximately 3% of the volume of the alveolar fluid.

For a tentative explanation of the different types of epithelial lesions, some peculiarities of the alveolar epithelium must be considered. Alveolar type I cells are very large and complex cells,[34] each forming thin cytoplasmic extensions that cover a surface 4000 to 5000 μm^2, an area that is about four times larger than that covered by an endothelial cell.[35] Accordingly, intercellular junctions are much more scarce in the epithelium than in the endothelium.[35] Furthermore, epithelial cell junctions have been shown to be much tighter than those of the endothe-

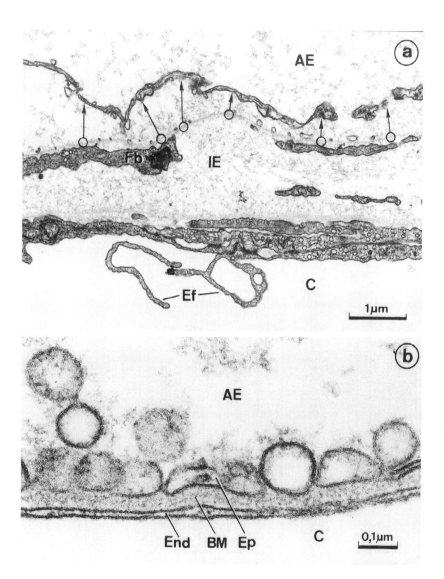

Figure 3. Epithelial lesions on the thick (a) and thin (b) side of the alveolar-capillary barrier. (a) Ruptured epithelial cell layer (arrow heads) scaled off from the basement membrane (circles). Note the copious interstitial edema. (b) Epithelial breaks on the thin side of the barrier. The vesicular fragmentation of the type I cell documents that the disruption occurred before fixation, that is, during high-pressure perfusion. AE = alveolar edema; IE = interstitial edema; Fb = fibroblast; Ef = endothelial flaps; C = capillary; End = endothelium; BM = basement membrane; Ep = epithelium.

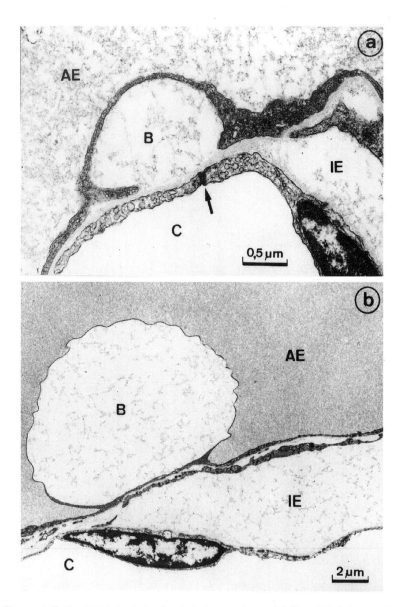

Figure 4. Epithelial blebs in hydrostatic lung edema. (a) Small bleb formed by an epithelial cell extension detached from the epithelial basement membrane on the thin part of the barrier. Arrow points to an open endothelial cell junction. (b) Larger bleb with a seemingly continuous wall on the thick side of the barrier. Note that the protein concentration of the bleb fluid is similar to that of interstitial edema but different from that of alveolar edema. AE = alveolar edema; B = bleb; IE = interstitial edema; C = capillaries.

lium.[36] These features may become important when the blood-gas barrier is subjected to stress from elevated capillary perfusion pressure. High and sudden stress may cause the barrier to break[2,3]; the endothelial layer by the opening of intercellular junctions, but the epithelial cell layer by cellular disruptions, as reflected by vesicular fragmentations. During moderate but persistent increases in microvascular pressure, endothelial and epithelial cells may react differently. Frequent and leaky endothelial junctions will let fluid pass into the interstitial space, thus causing a slow formation of interstitial edema that is prevented from seeping into the alveolar space by the presence of tight and infrequent epithelial junctions. As a consequence of the slowly increasing interstitial pressure, the cytoplasmic leaflets of type I cells will be put under continuously increasing shear stress; a focal loosening of their attachment to the basement membrane, ie, by disruption of some laminin bridges, will then cause the leaflet to become locally stretched under the direct effect of increased interstitial pressure. It is noteworthy that approximately 85% of the blebs are located at the thick part of the barrier where the interstitial edema accumulates. The extensibility of the epithelial leaflets is remarkable in that the surface area of the blebs may assume the total surface area of an epithelial type I cell. Thus, epithelial cells appear to have a higher degree of plasticity than hitherto thought, which in turn may explain in part the excellent barrier function of the epithelial cell layer. Occasionally, however, ruptured blebs can be observed, indicating the limits of plasticity of the attenuated epithelial cell extensions (Figure 5).

All of these findings add weight to the interpretations outlined above that hydrostatic pulmonary edema is not a simple uniform membrane model of passive fluid movement following pressure gradients. They rather point to complex pathological events including various alterations in structure and function of both cellular layers of the blood-gas barrier (in the experiments discussed above, the basement membrane was the sole barrier component without detectable discontinuities). Thus, hydrostatic pulmonary edema may have more pathogenetic events in common with permeability pulmonary edema than previously thought.

However, this insight does not resolve the complexity of mechanisms possibly involved; critical questions remain unanswered. Barrier lesions, and in particular epithelial blebs, are closely associated with abundant alveolar edema, but are virtually absent in air spaces without an appreciable accumulation of alveolar edema fluid, although these "dry" regions were adequately perfused, as judged by the excellent perfusion fixation of the tissue. Hence, one might argue that epithelial blebs are a sequel of the elimination of a protective factor, for example, the elimination of normal surface forces that oppose local bulging of the

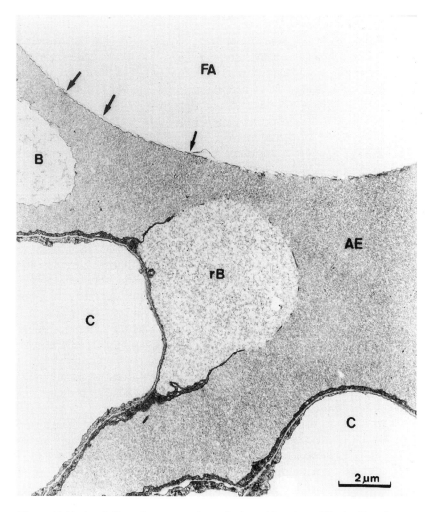

Figure 5. Hydrostatic pulmonary edema induced in a lung filled with a fluoro-carbon. Ruptured bleb (rB) in a pool of alveolar edema fluid. FA = alveolar space filled with fluorocarbon; B = intact bleb; AE = alveolar edema fluid; C = capillaries. Arrows point to surfactant material at the interface between fluorocarbon and edema fluid.

alveolar surface.[37] This ambiguity about the cause-effect relationship between alveolar flooding and epithelial lesions might reopen the question about the initial pathway of fluid escape, ie, whether alveoli are flooded by retrograde flow from leaks in the terminal airway epithelium,[18] or directly through gaps in the blood-gas barrier. The findings described above and recent investigations by other authors[2,3,23] certainly support the latter hypothesis. Additional evidence is given by a further observation: If hydrostatic pulmonary edema is produced in lungs that are inflated either by hexadecane or a fluorocarbon in order to prevent the spreading of edema fluid along the airways, edema fluid is found in the peripheral airspaces associated with bleb formations and epithelial discontinuities (Figure 5). In this context, ultrastructural findings in lungs of patients with hemodynamic pulmonary edema, and in particular, those with neurogenic edema as a particular form of acute high-pressure edema, are of interest in that numerous erythrocytes are found in the interstitial and alveolar edema fluid.[1] At some sites of the interstitium, they are firmly packed, forming interstitial hematomas (Figure 6). Thus, the "rusty" sputum and numerous iron-loaded macrophages expectorated by patients with lung congestion and edema appear to be of alveolar origin. The escape of blood cells from the capillaries into interstitial and alveolar spaces postulates pores or gaps in the basement membrane; these can be quite small considering the enormous plasticity of erythrocytes in transit, and they are probably of transient nature, which explains that discontinuities of the basement membrane cannot be detected on electron micrographs. However, all of these findings do not exclude extra-alveolar pathways of fluid escape in addition to alveolar leaks. The above-mentioned observations by Pietra[6] give grounds for suspicion that the pathogenesis of hydrostatic pulmonary edema is extremely complex.

It is stated above that hydrostatic edema and permeability edema may have some pathogenetic mechanisms in common. It is remarkable, however, that patients with hemodynamic pulmonary edema have a conspicuous absence of signs of inflammation, in contrast to those with permeability edema. Although in acute and severe hemodynamic edema, the sputum may show a tendency to coagulate, and small specks of fibrin can be observed in the alveoli, there are neither signs of intravascular coagulation, nor accumulations of polymorphonuclear leukocytes in capillaries, interstitial spaces, and alveolar spaces in spite of numerous cellular lesions and a direct contact of blood with denuded basement membranes. These observations indicate that it is not the type of barrier lesion per se, but rather the type and extent of injury to the blood-gas barrier, and the associated inflammatory reaction that makes the difference between both forms of pulmonary edema.

A further aspect of the complexity of hydrostatic pulmonary edema is the repair of the epithelial cell layer. A rapid clearance of the chest x-ray and return of normal lung function are observed in patients when pulmonary edema subsides. The question then is whether the enormous plasticity and adaptability of alveolar type I cells are also involved in the rapid repair response, and whether they thus circumvent the long-lasting repair mechanisms of type II cell proliferation and transdifferentiation associated with considerable lung function distur-

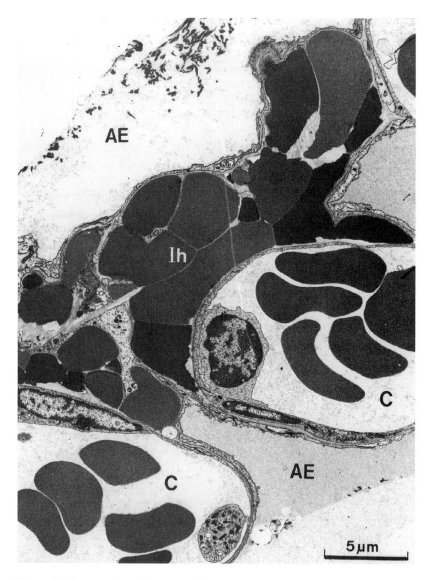

Figure 6. Neurogenic pulmonary edema in a patient after fatal head trauma. Abundant hemorrhagic interstitial and alveolar edema. Ih = interstitial hemorrhage; AE = protein-rich alveolar edema with fibrin specks; C = capillaries.

bances, as observed in permeability edema. Since it has been shown that the integrity of the alveolar epithelium plays a critical role in alveolar edema reabsorption,[38] the repair mechanisms in hemodynamic pulmonary edema must be further explored.

Summary

The formation and morphology of hydrostatic pulmonary edema appear to be complex, and there is sufficient evidence that the fluid and protein movement from the microvasculature into interstitial and alveolar spaces cannot be explained by uniform membrane models of fluid exchange. There is also good evidence that barrier leaks, and in particular leaks in the epithelial cell layer, play a role not only in permeability edema, but also in hydrostatic edema. It is likely that the differences between the two types of lung edema reflect the type and extent of injury to the cellular layers of the blood-gas barrier, whether or not there is a causative, associated, or ensuing inflammatory process.

References

1. Bachofen H, Bachofen M, Weibel ER. Ultrastructural aspects of pulmonary edema. *J Thorax Imag* 1988;3:1–7.
2. West JB, Tsukimoto K, Mathieu-Costello O, Prediletto R. Stress failure in pulmonary capillaries. *J Appl Physiol* 1991;70:1731–1742.
3. Tsukimoto K, Mathieu-Costello O, Prediletto R, Elliott AR, West JB. Ultrastructural appearances of pulmonary capillaries at high transmural pressures. *J Appl Physiol* 1991;71:573–582.
4. Bachofen H, Schürch S, Michel RP, Weibel ER. Experimental hydrostatic pulmonary edema in rabbit lungs. Morphology. *Am Rev Respir Dis* 1993; 147:989–996.
5. Bachofen H, Schürch S, Weibel ER. Experimental hydrostatic pulmonary edema in rabbit lungs. Barrier lesions. *Am Rev Respir Dis.* 1993;147: 997–1004.
6. Pietra GG, Johns LW. Confocal- and electron-microscopic localization of FITC-albumin in H_2O_2-induced pulmonary edema. *J Appl Physiol* 1996;80: 182–190.
7. Meyrick B, Brigham KL. Acute effects of Escherichia coli endotoxin on the pulmonary microcirculation of anesthetized sheep. Structure-function relationships. *Lab Invest* 1983;48:458–470.
8. Robin ED. Permeability lung edema. In: Fishman AP, Renkin EM (eds): *Pulmonary Edema.* Bethesda, MD: American Physiological Society; 1979; 217–229.
9. Newman JH. Sepsis and pulmonary edema. *Clin Chest Med* 1985;6: 371–391.
10. Montaner JSG, Tsang J, Evans KG, et al. Alveolar epithelial damage: A critical difference between high pressure and oleic acid-induced low pressure pulmonary edema. *J Clin Invest* 1986;77:1786–1796.

11. Staub NC. Pulmonary edema due to increased microvascular permeability to fluid and protein. *Circ Res* 1978;43:143–151.
12. Bachofen M, Bachofen H, Weibel ER. Lung edema in adult respiratory distress syndrome. In: Fishman AP, Renkin EM (eds): *Pulmonary Edema.* Bethesda, MD: American Physiological Society; 1979;241–252..
13. Albertine KH. Ultrastructural abnormalities in increased permeability pulmonary edema. *Clin Chest Med* 1985;6:345–369.
14. Velasquez M, Weibel ER, Kuhn C III, Schuster DP. PET-evaluation of pulmonary vascular permeability: A structure function correlation. *J Appl Physiol* 1991;70:2206–2216.
15. Lauweryns JM, Baert JH. The role of pulmonary lymphatics in the defenses of the distal lung: Morphological and experimental studies of the transport mechanisms of intratracheally instilled particles. *Ann N Y Acad Sci* 1974;221:244–275.
16. Bachofen M, Weibel ER. Alterations of the gas exchange apparatus in adult respiratory insufficiency associated with septicemia. *Am Rev Respir Dis* 1977;116:589–615.
17. Reidy MA, Schwartz SM. Endothelial regeneration. III. Time course of intimal changes after small defined injury to rat aortic endothelium. *Lab Invest* 1981;44:301–308.
18. Staub NC. Pathophysiology of pulmonary edema. In: Staub NC, Taylor AE (eds): *Edema.* New York: Raven Press; 1984;719–786.
19. Pietro GG, Szidon JP, Leventhal MM, Fishman AP. Hemoglobin traces in hemodynamic pulmonary edema. *Science* 1969;166:1643–1646.
20. Zumsteg TA, Havill AM, Gee MH. Relationships among lung extravascular fluid compartments with alveolar flooding. *J Appl Physiol* 1982;53: 267–271.
21. Mason GR, Effros RM. Flow of edema fluid into pulmonary airways. *J Appl Physiol* 1983;55:1262–1268.
22. Conhaim RL, Eaton A, Staub NC, Heath TD. Equivalent pore estimate for the alveolar-airway barrier in isolated dog lung. *J Appl Physiol* 1986; 60:513–520.
23. Conhaim RL. Airway level at which edema liquid enters the air space of isolated dog lungs. *J Appl Physiol* 1989;67:2234–2242.
24. Luchtel DL, Embree L, Guest R, Albert RK. Extra-alveolar veins are contiguous with, and leak fluid into, periarterial cuffs in rabbit lungs. *J Appl Physiol* 1991;71:1606–1613.
25. Pappenheimer JR, Renkin EM, Borrero LM. Filtration, diffusion and molecular sieving through peripheral capillary membranes: A contribution to the pore theory of capillary permeability. *Am J Physiol* 1951;167:13–46.
26. Fishman AP, Pietra GG. Hemodynamic pulmonary edema. In: Fishman AP, Renkin EM (eds): *Pulmonary Edema.* Bethesda, MD: American Physiological Society; 1979;79–96.
27. Gorin AM, Stewart PA. Differential permeability of endothelial and epithelial barriers to albumin flux. *J Appl Physiol* 1979;47:1315–1324.
28. Hook JR, Bastacky J, Conhaim RL, Staub NC, Hayes TL. A new method for pulmonary edema research: Scanning electron microscopy of frozen hydrated edematous lungs. *Scanning* 1987;9:71–79.
29. Wu DXY, Weibel ER, Bachofen H, Schürch S. Lung lesions in experimental hydrostatic pulmonary edema: An electron microscopic and morphometric study. *Exp Lung Res* 1995;21:711–730.
30. Staub NC. Pulmonary edema. *Physiol Rev* 1974;54:678–811.

31. Matthay MA. Pathophysiology of pulmonary edema. *Clin Chest Med* 1985;5:301–314.
32. Vreim CE, Snashall PD, Staub NC. Protein composition of lung fluids in anesthetized dogs with acute cardiogenic edema. *Am J Physiol* 1976;231: 1466–1469.
33. De Fouw DO. Morphologic study of the alveolar septa in normal and edematous isolated dog lungs fixed by vascular perfusion. *Lab Invest* 1980;42: 314–319.
34. Weibel ER. The mystery of "non-nucleated plates" in the alveolar epithelium of the lung explained. *Acta Anat* 1971;78:425–433.
35. Stone KL, Mercer RR, Gehr P, Stockstill B, Crapo JD. Allometric relationship of cell numbers and size in the mammalian lung. *Am J Respir Cell Mol Biol* 1992;6:235–243.
36. Schneeberger EE, Karnovsky MJ. The influence of intravascular fluid volume on the permeability of newborn and adult mouse lungs to ultrastructural protein tracers. *J Cell Biol* 1971;49:319–334.
37. Wilson TA, Bachofen H. A model for mechanical structure of the alveolar duct. *J Appl Physiol* 1982;52:1064–1072.
38. Matthay MA, Wiener-Kronisch JP. Intact epithelial barrier function is critical for the resolution of alveolar edema in humans. *Am Rev Respir Dis* 1990;142:1250–1257.

Chapter 3

Pressure, Flow, and Filtration in the Lung During Strenuous Exercise

John H. Newman, MD and Casilda I. Hermo, MD

Introduction

In the age of molecular biology, why study exercise? A glib but accurate answer might be that the molecules are put together in the first place so that we *can* exercise! A more compelling answer is that the study of exercise is pertinent to health and disease. The effects of exercise on lung circulation are not completely understood, and exercise, not rest, is the normal condition for most awake animals and humans. Most of the variables that we use in human biology are derived from basal conditions—vascular pressure, cardiac output, oxygen consumption, ventilation—and yet the simple act of going out to get the paper in the morning significantly and abruptly changes metabolism and cardiopulmonary function. In disease, modest demands on cardiac and lung reserve can result in severe symptoms and impaired function. The study of the limits of cardiac and pulmonary function in health are needed to judge the mechanisms and the degree of impairment during disease. Thus, the study of exercise is of fundamental importance.

The lung undergoes fantastic changes during exercise. In normal humans, cardiac output and, thus, pulmonary blood flow, can increase more than fivefold from 5 L at rest to 25 to 30 L/min during exhaustive exercise.[1,2] The manner in which the lung handles this flow has been the

From: Weir EK, Reeves JT (eds). *Pulmonary Edema*. Armonk, NY: Futura Publishing Company, Inc.; ©1998.

This work is supported by Grant No. HL 45107 from the National Institutes of Health, National Heart Lung and Blood Institute; and the St. Thomas Foundation.

subject of a number of studies, but important questions remain such as:
(1) what is capillary pressure during exercise, (2) how does the lung stay
dry despite the very high flow of blood, (3) what are the limits to exercise imposed by filtration, pulmonary and intracardiac pressures, (4)
what are the interactions of the lung and heart that impose these limits?

Data from published studies by Newman et al,[3,4] along with the pi-
oneering work of Coates and O'Brodovich[5-7] have shown massive increases in lung lymph flow during exercise, that are poorly explained.
Exercise lymph flows are 5 to 7 times baseline, levels that are ordinar-
ily seen only during lung injury and increased lung vascular permeability[8-10] or during exceedingly high levels of chronic left atrial hypertension (25 to 40 cm H_2O left atrial pressure [Figure 1]).[11-13] In
experiments where sheep are trotted to maximal effort, lymph flow returns rapidly to baseline levels after cessation of exercise, a strong indication that permeability is not altered. Lymph-to-plasma protein
(L/P) ratio actually decreases faster in lymph during exercise than it
does during acute left atrial hypertension,[12] which further reduces the

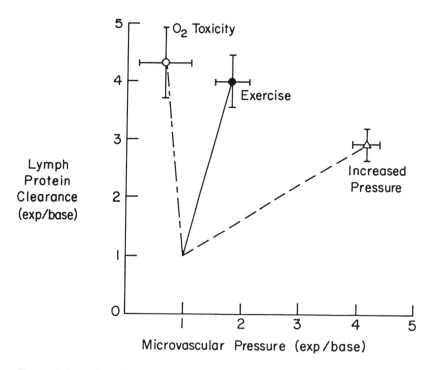

Figure 1. Lung lymph protein clearance during exercise is very high—some-
where between that of increased permeability (Oxygen toxicity) and that of
passive pulmonary congestion (increased pressure). Microvascular pressure
may be underestimated during exercise.

likelihood of a permeability change during exercise, but implicates microvascular hypertension.

Studies in humans summarized by Reeves et al[2] have shown that both pulmonary arterial pressure and pulmonary wedge pressure rise with incremental exercise. The wedge pressure rises markedly, in fact, achieving levels of 20 to 35 mm Hg with maximal effort.[14] One explanation is that left ventricular end-diastolic pressure and/or left atrial pressure rise during high flow. Direct left atrial pressure measurements have not been made in exercising humans, but it has been shown that left atrial pressure rises only minimally in the sheep during progressive exercise. It seems possible that the discrepancy between human data and sheep data is explained by the possibility that the wedged catheter is reading a more upstream pressure in humans.[15] Another possibility is that the limits of pericardial compliance are reached with progressive exercise, resulting in restricted filling and high diastolic chamber pressures.[16,17] This mechanism may explain the large differences in wedge pressure among humans and sheep, because in sheep the pericardium around the left atrium is usually removed at surgery. If pericardial restriction occurs, raising capillary pressure to edemagenic levels, then "cardiac limitation" in exercise may have a different origin in some humans than via a contractile limitation. Based on the human data and the lymph protein washdown observed in sheep, it is hypothesized that pulmonary capillary pressure is higher during exercise than is currently recognized. In vitro studies of pressure and flow relationships strongly support this hypothesis.[18] A supporting observation is that pericardial limitation may be the cause of high capillary pressures during the Mueller maneuver[16] and after high-volume infusion,[10] where the stroke volume of both ventricles increases by approximately 70 mL, possibly reaching pericardial limits.

Newman et al performed an experiment that tested the importance of the pericardium. They measured right ventricular (RV) mean pressure and wedge pressure via a Swan-Ganz catheter, before and after partial pericardiectomy in a sheep (Figure 2). They plotted the change in pressure of the RV and LA from rest to modest exercise. Left atrial (wedge) pressure rose by 8 cm with pericardium intact, but only by 1 to 2 cm H_2O after resection.[16] This is an extremely important issue not only for their work, but for concepts of cardiac limitation during exercise. If these experiments prove an important effect, pericardial compliance will have to be included in any explanation of the hemodynamics of strenuous exercise.

An important clinical goal is to discover how to better measure capillary pressure during exercise. Obviously, there is no way to directly measure capillary pressure in vivo. Micropuncture is limited to pleural vessels in animals under anesthesia,[19] as is the transthoracic

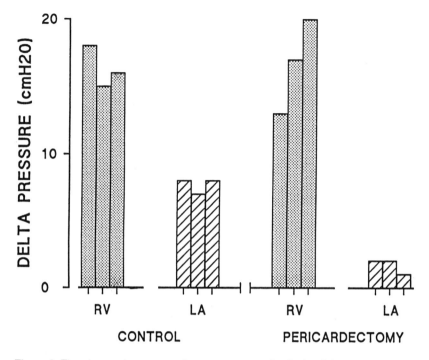

Figure 2. The change in pressure from rest to exercise in the right ventricle (RV) and left atrium (LA) in a sheep with and without intact pericardium.

window technique.[20] Estimations of capillary pressure using the Gaar equation are useful, but are known to be erroneous during arterial constriction such as with hypoxia[19,21]; with venoconstriction induced by sympathetic stimulation,[22] where the equation overestimates capillary pressure; or during the endotoxin reaction,[23] where venoconstriction raises capillary pressure far above LA pressure. Retrograde pulmonary venous catheters are difficult to place and have not been used during exercise. In vitro techniques such as isogravimetric capillary pressure are not feasible in vivo.[23]

Over the last 10 years, a number of investigators[21,24–29] have developed vascular occlusion techniques for more closely approximating lung capillary pressure in vitro and in vivo. The arterial bed is the resistor and the microvessels (presumably primarily capillaries) function as a slowly discharging capacitor. When flow is abruptly stopped by occlusion, pressure drops almost instantly through the larger resistance vessels, followed by slower exponential decay in pressure as the capillary bed empties. Plotting the two phases and extrapolating the capillary exponent back to the time of occlusion yields a close measure of capillary pressure. The feasibility of adapting this technique to exercise should be explored.

Another profound change that takes place during exercise is change in ventilation. At maximal exercise, a normal human can breathe at 100 to 180 L/min, compared to approximately 5 L/min, which is needed at rest.[30] Ventilation increases proportionately with oxygen consumption, until the anaerobic threshold, where ventilation increases steeply, more closely tracking carbon dioxide production and blood lactate. Exercise ventilation is achieved early by large increases in tidal volume and smaller increases in rate, followed by a plateau of tidal volume, but a continued increase in rate as exercise approaches maximum. Most of the muscular work of ventilation is via the inspiratory muscles, although some expiratory effort occurs during strenuous exercise; and the exhaled volume drops below functional residual capacity.[31,32] Thus, negative pressure ventilation is the major mode during exercise, but positive pressure oscillations occur and the pressure swings are greater at exercise than at rest. Several investigators have analyzed the effects of negative and positive pressure ventilation on lung vascular filtration and lung lymph flow at rest. They have found that negative pleural pressure and alveolar expansion increase the transvascular hydrostatic gradient, especially around extra-alveolar vessels, but that filtration and lymph clearance increase only by 30% to 50%, depending on the experimental conditions.[10,33–38]

Because of the small apparent effect of ventilation on lymph clearance at rest, it has been concluded that chest wall and lung motion have little to do with the clearance of filtered fluid in the lung. Most studies of ventilation on filtration and clearance were not made under the conditions of strenuous exercise, where the capillary bed is under a large blood volume and pressure load. Newman et al conducted preliminary experiments that independently reproduced the changes in vascular pressure and ventilation that occur with exercise (Figure 3). In sheep, each instrumented a with left atrial balloon catheter, they performed nasotracheal intubation so that they could measure ventilation, while they altered microvascular pressure. They measured lymph flow and ventilation at rest and during exercise using a Buxco lung mechanics computer (Buxco Co., Sharon, CT) They then reproduced the level of ventilation seen during exercise with the sheep at rest by adding dead-space via low-resistance ribbed ventilator tubing added to the endotracheal tube. Finally, they raised left atrial pressure to cause a microvascular pressure (Pmv) similar to that of exercise (P_{PA} 37 cm H_2O P_{LA} 24 cm H_2O) with the sheep *already hyperpneic*, and found a dramatic rapid increase in lymph flow comparable to that seen during exercise. This was unlike lymph flow during resting hyperpnea or resting left atrial hypertension alone. Thus, they concluded that the hyperpnea of exercise has a major impact on clearance of filtrate. How this occurs— whether by airway pressure or volume fluctuations, by the develop-

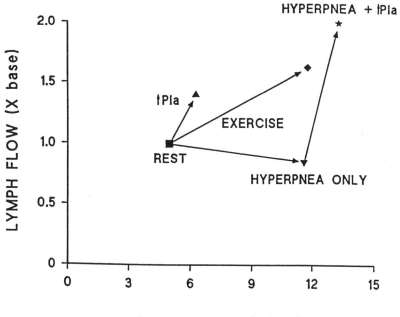

Figure 3. Pressures, minute ventilation, and lymph flow were first measured at rest and during exercise. Hyperpnea at rest was then induced by carbon dioxide rebreathing, with a small reduction in lymph flow. At rest again, left atrial pressure was raised for 35 minutes. Lymph flow rose modestly with no significant change in ventilation. The combination of hyperpnea and raised left atrial pressure at rest caused a large increase in lymph flow similar to exercise.

ment of negative interstitial pressure, or by augmented lymphatic pumping—is not clear.

Lymphatic function demands further study, both at rest and in exercise. Lymphatics are active conduits and can respond to autonomic stimuli.[10] It is suspected from preliminary experiments that increased lymphatic pumping contributes to lymph clearance during exercise. Lymphatic function has been reported by Drake et al[37–40] and in a number of unique publications.

In summary, there is a strong rationale for examining in detail capillary pressure and mechanisms of lymphatic clearance of filtered fluid during exercise. The basic information has relevance to many disparate situations including normal and exhaustive exercise, heart failure, high altitude pulmonary edema, neurogenic pulmonary edema, equine exercise pulmonary edema, and dyspnea in a variety of heart and lung disorders. Studies of acute pulmonary vasoconstriction that results from left atrial hypertension are relevant to chronic heart failure and transplant cardiology, where chronic reactive pulmonary hypertension can result in acute right heart failure in the donor heart post-transplantation.[8,41–44]

Experimental Model

Chronic Sheep Preparation

Catheters are placed in the main pulmonary artery, the left atrium, and the efferent duct of the caudal mediastinal lymph node. The tail of the node is ligated to minimize contamination by nonpulmonary lymph, and the diaphragm is scarified to reduce lymphatic drainage into the node from subdiaphragmatic tissues. Catheters are put into the superior vena cava and the thoracic aorta through neck vessels, and a #8 Cordis introducer (Cordis Co., Miami, FL) is placed in the jugular vein for later passage of a Swan-Ganz thermodilution catheter. A flat silastic balloon pressure catheter can be placed in the pericardial space, and another can be placed in the pericardial-pleural space. A 16 mm ultrasonic flow probe (T101 Ultrasonic Bloodflow Meter, Transonic Systems, Ithaca, NY) is placed around the main pulmonary artery for measurement of cardiac output. A #18 French Foley catheter is placed in the left atrium. An incision is made in the dome of the left atrium, the Foley is placed in the chamber, and the balloon is inflated with saline and pulled snug against the chamber wall. The Foley is then basket-sutured in place with Teflon pledgets. Sheep are nasally intubated with a #8 cuffed Portex tube via xylocaine topical anesthesia and bronchoscopic guidance.

Sheep are trained to run in a Quinton treadmill; training is much like human training, using interval runs of increasing speed and duration. Most sheep can trot at 2 to 2.5 mph for 45 minutes, and up to 6.0 mph for 5 to 10 minutes after appropriate training. For lymph measurements, the tip of the lymph catheter is held at or below the sternum to avoid artificial reductions in flow due to outflow resistance. Lymph is collected continuously, into a tube attached to a force transducer that is calibrated to measure lymph flow as a function of weight gain. This system allows very sensitive detection of rate and magnitude of change in lymph flow. For pressure measurements, we use transducers fixed to the chest near the level of the atria. Flow is acquired via an ultrasonic flow probe, integrated by the Transonic flow meter, and the output is fed into an AstroMed Electronic Recorder. The flow probe for each sheep is calibrated to cardiac output measured by thermal dilution. A #7.5 Swan-Ganz catheter is passed via the Cordis introducer into the pulmonary artery. Cardiac output is taken as the mean of 4 to 5 boluses of 5-mL iced saline. To vary cardiac output at rest, 1 mg isoproterenol is diluted in 100 mL of normal saline and delivered into the jugular vein by infusion pump at several rates to yield 1.5 to 2.5 × increased cardiac output (CO). The thermal dilution signal is assumed to be the true flow, and a regression line is made to normalize ultrasonic flow.

Hemodynamic Changes and Lung Lymph Clearance with Exercise

Pulmonary artery pressure rises to high levels during strenuous exercise (Figure 4).[4,48] Pulmonary artery pressures are at the level that may approach right ventricular afterload limits (40 to 50 cm H_2O). At the onset of constant rate of exercise, cardiac output rises quickly to new steady levels; pulmonary pressure rises more slowly to a peak and then decreases by 3 to 4 cm H_2O to steady state. Microvascular pressure rises more than does left atrial pressure. Pulmonary vascular resistance (PVR) decreases rapidly with exercise, and in two phases. The first phase is a 30% to 50% decrease over 20 to 40 seconds of exercise. This decrease is unaffected by intensity of exercise or by vasoactive media-

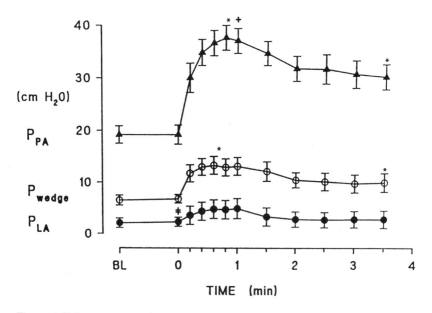

Figure 4. Pulmonary vascular pressures rise rapidly at the start of exercise. Pulmonary artery wedge pressure rises more than does left atrial pressure. True capillary pressure is unknown. The maximum pulmonary artery pressure may approach maximal stress on the right ventricle.

tors, which suggests that it is due to recruitment of capillaries of low critical opening pressure. A slower phase of reduction in resistance is influenced by mediators and is due to mechanical dilation of resistance vessels. Most of the reduction in resistance is in vessels upstream from small veins. Capillary pressure is still unknown. Capillary pressure is high during exercise (higher than estimated by the Gaar equation) because lymph flow is much higher than expected (Figure 5). Lymph/

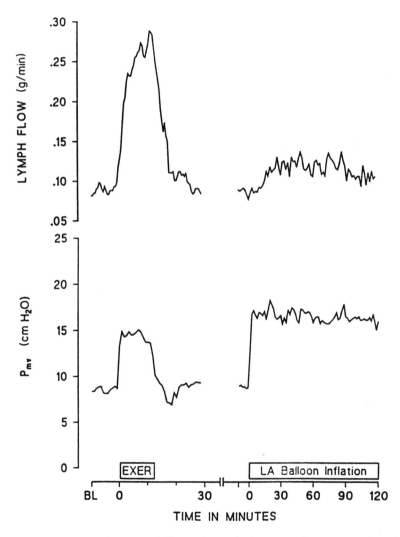

Figure 5. Lymph flows at similar estimated microvascular pressure in paired studies in sheep at rest and at exercise. Microvascular pressure was elevated by an indwelling balloon catheter in the left atrium.

plasma protein ratio drops rapidly, denoting hydrostatic effects, and lymph flow is higher during exercise than it is at comparable estimated capillary pressures induced by left atrial hypertension (Figure 6).

The focus of several experiments has been to determine how the lung stays dry during exercise.[3,4,50] Lymph flow rises rapidly with onset of exercise (up to 5 to 7 times baseline), but returns to baseline levels almost instantly at cessation of running; this suggests that the lung interstitium stays dry (nonedematous) despite high liquid transit (Figure 6). Permeability does not change because the L/P protein ratio returns quickly to resting levels. In experiments where sheep have been exercised for 40 minutes to 60 minutes at a lower pace, the return of the increased lymph flow to baseline has been somewhat delayed, suggesting that perhaps some residual excess interstitial fluid exists. This is a small amount and appears to clear over 5 to 15 minutes. Based on the rapid transients of increased and decreased lymph flow with onset and cessation of exercise, and the rapid decrease in L/P protein ratio that establishes high capillary pressure, it is believed that almost all of the increased filtrate is rapidly cleared during exercise, thus keeping the lung dry. Preliminary experiments with hyperpnea (Figure 3) suggest that a pumping mechanism exists during the hyperpnea of exer-

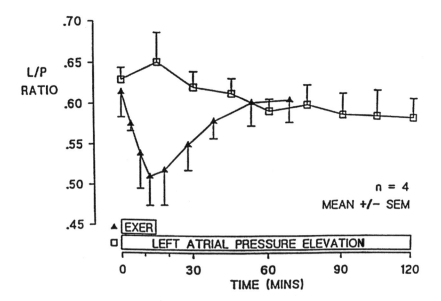

Figure 6. The lymph-to-plasma protein concentration (L/P) ratio decreases much more rapidly during exercise than during passive left atrial hypertension at a comparable baseline microvascular pressure. Microvascular pressure is elevated by means of an indwelling left atrial balloon.

cise that accelerates clearance. It is likely that prior experiments failed to show this mechanism because of insufficient hyperpnea and a lack of sufficient concomitant increase in filtration.

Several investigators have taken interest in the role of endogenous nitric oxide (NO) in exercise.[48,49] It is known that sympathetic activation occurs with exercise and that α-adrenergic constriction is balanced by β-adrenergic dilatation, resulting in neutral effects on tone. Newman and colleagues hypothesized that NO release would result from the increased shear across the endothelium during exercise, and that it would contribute to exercise-induced vasodilation. They found that the combination of unopposed α-activation during β-blockade and NO synthase inhibition resulted in extraordinary vasoconstriction of upstream vessels in the lung (Figure 7).[47] Because there were no lymph catheters in these experiments, inferences on capillary pressure could not be made. They then made a detailed study of the role of endogenous NO on the pulmonary circulation, using combinations of NO synthesis inhibition, L-arginine (substrate) infusion, and NO inhalation at rest, during hypoxic vasoconstriction and with exercise. The main findings were that NO plays a large role in reducing pulmonary vascular tone both at rest and during exercise, but that the vasodilation of exercise is not dependent on enhanced NO release.[48,49] One loose end is that NO synthase inhibition results in progressive increases in pulmonary artery pressure and resistance, suggesting that only tiny amounts of endogenous NO may have large effects on cGMP-induced vaso-relaxation.

Newman and colleagues recently made a novel observation, in part made possible by the selective nature of inhaled NO on the pulmonary circulation.[44,45] They tested the hypothesis that back pressure on the pulmonary circulation (clinically, either left heart failure or mitral valve disease) results in pulmonary vasoconstriction. This is an old idea, but they were stimulated by their observations of apparently excessive pulmonary hypertension in patients with heart failure.[41,43,46] In sheep at rest they inflated a left atrial balloon to 10 to 20 cm H_2O above baseline. Part of the response to left atrial hypertension was a reduction in PVR due to recruitment and/or distension of the bed. This they observed, but buried in this reduction in PVR was acute vasoconstriction, responsive to inhaled NO. PVR decreased to as low as 0.45 Wood units in some sheep with driving pressure across the pulmonary circulation ($Pa - P_{LA}$) of only 2 cm H_2O ($P_{PA} = 24$, $P_{LA} = 22$), with a cardiac output of 4.0 L/min[51] (see Table 1).

Newman and coworkers plan to pursue this observation, and wish to understand the mechanism by which vasoconstriction is elicited— whether it is by mediator release or by alteration in channel function. It is suspected that this phenomenon is present in the pulmonary hyper-

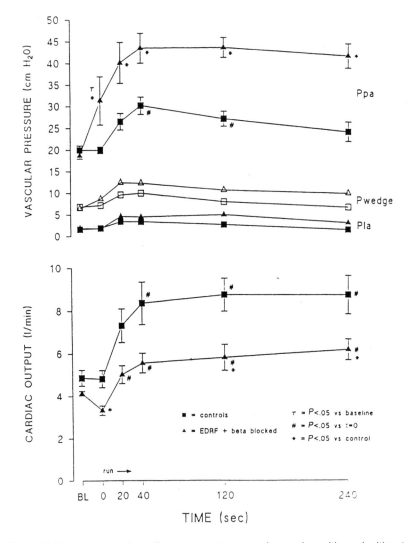

Figure 7. Pressures and cardiac output at rest and exercise with and without combined β-adrenergic and NO synthase blockade. Pulmonary artery pressures were almost double those of controls during exercise, despite a 3-liter reduction in cardiac output.

Table 1

Hemodynamic Measurements at Rest and During Left Atrial
Hypertension and the Response to Inhaled Nitric Oxide

Intervention	P_{PA} (cm H_2O)	P_{LA} (cm H_2O)	CO (L/min)	PVR	PSA (mm Hg)
Baseline + CG	18.7±0.99	3.7±0.8	5.0±0.3	2.9±0.3	91.5±5.1
Baseline + NO	15.7±0.8*	3.7±0.6	5.2±0.4	2.3±0.2	89.8±4.8
↑ Pla 10 + CG	24.5±1.6	13.7±0.6	4.4±0.3	2.4±0.4	89.6±4.4
↑ Pla 10 + NO	18.3±0.8*	14±0.6	4.6±0.3	1±0.1*	89.2±5.6
↑ Pla 20 + CG	34.7±0.8	24.2±0.9	4.6±0.3	2.3±0.3	85.0±3.5
↑ Pla 20 + NO	25.5±NO	25.5±0.9	4.6±0.2	0.6±0.1*	84.5±2.6

CG = control gas; NO = nitric oxide.
Values are the mean±SEM. *$P<0.05$ versus values without NO.

tension associated with chronic left heart failure and valvular disease, and perhaps in that hypertension associated with septal defects and high pulmonary flows.

References

1. Dempsey JA, Vidruk EH, Masterbrook SM. Pulmonary control systems in exercise. *Fed Proc* 1980;39:1498–1505
2. Reeves JT, Grover RF, Dempsey JA. Pulmonary circulation during exercise. In: Weir EK, Reeves JT (eds): *Pulmonary Vascular Physiology and Pathophysiology, Vol. 38.* New York: Marcel-Dekker, Inc.; 1989.
3. Cochran CP, King LS, Newman JH. Lung microvascular pressure and fluid filtration during exercise versus left atrial pressure elevation in sheep. *Am Rev Respir Dis* 1989;139(4):415.
4. Newman JH, Butka BJ, Parker RE, Roselli RJ. Effect of progressive exercise on lung fluid balance in sheep. *J Appl Physiol* 1988;64:2125–2131.
5. Coates GH, O'Brodovich H, Jerreries AL, Gray GW. Effects of exercise on lung lymph flow in sheep and goats during normoxia and hypoxia. *J Clin Invest* 1984;74:133–141.
6. O'Brodovich HM, Coates G. Effect of isoproterenol or exercise on pulmonary lymph flow and hemodynamics. *J Appl Physiol* 1986;60:38–44.
7. O'Brodovich H, Coates G. Effect of exercise on lung lymph flow in unanesthetized sheep with increased pulmonary vascular permeability. *Am Rev Respir Dis* 1986;134:862–866.
8. Edwards BS, Rodeheffer RJ. Prognostic features in patients with congestive heart failure and selection criteria for cardiac transplantation. *Mayo Clin Proc* 1992;67:485–492.

9. Newman JH, Loyd JE, English DE, Ogletree ML, Fulkersen WJ, Brigham KL. Effects of 100% oxygen on lung vascular function in awake sheep. *J Appl Physiol* 1983;54:1379–1386.

10. Taylor AE, Parker JC. Pulmonary interstitial spaces and lymphatics. In: *Handbook of Physiology. The Respiratory System. Circulation and Nonrespiratory Functions. Section 3, Vol. I.* Bethesda, MD: American Physiological Society; 1985;167–230.

11. Parker RE, Roselli RJ, Brigham KL. Effects of prolonged left atrial pressure elevations on protein transport in the unanesthetized sheep. *J Appl Physiol* 1985;58:869–874.

12. Parker RE, Roselli RJ, Brigham KL, Harris TR. Effects of graded increases in pulmonary vascular pressures on lung fluid balance in unanesthetized sheep. *Circ Res* 1981;49:1164–1172.

13. Roselli RJ, Parker RE, Harris TR. A model of unsteady state transvascular fluid and protein transport in the lung. *J Appl Physiol* 1984;56:1389–1402.

14. Groves BM, Reeves JT, Sutton JR, et al. Operation Everest II: Elevated high altitude pulmonary resistance unresponsive to oxygen. *J Appl Physiol* 1987;63:521–530.

15. O'Quin R, Marini JJ. Pulmonary artery occlusion pressure: Clinical physiology, measurement, and interpretation. *Am Rev Respir Dis* 1983;128:319–326.

16. Permutt S, Wise RA, Sylvester JT. Interaction between the circulatory and ventilatory pumps. In: Roussos C, Macklem PT (eds): *The Thorax, Part B, Vol. 29.* New York: Marcel Dekker; 1985.

17. Sullivan MJ, Cobb FR, Higginbotham MB. Stroke volume increases by similar mechanisms during upright exercise in normal men and women. *Am J Cardiol* 1991;67:1405–1412.

18. Younes M, Bhouty Z, Ali J. Longitudinal distribution of pulmonary vascular resistance with very high pulmonary blood flow. *J Appl Physiol* 1987;62:344–358.

19. Bhattacharya J. The lung microvascular pressure profile. *Am Rev Respir Dis* 1986;134:854–855.

20. Wagner WW Jr, Latham LP, Capen RL. Capillary recruitment during airway hypoxia: Role of pulmonary artery pressure. *J Appl Physiol* 1979;47:383–387.

21. Dawson CA, Linehan JH, Bronikowski TA. Pressure and flow in the pulmonary vascular bed. In: *Pulmonary Vascular Physiology and Pathophysiology, Vol. 38.* New York: Marcel Dekker, Inc.; 1989;51–105.

22. Dauber I, Weil J. Lung injury edema in dogs. Influence of sympathetic ablution. *J Clin Invest* 1983;72:1977–1981.

23. Parker RE, Brigham KL. Effects of endotoxemia on pulmonary vascular resistances in unanesthetized sheep. *J Appl Physiol* 1987;63:1058–1062.

24. Parker JC, Kvietys PR, Ryan KP, Taylor AE. Comparison of isogravimetric and venous occlusion capillary pressure in isolated dog lungs. *J Appl Physiol* 1983;55:964–968.

25. Cope DK, Allison RC, Parmentier JL, Miller JN, Taylor AE. Measurement of effective pulmonary capillary pressure using the pressure profile after pulmonary artery occlusion. *Crit Care Med* 1986;4:16–22.

26. Dawson CA, Linehan JH, Rickaby DA. Pulmonary microvascular hemodynamics. *Ann N Y Acad Sci* 1982;384:90–106.

27. Hakim TR, Maarek JI, Chang HK. Estimation of pulmonary capillary pressure in intact dog lungs using the arterial occlusion technique. *Am Rev Respir Dis* 1989;140:217–224.

28. Holloway H, Perry M, Downey J, Parker J, Taylor A. Estimation of effective pulmonary capillary pressure in intact lungs. *J Appl Physiol* 1983;54: 846–851.
29. Roselli RJ, Parker RE. Venous occlusion measurement of pulmonary capillary pressure: Effects of embolization. *J Appl Physiol* 1987;63: 2340–2342.
30. Pardy RL, Hussain SN, Macklem PA.The ventilatory pump in exercise. *Clin Chest Med* 1984;5(1):35–49.
31. Henke KG, Sharratt M, Pegelow D, Dempsey JA. Regulation of end expiratory lung volume during exercise. *J Appl Physiol* 1988;64:135–146.
32. Younes M, Kivinen G. Respiratory mechanics and breathing pattern during and following maximal exercise. *J Appl Physiol* 1984;57:1773–1782.
33. Albelda SM, Hansen-Flaschen JH, Lanken PN, Fishman AP. Effects of increased ventilation on lung lymph flow in unanesthetized sheep. *J Appl Physiol* 1986;60:2063–2070.
34. Gee MH, Williams DO. Effect of lung inflation on perivascular cuff fluid volume in isolated dog lung lobes. *Microvasc Res* 1978;17:192–201.
35. Giesbrecht GG, Ali F, Younes M. Short-term effect of tidal pleural pressure swings on pulmonary blood flow during rest and exercise. *J Appl Physiol* 1991;71:465–473.
36. Loyd JE, Nolop KB, Parker RE, Roselli RJ, Brigham KL. Effects of inspiratory resistance loading on lung fluid balance in awake sheep. *J Appl Physiol* 1986;60:198–203.
37. Drake RE, Adcock DK, Scott RL, Gabel JC. Effect of outflow pressure upon lymph flow from dog lungs. *Circ Res* 1982;50:865–869.
38. Drake RE, Allen SJ, Katz J, Gabel JC, Laine GA. Equivalent circuit technique for lymph flow studies. *Am J Physiol* 1986;251:H1090–H1094.
39. Drake RE, Laine GA, Allen J, Katz J, Gabel JC. Overestimation of sheep lung lymph contamination. *J Appl Physiol* 1986;61:1590–1592.
40. Gabel JC, Fallon KD, Laine GA, Drake RE. Lung lymph flow during volume infusions. *J Appl Physiol* 1986;60:623–629.
41. Haworth SG, Hall SM, Patel M. Peripheral pulmonary vascular and airway abnormalities in adolescents with rheumatic mitral stenosis. *Int J Cardiol* 1988;18:405.
42. Naeije R, Lipski A, Abramowicz M, et al. Nature of pulmonary hypertension in congestive heart failure. Effects of cardiac transplantation. *Am J Respir Crit Care Med* 1994;149:881–887.
43. Ohshima M, Yamazoe M, Tamura Y, et al. Immediate effects of percutaneous transvenous mitral commissurotomy on pulmonary hemodynamics at rest and during exercise in mitral stenosis. *Am J Cardiol* 1992;70: 641–644.
44. Frostell C, Fratacci MD, Wain JC, Jones R, Zapol WM. Inhaled nitric oxide: A selective pulmonary vasodilator reversing hypoxic pulmonary vasoconstriction. *Circulation* 1991;83:2038–2047.
45. Frostell CG, Blomqvist H, Hedenstierna G, Lundberg J. Zapol WM. Inhaled nitric oxide selectively reverses human hypoxic pulmonary vasoconstriction without causing systemic vasodilatation. *Anesthesiology* 1993; 78:427–435.
46. Roberts JD Jr, Lang P, Bigatello LM, Vlahakes GJ, Zapol WM. Inhaled nitric oxide in congenital heart disease. *Circulation* 1993;87:447–453.
47. Kane DW, Tesauro TA, Newman JH. Adrenergic modulation of pulmonary hemodynamics during strenuous exercise in sheep. *Am Rev Respir Dis* 1993;147:1233–1238.

48. Kane DW, Tesauro T, Koizumi T, Gupta R. Newman JH. Exercise induced pulmonary vasoconstriction during inhibition of NO synthase and beta adrenergic blockade. *J Clin Invest* 1994;93:677–683.
49. Koizumi T, Gupta R, Banerjee M, Newman JH. Changes in pulmonary vascular tone during exercise: Effects of NO synthase inhibition, L-arginine infusion and NO inhalation. *J Clin Invest* 1994;94:2275–2282.
50. Koizumi T, Johnston D, Bjertnaes L, Banerjee M, Newman JH. Clearance of filtrate during passive pulmonary capillary hypertension versus exercise: Role of hyperpnea. *Am J Respir Crit Care Med* 1994;149(4):A820.
51. Hermo CI, Koizumi T, Newman JH. Effect of inhaled NO on pulmonary vascular resistance during left atrial hypertension in sheep. *Circulation* 1994;90(4 Part 2):A1655.

Chapter 4

Lung Edema in Neonates

Candice D. Fike, MD

Introduction

The basic principles that govern lung fluid filtration are the same in newborn and adult animals. In lungs of both age groups, fluid is continuously filtered from the pulmonary circulation into the interstitial space and then returned to the intravascular compartment by the lymphatics. The bulk of fluid filtration in the lung occurs in the capillaries, and the rate that fluid is filtered out of the capillaries is determined largely by the balance between hydrostatic and protein osmotic pressures across the capillary bed. Although the determinants of lung fluid filtration are the same in newborn and adult animals, there is evidence that both the basal rate of lung fluid filtration and the change in rate of fluid filtration in response to a variety of physiological stimuli differ with postnatal age. For example, lung fluid filtration is greater per gram of lung tissue in newborn lambs and puppies than in mature sheep and dogs.[1,2] The rate of lung fluid filtration appears to increase more with elevations in pulmonary blood flow in newborn lambs than it does in mature sheep.[3,4] In addition, lung fluid filtration increases in response to alveolar hypoxia in newborn lambs, but does not in adult sheep.[5,6] In other words, lung fluid filtration increases more in response to a variety of physiological stimuli in newborns than in adults, such that the propensity for edema formation may be greater in newborns than adults. To improve our understanding of the pathogenesis of neonatal lung edema, it is important to determine the factors that contribute to the neonatal tendency for a high rate of lung fluid filtration.

From: Weir EK, Reeves JT (eds). *Pulmonary Edema*. Armonk, NY: Futura Publishing Company, Inc.; ©1998.

This work was supported by the American Heart Association and by NIH R29-HL-42883.

Microvascular Pressure Measurements

One of the major determinants of lung fluid filtration is capillary hydrostatic pressure. An explanation for age-related differences in lung fluid filtration rates could be that regulation of capillary hydrostatic pressures changes with postnatal age. Ideal testing of this hypothesis requires measurement of the hydrostatic pressure in alveolar septal wall capillaries of lungs of newborn and older animals. However, alveolar septal wall capillaries are not accessible for direct pressure measurements. Therefore, capillary hydrostatic pressure must be estimated from indirect methods.[7] For example, 20- to 80-μm diameter subpleural microvessels are present on the lung surface of many species, and the pressure in these subpleural microvessels can be measured by direct micropuncture. The pressure in these subpleural microvessels can then be used to estimate pulmonary capillary pressure.[8]

To determine whether microvascular pressures are regulated differently in lungs of newborns and adults, Fike and colleagues[9,10] first measured microvascular pressures under baseline conditions. The direct micropuncture technique was applied to isolated perfused lungs of rabbits of different postnatal ages: 12- to 72-hour-old rabbits, 5- to 15-day-old rabbits, and adult rabbits. They measured pressures in 20- to 80-μm diameter subpleural arterioles and venules at blood flow rates, approximating in vivo cardiac outputs for each age group (200 mL·min^{-1}·kg^{-1} for 12- to 72-hour-old rabbits and 5- to 15-day-old rabbits, and 100 mL·min^{-1}·kg^{-1} for the adult rabbits). During micropuncture, airway and left atrial pressures were held constant at the same level in all age groups. An airway pressure of 5 cm H_2O was used so that the pleura was taut enough for the pipette to puncture it, and zone 3 conditions (left atrial pressure of 9 cm H_2O > airway pressure of 5 cm H_2O) were used[11] to ensure maximal perfusion of the pulmonary capillary bed. They found that the pressure in 20- to 80-μm diameter arterioles tended to be higher in 12- to 72-hour-old rabbits compared to adult rabbits (Figure 1).[10] Assuming a linear drop in pressure between 20- and 80-μm-diameter arterioles and 20- and 80-μm-diameter venules, the mid-microvascular pressure (Pmv) can be used to approximate capillary pressure. Comparison of these values between age groups demonstrates no significant change in Pmv with postnatal age in rabbits: Pmv = 15.4±2.4 cm H_2O in 12- to 72-hour-old rabbits (n=10) versus 14.7±3.8 cm H_2O in 5- to 15-day-old rabbits (n=15) versus 15.1±2.8 cm H_2O in adult rabbits (n=7). This lack of a postnatal change in Pmv in rabbit lungs suggests that at a given left atrial pressure, the capillary pressure should be essentially the same in zone 3 lungs of each age group. However, if left atrial pressure decreases with postnatal age,

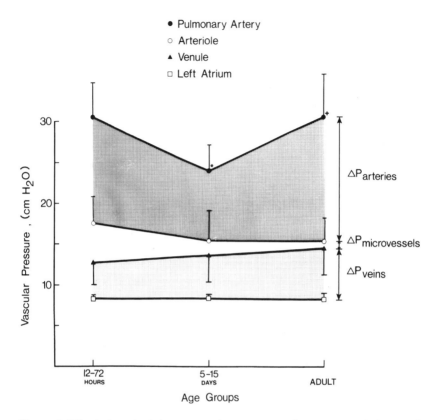

Figure 1. Effect of postnatal age on pulmonary vascular pressures in lungs of rabbits. *Different from value in 12- to 72-hour-old rabbits; +different from value in 5- to 15-day-old rabbits; one-way analysis of variance with Newman-Keuls multiple comparison test ($P<0.05$).

as has been found,[1] then capillary pressure should decrease concomitantly and may contribute to a maturational decrease in lung fluid filtration, such as has been observed to occur in sheep.[1]

The above conclusion regarding capillary pressures is only relevant for zone 3 lungs of the different age groups. It is possible that the relationship between microvascular, left atrial, and airway pressures differ with postnatal age such that Pmv might not be the same in zone 2 lungs of adult and newborn rabbits. To evaluate this possibility, Fike et al[12,13] measured the pressures in 20- to 80-μm diameter arterioles and 20- to 80-μm diameter venules in isolated perfused lungs of 5- to 15-day-old rabbits and adult rabbits as left atrial pressure was lowered below (zone 2) airway pressure. They found that under zone 2 conditions, microarteriolar pressures were the same, but microvenular pressures tended to be lower in newborn rabbits than in adult rabbits (Figure 2).[12,13] The reason for this age-related difference in venular pressures under zone 2 conditions is that the site of flow limitation, or the vascular waterfall effect,[14] appears to differ between these two age groups. That is, in 5- to 15-day-old rabbits, microvenular pressure continues to decrease when left atrial pressure decreases below airway pressure (Figure 2),[12] consistent with capillaries as the site of the vascular waterfall.[14] In contrast, in adult rabbits, microvenular pressures remain fairly constant as left atrial pressure decreases below airway pressure (Figure 2),[13] consistent with venules larger than 20 to 80 μm in diameter as the site of the vascular waterfall.[14] The relevance of these findings to lung fluid filtration is that with equivalent left atrial pressures under zone 2 conditions, Pmvs would tend to be higher in adult lungs than in newborn lungs (Figure 2). However, left atrial pressures may not be the same in the two age groups.[1] Also, the proportion of the lungs in zone 2 conditions may not be the same in the two age groups.[15]

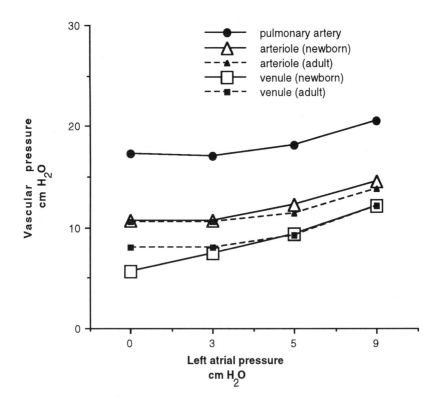

Figure 2. Effect of changing left atrial pressure from above (zone 3) to below (zone 2) an airway pressure of 5 cm H_2O on pulmonary vascular pressures in lungs of newborn (5- to 15-day-old) rabbits and adult rabbits.

Another issue to be considered is that Pmv may vary with height of the lung due to the influence of gravity.[11] Because of the markedly smaller lung size, the variability in Pmv due to height is much smaller in newborns than in adults. Some newborn animals, such as mice, are small enough that the use of one Pmv to represent fluid filtration for the entire lung is reasonable. However, in most adult animals, the height of the lung is large enough to cause a significant gradient in Pmv from the top of the lung to the bottom of the lung. Another problem is that the mass of the lung is not uniformly distributed with height.[16] For example, the high Pmv encountered at the bottom of the lung would have a small contribution to total lung fluid filtration if the effective lung mass at the bottom of the lung was small.

Also to be considered is the finding by Fike and colleague[10] that there is a measurable gradient in pressure across the microvascular bed that changes with postnatal age. In particular, 20- to 80-μm diameter arteriolar pressure is higher in 12- to 72-hour-old rabbits than in adult rabbits,[10] which could contribute to a higher rate of fluid filtration in lungs of the younger animals. Without knowledge of the contribution to total lung fluid filtration from these 20- to 80-μm diameter arterioles, estimates of postnatally related differences in fluid filtration rate across them cannot be made.

The above discussion points out some of the problems associated with using one Pmv to represent fluid filtration for the entire lung. To better estimate why rates of lung fluid filtration differ between newborns and adults, it is necessary to know how the distribution of Pmvs relative to zonal conditions and lung mass differs with postnatal age. The contribution to total lung fluid filtration from microvessels must also be determined. Nonetheless, by measuring microvascular pressure responses to different conditions and stimuli it is possible to evaluate whether regulation of microvascular pressures changes with postnatal age. This issue is discussed below.

Perimicrovascular Interstitial Pressure Measurements

The other hydrostatic pressure that is important for regulation of lung fluid balance is interstitial pressure. The issue of particular relevance to maturational differences in lung fluid flux is that even in the face of equivalent microvascular or capillary pressures, if lower pericapillary interstitial pressures were found in newborn lungs compared to adult lungs, then this would result in a higher rate of lung fluid filtration in newborn lungs. As with intravascular pressure measurements, the inaccessibility of the alveolar septal wall capillaries has led to the use of indirect estimates of the interstitial pressure surrounding these vessels.[17] To approximate the pressure in the interstitium surrounding the pulmonary capillaries, the alveolar liquid pressure (the pressure in the fluid that lines the alveolar wall) has been measured by direct micropuncture.[17-20] The assumption is that in edematous lungs, alveolar liquid pressure will equilibrate with pericapillary interstitial fluid pressure because interstitial flow resistance is likely to be small, and osmotic gradients across the alveolar epithelium are likely to be absent.[17] Because measurements of alveolar liquid pressure in living animals[20] have been similar to measurements in excised lungs with varying amounts of edema,[12,13,18-20] it seems reasonable to conclude that alveolar liquid pressure should reflect pericapillary interstitial pressure in nonedematous as well as in edematous lungs. In addition to alveolar liquid pressure measurements, the direct micropuncture technique has been used to measure lung liquid tissue pressures in the interstitium around 20- to 80-μm diameter subpleural microvessels.[12,13] For example, Fike et al[18] found no gradient between alveolar liquid pressure and the interstitial pressure of 20- to 80-μm diameter venules (perivenular interstitial pressure) in nonedematous to mildly edematous, perfused lungs of newborn rabbits. Nor did they find a gradient between the perivenular pressure and the interstitial pressure of 20- to 80-μm diameter arterioles (periarteriolar pressure) in perfused lungs of adult rabbits (Figure 3).[13] Based on the assumption that alveolar liquid pressure reflects pericapillary pressure, their findings lead them to conclude that measurements of perimicrovascular pressure reflect pericapillary pressure.

To evaluate whether perimicrovascular interstitial pressure, hence pericapillary interstitial pressure, differs between lungs of newborns and adults, Fike and colleagues[12,13] measured perivenular pressures by direct micropuncture in isolated perfused lungs of 5- to 15-day-old rabbits and adult rabbits. To evaluate the influence of changing vascular pressure and zonal conditions on perivenular interstitial pressure, they measured perivenular pressure at left atrial pressures above (zone 3) and below (zone 2) an airway pressure of 5 cm H_2O. Notably, perivenular interstitial pressures were similar in lungs of 5- to 15-day-old rabbits and adult rabbits at the airway and left atrial pressures studied (Figure 3).[12,13] Moreover, changing left atrial pressure by 10 cm H_2O, ie, changing from zone 3 to zone 2 conditions, had minimal effect on perivenular interstitial pressure in lungs of either age group (Figure 3).[12,13] Unlike the finding of a gradient of pressure across the microvascular bed that is influenced by zonal conditions and postnatal age, these results provide no evidence that at inflation pressures near functional residual capacity, postnatal differences in perivenular, hence pericapillary interstitial pressures, contribute to maturational differences in lung fluid flux.

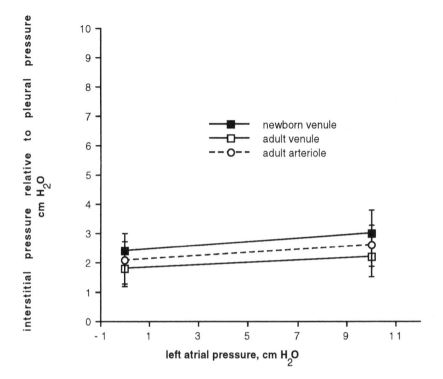

Figure 3. Effect on pulmonary perimicrovascular interstitial pressures of changing left atrial pressure from above (zone 3) to below (zone 2) an airway pressure of 5 cm H_2O in lungs of newborn (5- to 15-day-old) rabbits and adult rabbits.

Regulation of Perimicrovascular Interstitial Pressure

It should be noted that there are situations in which pericapillary interstitial pressure might differ between newborns and adults. For example, Fike and colleagues[18] found that alveolar liquid pressure is lower in lungs of 1-to 15-day-old rabbits than in adult rabbits at inflation pressures near total lung capacity. This age-related difference in the effect of lung inflation on alveolar liquid pressures may be due to either a larger surface tension or smaller radius of curvature of the alveolar air-liquid interface in the newborn lung, according to the Laplace relationship. In other words, due to age-related differences in the influence of lung inflation on alveolar liquid pressure (ie, pericapillary interstitial pressure), newborns may be more likely than adults to develop lung edema under conditions of positive pressure ventilation.

Regulation of Microvascular Pressures

The finding by Fike and colleagues[10] of a gradient in microvascular pressure that changes with postnatal age, raises the question of how the microarteriolar and microvenular pressures are controlled and whether these pressures are controlled similarly in lungs of newborn and adult animals. To evaluate maturational differences in regulation of pulmonary microvascular pressures, they performed studies to determine if the sites of pulmonary vasoconstriction in response to the vasoactive stimulus, alveolar hypoxia, changed with postnatal age in rabbits.[21,24] Their interest in evaluating the response to hypoxia stems from the fact that children appear to be more susceptible than adults to the development of pulmonary edema at high altitude.[22,23] To evaluate microvascular pressure responses to hypoxia, they measured pressures in 20- to 80-μm diameter arterioles and venules in isolated perfused lungs of 12- to 72-hour-old rabbits, 7- to 23-day-old rabbits, and adult rabbits that were inflated sequentially with normoxic and hypoxic gas mixtures.[21,24]

Their results showed that 20- to 80-μm diameter arteriolar pressure responses to hypoxia differed with postnatal age. Specifically, 20- to 80-μm diameter arteriolar pressures increased by 1.4 ± 0.3 cm H_2O with hypoxia in lungs of 12- to 72-hour-old rabbits, did not change with hypoxia in lungs of 7- to 23-day-old rabbits, and decreased by 1.3 ± 1.1 cm H_2O with hypoxia in lungs of adult rabbits.[21,24] In contrast to this decrease in magnitude of hypoxic response with postnatal age, the magnitude of hypoxic response of pulmonary arteries larger than 20 to 80 μm in diameter increased with postnatal age.[21,24] Perhaps most importantly, 20- to 80-μm diameter venular pressures did not change with hypoxia in lungs of any age group.[21,24] The lack of an age-related difference in 20- to 80-μm diameter venular responses to hypoxia does not support the idea that larger increases in capillary pressure explain hypoxia-related differences in lung edema formation between newborns and adults. Yet, even small changes in capillary pressure can alter lung fluid filtration due to the large surface area that can be involved. It is possible that an increased rate of lung fluid filtration might result from an increase in pressure in vessels located downstream from 20- to 80-μm diameter arterioles, but upstream from 20- to 80-μm diameter venules, such as occurred with hypoxia in 12- to 72-hour-old rabbit lungs.[21]

Partly because of differences in the amount of capillary surface area that might be affected, venular constriction may have the potential to have a greater impact on the regulation of lung fluid filtration than does arteriolar constriction. Therefore, Fike and colleagues wanted to know whether regulation of 20 to 80 μm venous pressures by stimuli other than hypoxia might differ with postnatal age. For these studies,[25] they measured 20- to 80-μm diameter venular pressure in isolated lungs of 12- to 72-hour-old rabbits and adult rabbits either before and during serotonin infusions or before and after nitric oxide (NO) synthesis inhibition with N^w nitro-L-arginine. Serotonin was chosen as a vasoactive stimulus because it is a smooth-muscle constrictor released by activated platelets, and it may mediate some of the hypertensive responses in disease states such as sepsis. Inhibition of NO synthesis is of interest because even though numerous studies have provided evidence that NO is important in regulating pulmonary arterial pressure,[26–28] the role of NO in regulating venous and microvascular pressures has received less attention. The results found by Fike and coworker[25] demonstrated no maturational differences in 20- to 80-μm diameter venular responses to serotonin (in six newborns: venular pressure was 11.1 ± 0.5 cm H_2O versus 10.9 ± 0.4 cm H_2O respectively, before and during infusion of serotonin; in nine adults: venular pressure was 13.6 ± 1.7 cm H_2O versus 13.1 ± 2.1 cm H_2O respectively, before and during infusion of serotonin). In contrast, the role of NO in regulating venous pressures was influenced by postnatal age. Specifically, in lungs of adult but not newborn rabbits, 20- to 80-μm diameter venular pressures increased with NO inhibition.[25] Moreover, in some additional studies Fike and coworker found that after NO inhibition, serotonin infusion caused an increase in 20- to 80-μm diameter venular pressures in lungs of adult rabbits, but not in lungs of newborn rabbits.[25] Thus, NO appears to modulate both basal venous tone and venous responses to serotonin in an age-dependent fashion in rabbits. Overall, Fike and colleague's findings in rabbits do not support the idea that maturational differences in regulation of microvenular pressures contribute to a greater tendency for lung edema formation in newborns than in adults. However, they find that age-related differences in regulation of microarteriolar pressure in rabbits could contribute to developmental differences in lung fluid filtration rates if increased pressure in small arterioles reflects increased pressure in part of the capillary bed and/or if the contribution to lung fluid filtration from these small arterioles is physiologically significant.

An obvious concern is whether results in rabbits can be extrapolated to other species. To evaluate maturational differences in regulation of pulmonary microvascular pressures in another species, Fike and colleagues performed studies to determine if the vascular sites of pulmonary constriction in response to either alveolar hypoxia or to NO synthesis inhibition differed with postnatal age in piglets.[29–31] They chose piglets because postnatal changes in their pulmonary circulation occur over a short time period and follow a pattern similar to that of humans.[32] To evaluate differences in hypoxic responses, they measured pulmonary vascular pressures in isolated perfused lungs of 3- to 8-day-old piglets and 11- to 15-day-old piglets that were inflated sequentially with normoxic and hypoxic gas mixtures.[29,30] To evaluate the role of NO in other studies they measured pulmonary vascular pressures before and after addition of the NO synthesis inhibitor, N^{w}nitro-L-arginine methyl ester (L-NAME), to the perfusate of lungs of both age groups.[31]

Fike and colleague found that both pulmonary arterial pressure and 20- to 80-μm diameter venular pressure increased with hypoxia in lungs of younger (3- to 8-day-old) piglets; whereas for older (11- to 15-day-old) piglets the pulmonary arterial pressure response to hypoxia was so small and inconsistent, that 20- to 80-μm diameter venular pressures were not measured.[29,30] In fact, the hypoxia-induced increase in pressure across the venular compartment of younger piglets (4.7±4.1 cm H_2O) was greater than the hypoxia-induced increase in pressure across the entire pulmonary circulation of the older piglets (1.9±4.0 cm H_2O). Therefore, the increase in venous pressure, hence capillary pressure, must have been greater with hypoxia in the younger piglet in than the older piglets. Their findings also suggest that NO plays a greater role in regulating microvenular pressures in younger piglets than in older piglets.[31] This conclusion is based on their finding that with NO inhibition, both pulmonary arterial and microvenular pressures increased by a greater amount in lungs of the younger piglets than in lungs of the older piglets (Figure 4).[31] These findings are consistent with the idea that NO production is an important mechanism for maintaining of low venous pressure, hence providing protection against edema formation, in lungs of newborns. Thus, in contrast to findings in rabbits, results of studies in piglets support the idea that maturational differences in regulation of microvenular pressures may contribute significantly to a greater tendency for lung edema formation in newborns than in older animals.

In further attempts to improve their understanding of the susceptibility of newborns to lung edema formation, Fike and colleague evaluated the influence of chronic hypoxia on the regulation of microvenular pressures in newborns.[30,31] Their interest in chronic hypoxia stems from the fact that infants with a variety of cardiopulmonary disorders suffer from prolonged episodes of hypoxia. For these studies, they raised newborn piglets in hypoxic chambers or control chambers for 5 days or 10 days. Using isolated lungs, they evaluated pulmonary microvenular pressure responses to acute hypoxia by measuring 20- to 80-μm diameter venular pressures during sequential inflation with normoxic and hypoxic gas mixtures.[30] In other lungs, they determined whether regulation of microvenular pressures by NO was altered by measuring 20- to 80-μm diameter venular pressures before and after NO synthesis inhibition with L-NAME.[31] They found that newborn

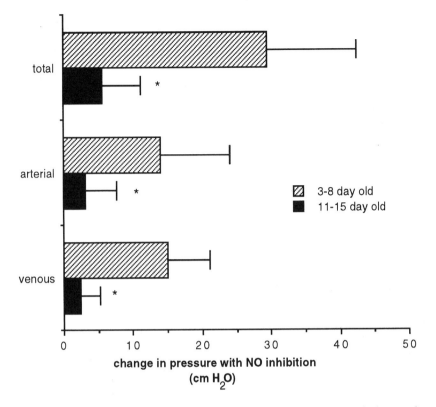

Figure 4. Effect of NO inhibition on pulmonary vascular pressures in lungs of 3- to 8-day-old piglets and 11- to 15-day-old piglets. Total = pressure gradient from pulmonary artery to left atrium; arterial = pressure gradient from pulmonary artery to 20- to 80-μm diameter venule; venous = pressure gradient from 20- to 80-μm diameter venule to left atrium. *Different from value in 3- to 8-day-old piglet, unpaired t test (*P*<0.05).

piglets developed pulmonary hypertension, and that the degree of pulmonary hypertension progressed with length of exposure to chronic hypoxia.[30] Notably, 20- to 80-μm diameter venular pressures were not elevated in the chronically hypoxic animals, indicating that the vascular sites of development of pulmonary hypertension involved arteries and not veins.[30] They also found that 20- to 80-μm diameter venular responses to acute hypoxia were augmented in the piglets exposed to hypoxia for the shorter (5 days), but not the longer (10 days), time period.[30] Another finding was that the 20- to 80-μm diameter venular responses to NO inhibition were not altered after 5 days of hypoxia, but were blunted in lungs of piglets exposed to 10 days of hypoxia.[31] Thus, regulation of microvenular pressures was altered by exposure to chronic hypoxia. With relatively short periods of chronic hypoxia, altered venous responses to some stimuli, such as acute hypoxia, might lead to a greater tendency for edema formation. With more prolonged exposure to hypoxia, the augmented tendency to increase microvenular pressure might not be present. Only with the longer exposure to chronic hypoxia does the role of NO in maintaining low microvenous pressure appear to be altered. Indeed their findings suggest that NO production is decreased with the longer exposure to chronic hypoxia, a finding that has important implications regarding the role of NO production and the development of neonatal pulmonary hypertension.[31]

Summary

Postnatal differences in the regulation of microvascular and perimicrovascular interstitial pressures help explain the susceptibility of newborns to development of pulmonary edema. Findings in rabbits suggest that a higher pressure on the arterial side of the microvascular bed and a propensity to increase microarteriolar pressures in response to physiologically relevant stimuli are factors that may contribute to the tendency for newborns to develop lung edema. Lower perimicrovascular interstitial pressures may make newborns more likely than adults to develop lung edema under conditions of positive pressure ventilation. Fike and colleagues' findings in piglets support the idea that large microvenular pressure responses may promote neonatal lung edema formation and that production of NO may be an important mechanism to maintain low microvenous pressures. Studies in piglets also indicate that this proclivity to elevate microvenular pressures may be augmented by a few days' exposure to chronic hypoxia. A future goal is to determine the mechanisms for the maturational differences in regulation of microvascular pressures in order to develop better therapies for the treatment and prevention of lung edema in neonates.

References

1. Bland RD, Bressack MA, Haberkern CM, Hansen TN. Lung fluid balance in hypoxic, awake newborn lambs and mature sheep. *Biol Neonate* 1980; 38:221–228.
2. Levine OR, Rodriguez-Martinez F, Mellins RB. Fluid filtration in the lung of the intact puppy. *J Appl Physiol* 1973;34:683–686.
3. Coates G, O'Brodovich H, Jeffries AL, Gray GW. Effects of exercise on lung lymph flow in sheep and goats during normoxia and hypoxia. *J Clin Invest* 1984;74:133–141.
4. Feltes T, Hansen TN. Effects of an aorticopulmonary shunt on lung fluid balance in the young lamb. *Pediatr Res* 1989;26:94–97.

5. Bland RD, Demling RH, Selinger SL, Staub NC. Effects of alveolar hypoxia on lung fluid and protein transport in unanesthetized sheep. *Circ Res* 1977;40:269–274.
6. Bressack M, Bland RD. Alveolar hypoxia increases lung fluid filtration in unanesthetized newborn lambs. *Circ Res* 1980;46:111–116.
7. Dawson CA, Linehan JH, Rickaby DH. Pulmonary microcirculatory hemodynamics. *Ann N Y Acad Sci* 1982;384:90–106.
8. Bhattacharya J, Staub NC. Direct measurement of microvascular pressures in the isolated perfused dog lung. *Science* 1980;210:327–328.
9. Fike CD, Lai-Fook SJ, Bland RD. Microvascular pressures measured by micropuncture in lungs of newborn rabbits. *J Appl Physiol* 1987;63: 1070–1075.
10. Fike CD, Kaplowitz MR. Longitudinal distribution of pulmonary vascular pressures as a function of postnatal age in rabbits. *J Appl Physiol* 1991;71:2160–2167.
11. West JB, Dollery CT, Naimark A. Distribution of blood flow in isolated lung: Relation to vascular and alveolar pressures. *J Appl Physiol* 1964;19: 713–724.
12. Fike CD, Lai-Fook SJ. Effect of airway and left atrial pressures on microcirculation of newborn lungs. *J Appl Physiol* 1990;69:1063–1072.
13. Fike CD, Kaplowitz MR. Effect of airway and left atrial pressures on microvascular and interstitial pressures in adult lungs. *J Appl Physiol* 1993;74: 2112–2120.
14. Permutt S, Bromberger-Barnea R, Bane HN. Alveolar pressure, pulmonary venous pressure, and the vascular waterfall. *Med Thorac* 1962; 19:239–260.
15. Nelin LD, Wearden ME, Welty SE, Hansen TN. The effect of blood flow and left atrial pressure on the DLCO in lambs and sheep. *Resp Physiol* 1992;88:333–342.
16. Staub NC. The forces regulating fluid filtration in the lung. *Microvasc Res* 1978;15:45–55.
17. Lai-Fook SJ. Mechanics of lung fluid balance. *Crit Rev Biomed Eng* 1986;13: 171–200.
18. Fike CD, Lai-Fook SJ, Bland RD. Alveolar liquid pressures in newborn and adult rabbit lungs. *J Appl Physiol* 1988;64:1629–1635.
19. Ganesan S, Lai-Fook SJ, Schurch S. Alveolar liquid pressures in nonedematous and kerosene-washed rabbit lungs by micropuncture. *Respir Physiol* 1989;78:281–296.
20. Ganesan S, Lai-Fook SJ. Alveolar liquid pressure measured in the intact rabbit chest by micropuncture. *J Appl Physiol* 1993;75:1525–1528.
21. Fike CD, Kaplowitz MR. Developmental differences of the vascular response to hypoxia in lungs of rabbits. *J Appl Physiol* 1994;77:507–516.
22. Hultgren HN, Grover RF. Circulatory adaptation to high altitude. *Ann Rev Med* 1968;19:119–152.
23. Scoggin CH, Hyers TM, Reeves JT, Grover RF. High-altitude pulmonary edema in the children and young adults of Leadville, Colorado. *New Engl J Med* 1977;297:1269–1272.
24. Fike CD, Lai-Fook SJ, Bland RD. Microvascular pressures during hypoxia in isolated lungs of newborn rabbits. *J Appl Physiol* 1988;65:283–287.
25. Fike CD, Kaplowitz MR. Developmental differences in the effect of N^w nitro-L-arginine on venular responses to serotonin (5-HT) in rabbit lungs. *FASEB J* 1993;7:A769.

26. Abman SH, Chatfield BA, Hall SL, McMurtry IF. Role of endothelium-derived relaxing factor during transition of pulmonary circulation at birth. *Am J Physiol* 1990;259:H1921–H1927.
27. Shaul PW, Farra MA, Magness RR. Pulmonary endothelial nitric oxide production is developmentally regulated in the fetus and the newborn. *Am J Physiol* 1993;265:H1056–H1063.
28. Zellers TM, Vanhoutte PM. Endothelium-dependent relaxations of piglet pulmonary arteries augment with maturation. *Pediatr Res* 1991;30: 176–180.
29. Fike CD, Kaplowitz MR. Pulmonary venous pressure increases during alveolar hypoxia in isolated lungs of newborn pigs. *J Appl Physiol* 1992; 73:552–556.
30. Fike CD, Kaplowitz MR. Effect of chronic hypoxia on pulmonary vascular pressures in isolated lungs of newborn pigs. *J Appl Physiol* 1994;77: 2853–2862.
31. Fike CD, Kaplowitz MR. Chronic hypoxia alters nitric oxide-dependent pulmonary vascular responses in lungs of newborn pigs. *J Appl Physiol* 1996;81:2078–2087.
32. Rendas A, Branthwaite M, Reid L. Growth of the pulmonary circulation in normal pig-structural analysis and cardiopulmonary function. *J Appl Physiol* 1978;45:806–817.

Chapter 5

Aquaporins, Caveolae, and Capillary Permeability

Jan E. Schnitzer, MD

The luminal cell surface of the endothelium is exposed directly to the circulating blood, and represents a key barrier to the movement of circulating molecules and cells from the blood to the interstitium and underlying tissue cells. Several pathways exist for the transport of plasma molecules across continuous endothelium: (1) intercellular junctions are highly regulated structures that form the paracellular pathway for the pressure-driven filtration of water and small solutes, (2) noncoated plasmalemmal vesicles (also called caveolae) transcytose blood macromolecules apparently by shuttling their blood-derived molecular cargo from the luminal to antiluminal aspect of the endothelium, and (3) transendothelial channels may form transiently in very attenuated regions of the cell by the fusion of two or more caveolae, each located on apposing plasma membranes, to provide a direct conduit for the exchange of both small and large plasma molecules (see Schnitzer[1] for review). Capillary permeability is dependent not only on the structure of these transport pathways, but in many vascular beds it is also dependent on the interaction of serum proteins such as albumin and orosomucoid with the endothelial glycocalyx.[1-6] This interaction with serum appears to be required to maintain "normal" endothelial cell barrier function and capillary permeability.

In most organs, the endothelium is the critical barrier preventing the passage of molecules and cells circulating in the blood to the underlying tissue cells. When this barrier is disrupted, and as the endothelium becomes dysfunctional, tissue homeostasis is disturbed and various pathologies may ensue including atherosclerosis, cerebral strokes, coagulopathies, ischemia, diabetic microangiopathy, and even

From: Weir EK, Reeves JT (eds). *Pulmonary Edema*. Armonk, NY: Futura Publishing Company, Inc.; ©1998.

hypertension. Conversely, the endothelium must overcome its inherent necessary restrictiveness by using specific transport mechanisms to provide essential nutrients to the underlying tissue cells in accordance with their particular metabolic requirements. It has been rather difficult to define the interactions between the endothelial cell surface and circulating blood molecules, especially with regards to transvascular transport. The development of techniques for isolating and growing endothelial cells in culture allowed some important characterization of these processes. Unfortunately, it is quite evident that endothelial cells change when grown in vitro, creating an apparently "dedifferentiated" phenotype much different, both morphologically and functionally, from that found in vivo. For instance, many continuous endothelia lose most of their caveolae when grown in culture.[3,7] Hence, it is necessary to refocus the attention of researchers to the endothelium as it exists in its native state in tissue.

A process has been developed for purifying directly from tissue not only the luminal endothelial cell surface membrane, but also the plasmalemmal transport vesicles, called caveolae, which carry molecules into and/or across the endothelium.[8] Briefly, the endothelial cell plasma membrane, which is directly in contact with the circulating blood, represents the critical interface for specific transport, and can be isolated with use of an in situ silica-coating procedure followed by tissue homogenization and centrifugation. Furthermore, investigators have separated the caveolae from this membrane by physically shearing them off the plasmalemma and then purifying them by centrifugation as low-density vesicles in a sucrose gradient. With use of these membrane fractions, investigators have begun to carry out "molecular mapping" studies to define the molecules that comprise the endothelial cell surface and its transport structures. In combination with functional transport assays, key proteins involved in the specific transport of water and macromolecules such as albumin have been identified in certain endothelia. Some of these findings are discussed in this chapter.

Caveolae in Endothelium

Protein transport by specific vesicular carriers is a fundamental cellular process found in a variety of cells that forms the basis of intracellular trafficking, receptor-mediated endocytosis, and transcytosis. Clathrin-coated vesicles, the best characterized of the vesicular carriers, provide a specific delivery system for many ligands into and across cells. Caveolae also appear to deliver ligands, including cholera toxin, tetanus toxin, and protein conjugated to colloidal gold particles, to specific destinations, such as endosomes, within the cell.[9–13] With electron microscopy, caveolae are recognized in many cell types as invaginated pits or vesicles that do not have a thick electron-dense fuzzy coat (distinct for coated vesicles), and have a rather consistent diameter of ~800Å. Their cytoplasmic surfaces have bipolar-oriented, thin striations that may be formed from caveolin polymerization.[14,15] Although the existence of caveolae in many cells, especially endothelium, has been known for over 40 years, it has been somewhat problematic to conclusively define their precise function(s).

Ultrastructural studies with orosomucoid and various albumins conjugated to gold provide evidence that caveolae may be involved not only in receptor-mediated endocytosis, but also in transcytosis.[10,16–18] Native monomeric albumin is transcytosed via caveolae but, unlike the modified albumins, apparently avoids accumulation within lysosomes.[18] It appears that endothelia of the continuous type found in many organs such as lung, heart, and skeletal muscle have a very abundant population of caveolae that function in the endocytosis or transcytosis of select membrane-bound ligands.[1] In the last few years, specific proteins that permit or facilitate the select transendothelial transport of insulin[19] and blood carrier proteins such as albumin[20,21] and transferrin[22] have been identified on the endothelial cell surface. It has been presumed that this specific transport is mediated by the abundant population of caveolae found in certain endothelia. However, only albumin has been shown by immunoelectron microscopy to bind and accumulate preferentially within caveolae for apparent transcytosis and release to the interstitium.[18]

In all of these studies, the select labeling within caveolae has been interpreted as indicative of specific discrete transport by caveolae. Yet, they are based primarily on ultrastructural examination, which unfortunately cannot prove definitively that caveolae function in transport. Caveolae exist as a racemose structure with many vesicles linked to each other in a chain to form a grape-like branching "cave" that penetrates deep into the cell. Conventional sections of these structures for electron microscopy can be quite misleading. They can show approximately 50% of the noncoated vesicles apparently free in the cytoplasm, while serial ultrathin sectioning reveals that only 1% or less of them are actually free and unattached to other membranes.[23] The additional discovery that aldehyde fixation artefactually increases the number of noncoated invaginations creates even more confusion.[24] Thus, many investigators have concluded that caveolae are not dynamic vesicular carriers but rather fixed permanent invaginations incapable of budding. With this in mind, potocytosis was proposed as an alternative way to move molecules into cells without the need for caveolae to bud off the cell surface.[25] It appears that past methodologies cannot resolve this issue and, therefore, other new approaches will be required to define whether caveolae are dynamic traffickers or static microdomains on the cell surface.

To address this recurrent unresolved controversy, in the last few years, Schnitzer and colleagues[8,10,13,21,26,27,68] have developed new strategies for assessing the function of caveolae in endothelial transport by examining the molecular aspects of this putative transport pathway and searching for specific pharmacological inhibitors. Caveolae have been purified to homogeneity from endothelium in rat lung tissue, which has allowed extensive molecular characterization of these invaginated plasmalemmal structures. In addition, various assays have been developed for measuring endothelial transport including in situ assays by perfusing tissue, intact and permeabilized cultured cells (transcytosis and endocytosis), and most recently, reconstituted cell-free systems.[10,12,13,21,28] Some of their recent findings in this area are discussed below.

Caveolae as Specific Transport Vesicles

The recent identification of two pharmacological agents that inhibit the apparent endocytosis and transcytosis of select ligands that preferentially bind within caveolae has bolstered the case for caveolae as carrier vesicles. Cholesterol-binding agents, such as filipin, that remove cholesterol from the plasma membrane cause caveolae to disassemble, which reduces the cell surface density of caveolae and thereby produces a significant reduction in the scavenger endocytosis of modified albumins, transcytosis of insulin and native albumin, and even transcapillary permeability of albumin in the rat lung.[10] Such transport by caveolae is also sensitive to alkylation with N-ethylmaleimide (NEM),[28,29] suggesting by analogy with other vesicular carrier systems, a dependence on specific NEM-sensitive factors that mediate caveolae formation, docking, and/or fusion with target membranes. Transport by discrete vesicular carriers is well established for intracellular membrane trafficking largely because of recent discoveries about the molecular mediators of vesicle formation, docking, and fusion. A general mechanism sensitive to NEM is required for the transport of a divergent group of vesicular carriers ranging from the specialized synaptic vesicles to the more common exocytic and endocytic carriers. It is becoming clear from the molecular mapping of endothelial cell caveolae purified from rat lungs, that they do contain the molecular machinery required for them to be specific discrete carrier vesicles.[8,27,28] Caveolae are indeed like other carrier vesicles and use similar NEM-sensitive molecular machinery for transport.[8,27,28] Caveolae have key proteins that mediate different aspects of vesicle formation, docking, or fusion including the vSNARE, VAMP, or cellubrevin; small and large GTP-binding proteins; the calcium-dependent lipid-binding protein, annexin; and the NEM-sensitive factor, NSF, along with SNAP.[27]

The purified caveolae are also likely to be transport vesicles because they contain not only the important blood carrier protein, albumin, which appears to be transcytosed by endothelial caveolae in situ,[18,30] but also albondin, which mediates albumin's specific binding and transport in endothelium.[21] Native albumin interacts with the endothelial cell surface and localizes preferentially within caveolae for apparent transport into or across the endothelium. Many continuous endothelia appear to have albumin-binding sites for specific transcytosis via an abundant population of caveolae. Ligands bound to albumin, such as fatty acids, may increase its endothelial binding and transcytosis,[31] in agreement with albumin's nutritional role as a blood carrier protein. Antibodies raised to albondin inhibit the specific endothelial transport and capillary permeability of albumin and also inhibit the binding of albumin both to the endothelial cell surface in culture and to its equivalent in situ, the purified luminal endothelial cell membrane. Normally, in the presence of nonimmune immunoglobulin G (IgG) as a control, bovine serum albumin (BSA) perfused in situ binds the endothelial cell surface, as detected in the luminal membranes purified afterwards from the lung tissue using the silica-coating methodology. Moreover, purification of the caveolae from this membrane reveals that about 85% of the bound BSA is found in the purified caveolae. Anti-albondin IgG, before and during the in situ BSA perfusion, inhibits BSA binding to both the purified cell membrane and caveolae by more than 90%.[31a] Approximately 75% to 80% of albondin is concentrated in the caveolae, whereas 20% to 25% remains free at the cell surface. Ultimately, in these experiments, the anti-albondin IgG inhibited BSA transport and accumulation in the total lung tissue by nearly 75%. It appears that albondin expressed primarily within caveolae may facilitate the efficient delivery across the endothelium of albumin, as a carrier for its ligands to meet the nutritional requirements of the underlying tissue cells.

Fission or Budding of Caveolae

In order to assess possible budding of caveolae directly from the endothelial cell plasma membrane, Schnitzer and colleagues[13] have developed a reconstituted, cell-free, in vitro assay and a permeabilized cultured endothelial cell system. If caveolae are not static but rather dynamic structures capable of budding from the cell surface to form discrete vesicles that transport their cargo into or across the cell, then it should be possible to detach caveolae from plasma membranes without the need of physical disruption (as used in our purification procedure) but rather under physiological conditions that require only the proper reconstitution of pertinent cytosolic factors. GTP, in the presence of cytosol plus adenosine triphosphate (ATP), stimulates the release of caveolae from the purified silica-coated endothelial cell plasma membranes and from the surface of permeabilized bovine microvascular endothelial cells.[13] The caveolar marker protein, caveolin, is released from these membranes in a concentration- and time-dependent manner with a maximal response of approximately 80% to 90% and an apparent median effective dose (ED_{50}) of 30-μmol/L GTP. By contrast, the signal for other plasmalemmal marker proteins not present in caveolae, such as angiotensin converting enzyme (ACE) and the glycosylphosphatidyl inositol- (GPI) anchored protein, 5'nucleotide (5'NT), remains constant. This caveolar fission specifically requires GTP hydrolysis because other high-energy nucleotides and the nonhydrolyzable GTP analogue GTPγS are ineffective. In fact, GTPγS prevents the budding of caveolae and the endocytosis of cholera toxin, which binds in caveolae.[13] The caveolin-rich vesicles specifically released by GTP hydrolysis are easily isolated by sucrose gradient centrifugation as a low-density vesicular fraction. The released free caveolar vesicles are transport vesicles rich in VAMP, albondin, and G_{M1}, but lacking GPI-anchored proteins 5'NT and urokinase-plasminogen activator receptor. Thus, caveolae can indeed bud directly from endothelial cell plasma membranes via a process requiring GTP hydrolysis. Schnitzer and colleagues interpret this GTP induction to reflect the involvement of specific GTPase(s), and are attempting to identify the responsible GTPase. Recent data indicate that dynamin may be the GTPase mediating caveolar fission.[31b]

Caveolae are genuine trafficking organelles capable of budding from the plasmalemma to form discrete carrier vesicles that contain the molecular machinery necessary for regulated specific transport. By purification of caveolae to homogeneity directly from luminal endothelial plasmalemma derived from rat lungs, it has been demonstrated that caveolae represent: (1) specific microdomains on the endothelial cell surface that have their own molecular topography that consists of certain preferentially distributed proteins, including caveolin, albondin, VAMP and G_{M1}, but not other cell surface proteins, and (2) transport vesicles with the necessary specific molecular machinery for the select binding and transcytosis of albumin. More recently Liu and colleagues found that caveolae contain many key signaling molecules including select kinases (platelet-derived growth factor [PDGF] receptors, protein kinase C [PKC], PI3-kinase and src-like kinases), phospholipase C, sphingomyelin, and even phosphoinositides.[32] More importantly, they contain most of the intrinsic tyrosine kinase activity of the plasma membrane, and they function as signal-transducing subcompartments of the plasma membrane. As signal-transducing organelles, caveolae organize a distinct set of signaling molecules to permit direct regionalized signal transduction within their boundaries. Disruption of the molecular organization of caveolae prevents efficient transduction of signals from the cell surface. Mechanical stimuli on the endothelial cell surface may transduce signals into the cell via caveolae,[33] suggesting a role for caveolae as mechanotransduction centers. Experiments must now be performed to define the precise role of these and other caveolar proteins in the regulation of transport.

Aquaporin and Water Transport in Endothelium

Water transport across endothelium of the continuous type, found in the microvessels of many organs such as lung, has been thought to occur almost completely via the paracellular pathway through intercellular junctions. Direct transmembrane and transcellular transport has been considered to be minimal. With the development of a methodology for purifying luminal endothelial cell plasma membranes directly from tissue, as described above, Schnitzer et al have discovered that the water channel protein, aquaporin-1, is expressed on the endothelial cell surface in vivo at levels comparable to the plasma membranes of other aquaporin-1-expressing cells such as the erythrocyte and renal epithelial cells.[34] Aquaporin-l forms a transmembrane water channel as a multisubunit oligomer comprised of four 28-kd protein subunits that are identical except that only one has a large N-linked glycan.[35,36] It has a rather diverse tissue distribution and is expressed on the surface of many fluid-transporting cells including various secretory or resorptive epithelia of the colonic crypts, choroid plexus, ciliary body, iris, lung alveolus, sweat gland, and gallbladder.[35–38] Some staining of endothelium by in situ hybridization or antibodies has been noted.[36–38]

Schnitzer and Oh found that although they are barely detectable in the initial rat lung homogenates, both the nonglycosylated and glycosylated form of aquaporin-1 are amply present in the purified silica-coated membranes.[34] Surprisingly, aquaporin-1 is found concentrated, but not exclusively, in caveolae. Mass balance calculations show that about 70% of aquaporin on the cell surface are in the caveolae and the remaining 30% are distributed over the rest of the plasmalemma. Dual-labeling immunofluorescence performed on bovine lung microvascular endothelial cells grown in culture provides further confirmation of these findings by showing that aquaporin-1 and the caveolar structural protein, caveolin , colocalize on the cell surface. Thus, physiologically relevant levels of aquaporin expression may indeed exist on endothelia, mostly within caveolae.

Water channel proteins embedded in plasma membranes can mediate the transmembrane and transcellular transport of water at physiologically relevant flow rates. Endothelia can express aquaporin-1 at levels comparable to other cells shown to mediate selective transmembrane water transport. For erythrocytes and certain renal epithelia, it has been clearly demonstrated that mercurial alkylating agents such as $HgCl_2$ effectively inhibited transmembrane and transcellular transport of water, but not other solutes, by modifying the Cys-189 residue of aquaporin-1. When the effects of these known inhibitors of aquaporin-1-mediated water transport were tested on the uptake of tritiated water perfused through the rat lung microvasculature in situ, it was found that $HgCl_2$ significantly reduced the water transport by approximately 60% inhibition at about 0.03 mmol.[34] The effects of $HgCl_2$ on the transport of small, presumably paracellular tracers such as SO_4 and inulin were negligible, consistent with $HgCl_2$ not causing a general redistribution of vascular transport or a general increase in endothelial barrier function by "tightening" intercellular junctions. $HgCl_2$ appeared to rather specifically and reversibly inhibit the tissue uptake of water.

The lipid composition of membranes can significantly affect the ability of water to cross the bilayer. Some membrane lipids, such as cholesterol and sphingomyelin, prevent such water transport. Interestingly, lipid analysis of the purified caveolae reveals that caveolae contain much of the sphingomyelin found in the plasma membrane,[32] suggesting that water- and solute-transmembrane transport in caveolae should be quite small except through selective pathways such as aquaporin.

Continuous endothelia may express aquaporin-1 in order to facilitate the direct transcellular transport of water. Interestingly, caveolae may play an important role in the transvascular transport of water not only by containing these specific water channels but also by increasing the total membrane surface area available for this transport. A reevaluation of the current dogma, that under all conditions nearly all transport of water is paracellular through intercellular junctions, may be necessary. It, logically, has been assumed in the past that most water transport does not occur directly across the endothelial cell membrane because normally the hydrophobicity of lipid bilayers prevents such transmembrane transport. This logic also prevailed for a number of years, in the modeling of transepithelial transport. For some epithelial cell barriers, the paracellular pathway for water transport is still well accepted, but in the case of certain renal epithelial barriers expressing aquaporins, the transport seems to be selectively transcellular. Especially with osmotic gradients as a driving force, aquaporin may provide a direct transcellular route for water transport. It may also function in endothelial cell volume regulation. This may also be true for certain endothelia, primarily, if not solely, endothelia of the continuous type expressing aquaporin and not endothelia of the fenestrated or sinusoidal type, where obvious membrane discontinuities exist for less selective transport of water and other solutes. Sinusoidal and fenestrated endothelia have open extramembranous passageways for direct water transport through either obvious gaps between the cells or circular "windows" of about 100 nm in diameter, called fenestrations. Conversely, continuous endothelia do not have such distinct membrane discontinuities. Consistent with this idea, aquaporin-1 is expressed in rat lungs and heart, but not in cortical brain or liver. This newly discovered pathway deserves future attention in microvascular research.

Because albondin and albumin also reside in caveolae, the possibility exists that binding of albumin to albondin could influence water transport via aquaporin, possibly through protein phosphorylation. This speculation provides an alternative mechanism for the effect of albumin on water conductivity as part of the "serum effect."

The Future

The field of capillary permeability and endothelial cell transport processes appears to be headed into a new era of research, focusing appropriately on the characterization of transport at the molecular level where more specific effectors and mechanisms can be defined in more definitive and testable terms. Although investigators are only beginning to unravel the mysteries of the processing system at the endothelial cell surface, the current data implicate a regulated mechanism for the transport of molecules as ubiquitous and small as water, as well as the much larger and less plentiful macromolecules. It may be necessary to begin to reevaluate the current dogma about the pathways relevant to transport across continuous endothelia, and to incorporate the physiologically significant contribution of these newly defined pathways into the current models of transcapillary exchange.

References

1. Schnitzer JE. Update on the cellular and molecular basis of capillary permeability. *Trends Cardiovasc Med* 1993;3:124–130.
2. Curry FE. Effect of albumin on the structure of the molecular filter at the capillary wall. *Fed Proc* 1985;44:2610–2613.
3. Schnitzer JE, Carley WW, Palade GE. Specific albumin binding to microvascular endothelium in culture. *Am J Physiol* 1988;254:H425–H437.
4. Schneeberger EE, Hamelin M. Interaction of serum proteins with lung endothelial glycocalyx: Its effect on endothelial permeability. *Am J Physiol* 1984;247:H206–H217.
5. Schnitzer JE, Pinney E. Quantitation of specific binding of orosomucoid to cultured microvascular endothelium: Role in capillary permeability. *Am J Physiol* 1992;263:H48–H55.

6. Haraldsson B, Rippe B. Orosomucoid as one of the serum components contributing to normal permselectivity in rat skeletal muscle. *Acta Physiol Scand* 1987;129:127–135.

7. Schnitzer JE, Siflinger-Birnboim A, Del Vecchio PJ, Malik AB. Segmental differentiation of permeability, protein glycosylation, and morphology of cultured bovine lung vascular endothelium. *Biochem Biophys Res Comm* 1994;199:11–19.

8. Schnitzer JE, McIntosh DP, Dvorak AM, Liu J, Oh P. Separation of caveolae from associated microdomains of GPI-anchored proteins. *Science* 1995; 269:1435–1439.

9. Montesano R, Roth J, Robert A, Orci L. Non-coated membrane invaginations are involved in binding and internalization of cholera and tetanus toxins. *Nature* 1982;296:651–653.

10. Schnitzer JE, Oh P, Pinney E, Allard A. Filipin-sensitive caveolae-mediated transport in endothelium: Reduced transcytosis, scavenger endocytosis, and capillary permeability of select macromolecules. *J Cell Biol* 1994;127:1217–1232.

11. Trans D, Carpentier J-L, Sawano F, Gorden P, Orci L. Ligands internalized through coated or non-coated invaginations follow a common intracellular pathway. *Proc Natl Acad Sci U S A* 1987;84:7957–7961.

12. Schnitzer JE, Bravo J. High affinity binding, endocytosis and degradation of conformationally-modified albumins: Potential role of gp30 and gp18 as novel scavenger receptors.J Biol Chem 1993;268:7562–7570.

13. Schnitzer JE, Oh P, McIntosh DP. Role of GTP hydrolysis in fission of caveolae directly from plasma membranes. *Science* 1996;274:239–242.

14. Peters K-R, Carley CC, Palade GE. Endothelial plasmalemmal vesicles have a characteristic stripped bipolar surface structure. *J Cell Biol* 1985;101: 2233.

15. Rothberg KG, Heuser JE, Donzell WC, Ying Y-S, Glenney JR, Anderson RGW. Caveolin, a protein component of caveolae membrane coats. *Cell* 1992;68:673–682.

16. Ghitescu L, Fixman A, Simionescu M, Simionescu N. Specific binding sites for albumin restricted to plasmalemmal vesicles of continuous capillary endothelium: Receptor-mediated transcytosis. *J Cell Biol* 1986;102:1304–1311.

17. Predescu D, Palade GE. Plasmalemmal vesicles represent the large pore system of continuous microvascular endothelium. *Am J Physiol* 1993;265: H725–H733.

18. Milici AJ, Watrous NE, Stukenbrok H, Palade GE. Transcytosis of albumin in capillary endothelium. *J Cell Biol* 1987;105:2603–2612.

19. King GL, Johnson SM. Receptor-mediated transport of insulin across endothelial cells. *Science* 1985;227:1583–1586.

20. Schnitzer JE, Sung A, Horvat R, Bravo J. Preferential interaction of albumin binding proteins, gp30 and gp18, with modified albumins: Presence in many cells and tissues with a possible role in catabolism. *J Biol Chem* 1992;264:24544–24553.

21. Schnitzer JE, Oh P. Albondin-mediated capillary permeability to albumin: Differential role of receptors in endothelial transcytosis and endocytosis of native and modified albumins. *J Biol Chem* 1994;269:6072–6082.

22. Jeffries WA, Brandon MR, Hunt SV, Williams AF, Gatter KC, Mason DY. Transferrin receptor on endothelium of brain capillaries. *Nature* 1984;312: 162–163.

23. Bundgaard M, Frokjaer-Jensen J, Crone C. Endothelial plasmalemmal vesicles as elements in a system of branching invaginations from the cell surface. *Proc Natl Acad Sci U S A* 1979;76:6439–6442.

24. Wagner RC, Andrews SB. Ultrastructure of the vesicular system in rapidly frozen capillary endothelium of the rete mirabile. *J Ultrastructure Res* 1985;90:172–182.

25. Anderson RGW, Kamen BA, Rothberg KG, Lacey SW. Potocytosis: Sequestration and transport of small molecules by caveolae. *Science* 1992; 255:410–411.

26. Schnitzer JE, Oh P, Jacobson BS, Dvorak AM. Caveolae from luminal plasmalemma for rat lung endothelium: Microdomains enriched in caveolin, Ca^{2+}-ATPase and inositol trisphosphate receptor. *Proc Natl Acad Sci U S A* 1995;92:1759–1763.

27. Schnitzer JE, Liu J, Oh P. Endothelial caveolae have the molecular transport machinery for vesicle budding, docking and fusion including VAMP, NSF, SNAP, annexins and GTPases. *J Biol Chem* 1995;270:14399–14404.

28. Schnitzer JE, Oh P, Pinney E, Allard J. NEM inhibits transcytosis, endocytosis and capillary permeability: Implication of caveolae fusion in endothelia. *Am J Physiol* 1995;37:H48–H55.

29. Predescu D, Horvat R, Predescu S, Palade GE. Transcytosis in the continuous endothelium of the myocardial microvasculature is inhibited by N-ethylmaleimide. *Proc Natl Acad Sci U S A* 1994;91:3014–3018.

30. Ghitescu L, Bendayan M. Transendothelial transport of albumin: A quantitative immunocytochemical study. *J Cell Biol* 1992;117:745–755.

31. Galis Z, Ghitescu L, Simionescu M. Fatty acid binding to albumin increases its uptake and transcytosis by the lung capillary endothelium. *Eur J Cell Biol* 1988;47:358–365.

31a. Schnitzer JE, Liu J, Oh P. Purification of endothelial caveolae reveals the molecular machinery for fusion-dependent albondin-mediated transcytosis of albumin. *Microcirculation* 1995;2:93.

31b. Oh P, Schnitzer, JE. Dynamin-mediated fission of caveolae from plasma membranes. *Mol Biol Cell* 1996;7:83a.

32. Liu J, Oh P, Horner T, Rogers RA, Schnitzer JE. Organized cell surface signal transduction in caveolae distinct from GPI-anchored protein microdomains. *J Biol Chem* 1997; 272(11):7211–7222.

33. Sung A, Rizzo V, Oh P, Schnitzer JE. Rapid mechanotransduction occurs in situ at the endothelial cell surface primarily in caveolae. *Mol Biol Cell* 1996;7:276a.

34. Schnitzer JE, Oh P. Aquaporin-1 in plasma membrane and caveolae provides mercury-senstive water channels across lung endothelium. *Am J Physiol* 1996;270:H416–H422.

35. van Os CH, Deen PMT, Dempster JA. Aquaporins: Water selective channels in biological membranes. Molecular structure and tissue distribution. *Biochim Biophys Acta* 1994;1197:291–309.

36. Hasegawa H, Lian S-C, Finkbeiner WE, Verkman AS. Extrarenal tissue distribution of CHIP28 water channels by in situ hybridization and antibody staining. *Am J Physiol* 1994;266:C893–C903.

37. Folkesson GH, Matthay MA, Hasegawa H, Kheradmand F, Verkman AS. Transcellular water transport in lung alveolar epithelium through mercury-sensitive water channels. *Proc Natl Acad Sci U S A* 1994;91:4970–4974.

38. Nielsen S, Smith BL, Christensen EI, Agre P. Distribution of the aquaporin CHIP in secretory and resportive epithelia and capillary endothelia. *Proc Natl Acad Sci U S A* 1993;90:7275–7279.

Chapter 6

Mechanisms of Edema Clearance

Yves Berthiaume, MD, MSc

Considerable progress has been made in understanding the patho-physiology of pulmonary edema over the last 20 years. Until recently, most of the attention was focused on the function and dysfunction of the pulmonary endothelium during lung injury. However, the structure and function of the alveolar epithelium are also important determinants in lung injury.[1] The alveolar epithelium is not only an important barrier to alveolar flooding but is also the most likely site of fluid reabsorption.[2] Reabsorption of liquid is an essential component in the resolution process of pulmonary edema and may have a significant impact on the prognosis of patients with this condition.[3] The mechanisms of alveolar liquid clearance are only partially understood at this moment, but most of the data strongly suggest that it depends on active sodium transport across the alveolar epithelium.[2]

Clearance Across the Alveolar Epithelium

Solute Transport

The alveolar epithelial barrier has a very low permeability to almost every hydrophilic molecule. The clearance of liquid, protein, and solute across the alveolar epithelium is slower than it is across the capillary endothelium.[4] Since the late 1970s, many laboratories have been able to show, using *in* and *ex* vivo models, that not only is the alveolar epithelium a tight epithelium but that it is also actively involved in the

This work was supported by a grant from the Medical Research Council of Canada (MT-10273). Dr. Berthiaume is a senior clinical investigator from Fonds de la Recherche en Santé du Québec (FRSQ).

transport of ions and solutes. Three different experimental approaches have led to demonstrations of active ion transport in the lung.

The first experimental strategy involved a model of alveolar flooding where autologous serum or an isotonic fluid containing trace amounts of albumin was instilled into the airspaces of the lung. Fluid clearance was then measured by determining the excess amount of water in the experimental lung compared to a control lung with use of a modified gravimetric method[5] or by measurement, over time, of the changes in concentration of a nonpermeable molecule (like albumin) instilled in the lung with the fluid.[6] With this experimental approach, it was established that liquid clearance was faster than protein clearance (Figure 1), so that the solution remaining in the airspaces became more concentrated as the liquid was removed.[5,7] Since this clearance of water in the face of rising osmotic pressure could not be explained by changes in hydrostatic or osmotic forces across the alveolar epithelium, it was proposed that active transport of ions could be responsible.[5,7] This clearance of liquid with rising protein concentration has been seen in the lungs of many species such as sheep,[5] dogs,[8] rats,[9] and rabbits,[10] as well as humans.[11]

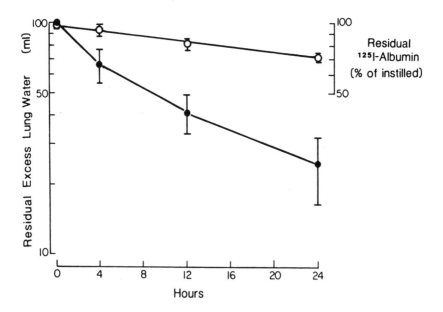

Figure 1. Removal rate of 100 mL excess water and ^{125}I-albumin over 24 hours. Solid circles = means ± SD of residual water left in serum-instilled lobe at 4 hours, 12 hours, and 24 hours; open circles = means ± SD of residual ^{125}I-albumin in experimental lung expressed as percent of total instilled ^{125}I-albumin at 4 hours, 12 hours, and 24 hours. Data from Reference 7.

Although these data suggest the presence of active ion transport, further support of this hypothesis came from experiments where lung liquid clearance was studied in the presence of inhibitors of ion transport (Table 1). Ouabain, a Na^+-K^+-ATPase inhibitor, significantly decreased Na^+ transport[12,13] and fluid absorption[11,13,14] in isolated lungs, indicating that transepithelial ion transport is important in this process. The presence of an active ion transport mechanism was further confirmed by Serikov et al,[15] who studied the effect of an increase in temperature on alveolar lung liquid clearance in isolated perfused goat lungs. In 4 hours, they saw a 26% increase in protein concentration over baseline, similar to the result observed in sheep.[6] However, when temperature of the perfusate was decreased to 18°C, there was no change in alveolar protein concentration, suggesting that alveolar liquid clearance had been inhibited. These results confirm that liquid clearance is not dependent so much on passive diffusion as it is dependent on an active transport process.

Investigation has since focused on Na^+ transport since it has been shown to be the dominant ion transport mechanism in alveolar type II cells,[16] and most liquid reabsorption is believed to occur in distal airways, mainly in the alveoli.[2] Amiloride, a drug well known to interfere with Na^+ transport,[16] decreases lung liquid clearance by 40% to 75% in different species (Table 1).[9–11,13,17] The potential role of Na^+ in this process is also confirmed by the fact that not only is liquid reabsorption inhibited by amiloride but unidirectional Na^+ movement from the

Table 1

Lung Liquid Clearance in the Presence of Inhibitors of Ion Transport

Model	Inhibition of liquid clearance		Inhibition of Na^+ transport		Reference
	Amiloride	Ouabain	Amiloride	Ouabain	
Isolated rat lung			+	+	12
Isolated rat lung	+	+	+	+	13
In situ rat lung	+		+		18
In situ sheep lung		+			14
Rabbit in vivo	+				10
Rat in vivo	+				9
Resected human lung	+	+			11

alveoli to the circulation is also inhibited by amiloride[12,13] and ouabain[12,13] (Table 1). Finally, this relationship between lung liquid clearance and Na[+] transport is further established by the demonstration that when Na[+] is replaced by choline in the alveolar instillate, there is a complete inhibition of fluid reabsorption.[18]

Additional support for the hypothesis came from experiments performed on fetal and adult animals where lung liquid absorption was modulated by β-adrenergic agonist. The fetal lung is a fluid-filled organ, and the presence of liquid in the lung is necessary for its normal development.[19] Around birth, at the time when the lung becomes the major organ involved in gas exchange with the surrounding environment, the presence of liquid must be decreased significantly so that liquid reabsorption becomes the major function of the distal airway epithelium.[19] In the latter part of the third trimester, intravenous infusions of a β-adrenergic agonist [19] are associated with decreased fluid secretion and increased fluid reabsorption. This effect of the beta-adrenergic agonist is inhibited by amiloride, suggesting that the process is also dependent on active Na[+] transport.[19] In adult animals, administration of a β-adrenergic agonist also enhances lung liquid clearance[6,20] (Figure 2) and Na[+] transport.[12,20] This effect of the β-adrenergic agonist is also inhibited by amiloride (Figure 2), suggesting once again that liquid reabsorption from airspaces of the lung is largely dependent on Na[+] transport.[6,12,20]

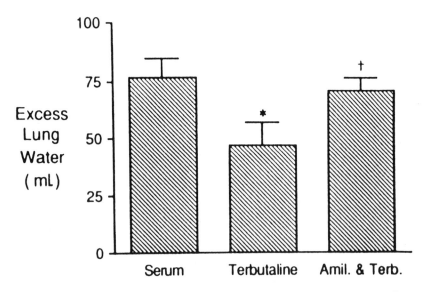

Figure 2. Excess lung water when serum alone, serum mixed with terbutaline, or serum mixed with terbutaline and amiloride was instilled. *Statistically different from the value of serum alone; †statistically different from the value for terbutaline. Data from Reference 6.

Water Transport in the Lung

Until recently, it was generally accepted that liquid movement across the alveolar epithelium was an intercellular process secondary to the osmotic gradient generated by solute transport across the alveolar epithelium.[17] However, the existence of specialized water-transporting proteins has now been proposed in erythrocytes, certain kidney tubules and, more recently, in the lung,[21] which could mean that water movement, occurs not only in the paracellular pathway but also through a transcellular process. With use of in situ hybridization, Hasegawa et al[22] have shown diffuse expression of CHIP28 (AquaPorin-1, AQP-1) transcript in the perialveolar region. Subsequently, a mercurial-insensitive water channel (MIWC, AQP-4) was cloned from a lung cDNA library, and two other proteins, glycerol intrinsic protein (GLIP; AQP-3) and AQP-5, were cloned from other sources and then found to be expressed in the trachea and/or lung.[21] MIWC and GLIP are expressed in the basolateral membrane of tracheal epithelia, and MIWC, but not GLIP, is expressed throughout large and small airways.[21] CHIP28 is expressed predominantly in perialveolar capillaries and to a lesser extent on the alveolar epithelium.[23] The potential role of these water transport proteins in lung liquid clearance was established recently by the study of water channel transcript expression in the developing and postnatal lung with use of RNase protection assay.[21] Transcripts encoding CHIP28, MIWC, and AQP-5 are expressed at relatively low levels in the lung before birth. CHIP28 mRNA increases strongly just after birth and remains elevated. MIWC mRNA increases strongly between *days 1* and *2* after birth and decreases slightly over the first week. In contrast, AQP-5 mRNA increases slowly and progressively over the first week. These changes in water channel expression parallel changes in expression of the Na^+ channel around birth.[24]

Although analysis of protein expression in the lung suggests potential roles of these proteins in lung liquid clearance, there are actually very few studies that have tried to define their physiological and functional significance. More than 20 years ago, Effros[25] demonstrated rapid translocation of solute-free water into the vascular space after injection of a hypertonic solution into the perfusate of isolated perfused lungs. However, direct evidence for the existence of specific transcellular water pathways in the lung was not available until recently (Figure 3). An in situ-perfused sheep lung model was used to measure transalveolar osmotic water permeability.[23] Hypertonic fluid (900 mOsm) was instilled bronchoscopically into the airspaces, and the time course of water movement from capillary to airspace was deduced from the dilution of instilled radiolabeled

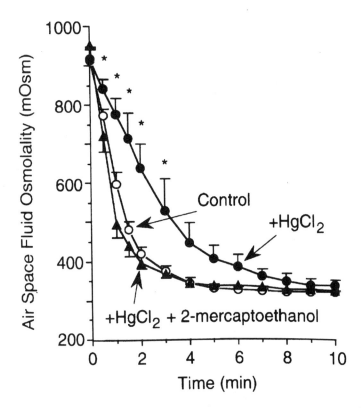

Figure 3. Transepithelial osmotic water permeability in intact sheep lung. Lungs were instilled with hyperosmotic saline (900 mOsm), and serial alveolar fluid samples were withdrawn and assayed for osmolality. Halftimes for osmotic equilibration were (in min): 0.85±0.1 (control), 2.7±0.4 (HgCl$_2$), and 0.7±0.1 (HgCl$_2$ + 2-mercaptoethanol). Each data point is the mean ± SE of measurements performed 3 to 6 times. *Significantly different ($P<0.05$) from the control value. Data from Reference 23.

albumin and from airspace fluid osmolality.[23] In control lungs, osmotically induced water movement was rapid and had an apparent P_f of 0.02 cm/s, similar to that seen in erythrocytes (Figure 3). Water permeability in the contralateral lung was inhibited reversibly by 70% by HgCl$_2$. These results indicate that mercurial-sensitive water channels facilitated transcellular movement of water between the airspace and capillary compartments in the lung. Despite the strong expression of several water channels in the lung and the physiological demonstration that they can participate in water movement in the lung, no study has yet associated lung liquid clearance with these channels.

Alveolar and Lung Protein Clearance

Edema fluid is not only composed of water and solutes, it also contains a significant quantity of proteins.[17] Hence, resolution of pulmonary edema also depends on protein clearance from the airspace. Protein clearance from airspaces of the lungs is slow. Tracer albumin instilled into the lungs of anesthetized sheep,[5] dogs,[26] and rabbits,[10] as well as in unanesthetized sheep[7,27] (Figure 1) and isolated perfused dog lungs[28] leaves that organ at a rate of 1% to 2% per hour over periods ranging from 4 hours to 144 hours. This slow rate of protein clearance contrasts with the rapid rate of alveolar liquid clearance. Rabbits remove 64% of liquid from the airspaces in 4 hours,[10] while sheep clear 29%[6] and dogs 15%.[8] Protein is rapidly eliminated from the lung once it moves from the alveoli to the interstitium, since the halftime for albumin clearance from the lung (T 1/2 = 55 h) is only slightly greater than the halftime for clearance from the alveoli (T 1/2 = 49 h) in sheep.[27]

Multiple mechanisms may be involved in protein clearance from the alveolar space: clearance by the mucociliary escalator, ingestion and degradation of protein by macrophages, diffusion of intact protein between epithelial cells, and transcytosis across epithelial cells. Although it has been suggested that protein can leave the alveoli by the mucociliary escalator, available experimental data do not support this hypothesis.[29] Macrophages have a large capacity to internalize and degrade macromolecules.[29] Are they important as an alveolar clearance pathway in the uninjured lung? After 100 mL of autologous serum was instilled into live sheep lungs, the number of macrophages in the airspaces increased tenfold over 24 hours, but the rate of alveolar and lung protein clearance remained constant.[7,27] Furthermore, tracer protein clearance curves were the same, whether the instilled solutions were crystalloid or protein-containing, even though crystalloid solutions are less chemotactic for macrophages. Nevertheless, it can be hypothesized that macrophages might be important in long-term clearance of alveolar protein, especially if the protein is precipitated in the airspaces. A small quantity of tracer protein is associated in longer intervals with alveolar macrophages in sheep[27] and in shorter intervals in rabbits.[30] Morphological observations also indicate that alveolar macrophages engulf some of the protein.[27] If ingestion and digestion of proteins by macrophages are the major route of protein clearance, one would expect to see a dissociation of tracer from the protein. However, most experimental evidence suggests that proteins leave the lung as intact molecules.[7,27,31] Thus, although macrophages can phagocytize protein, their overall quantitative contribution to protein clearance when proteins are in solution is relatively minor.

The majority of movement of proteins across the alveolar epithelium should then occur by endocytosis through epithelial cells or by diffusion between them. Intracellular vesicles are numerous in alveolar epithelial cells,[29] but electron microscopic studies have not consistently shown that vesicles are involved in transporting negatively charged protein out of the alveolar space.[32] Physiological studies have also failed to clearly demonstrate the role of trancytosis in protein clearance. Kim and colleagues[33] reported that albumin permeability of bullfrog alveolar epithelium was greater in the apical to basolateral direction than in the opposite direction. Since permeability would be equal in both directions for a passive process such as diffusion, they suggested that protein transport may involve an active process such as vesicular transport. This hypothesis is also supported by experiments where cooling of the lung from 38°C to 30°C significantly decreased the clearance of [^{125}I]-albumin,[15] while there was no change in mannitol transport (a marker of diffusion) at 30°C. However, Hastings et al[34] have measured the clearance of [^{125}I]IgG and [^{131}I]albumin instilled into the lungs of anesthetized rabbits in the presence or absence of 3×10^{-5}mol monensin. This drug inhibits endocytosis and lysosomal degradation of a variety of proteins in cell culture and tissue slice systems[34] by suppressing vesicle acidification. Monensin did not inhibit alveolar protein clearance, suggesting that endocytosis may not be quantitatively important for alveolar protein clearance.[34]

If protein diffusivity is important in alveolar protein clearance, it should be inversely proportional to protein size. Effros and Mason[35] collected published lung clearance rates for different sized solutes from many sources and found a consistent inverse relationship with molecular weight. Hastings[30] also found that alveolar clearance of [^{125}I]IgG and [^{131}I]albumin varied as predicted by molecular size in anesthetized rabbits and sheep. Folkesson and coworkers[36] reported that the amount of instilled bovine immunoglobulin G (IgG), bovine albumin, and l-deamino-cysteine-8-D-argininevassopressin (dDAVP) (MW 1067) transferred out of rat lungs in vivo followed an inversely exponential relationship to molecular weight. This would be consistent with diffusion, but does not rule out other mechanisms alone or in concert with diffusion.

In summary, alveolar protein clearance from the uninjured lung is a slow process. The most likely clearance mechanisms are endocytosis of proteins through alveolar epithelial cells and/or diffusion of proteins between cells.

Interstitial Liquid Clearance

Although the primary barrier to alveolar liquid clearance is the epithelial barrier, it is important to identify the major pathways for clearance of liquid once it has reached the interstitial space. Some indications of the major route of liquid clearance from the interstitial space can be obtained from the sheep model of alveolar flooding, where lung lymph flow is measured.[5] Lung lymph flow increased and the lymph/plasma protein ratio declined over 4 hours after instillation of a protein solution into the airspaces of one lower lobe; the increase in lymph flow accounted for 10% to 20% of the clearance of alveolar liquid transported to the interstitium.[5,6] In later studies, alveolar clearance was accelerated by terbutaline, and lung lymph also increased to higher levels, always with a fall in lymph protein concentration.[6] Some of the increase in lymph flow was due to a local increase in blood flow and vascular filtration.[6] This was supported by the changes in lung lymph flow that occurred with intravenous nitroprusside alone, which did not affect alveolar liquid clearance, or those changes that occurred when amiloride plus terbutaline were added to the instilled serum, blocking the enhanced alveolar liquid clearance but not the local increase in pulmonary blood flow.[6]

These observations suggest that the most likely clearance pathway for removal of excess interstitial fluid is the circulation. To test this hypothesis, Jayr and Matthay[37] studied lung liquid clearance in the absence of pulmonary blood flow. Occlusion of the pulmonary circulation did not decrease lung liquid clearance, but persistent bronchopulmonary anastomotic flow that averaged 42 mL/min was measured. With occlusion of the bronchoesophageal artery, blood flow fell to 12 mL/min, but alveolar lung liquid clearance continued at a normal rate, suggesting that a minimal amount of blood flow is necessary for lung liquid clearance.[37] To test the hypothesis further, Sakuma et al[14] developed an experimental model in which all blood flow was removed by ligating the inflow and outflow of the pulmonary circulation. In this preparation, there was also a small increase in lymph flow following liquid instillation but it represented only 10% of the measured lung liquid clearance. This suggests that most of the liquid cleared from the lung was by bulk flow into the pulmonary vascular space. This hypothesis is further supported by the observation that protein concentration in pulmonary artery blood declined after serum instillation in the lung (Table 2).[14] Since both inflow and outflow pulmonary vessels were ligated, this decrease of protein concentration in pulmonary artery blood suggests that interstitial fluid was absorbed in the stagnant circulation. The absence of lung liquid clearance in this experimental model also demonstrates the importance of the circulation in this process (Table 2). Thus, diffusion of low-protein-containing interstitial fluid into the circulation is the major mechanism for clearance. Under some pathological conditions, the pleural space can also serve as an important clearance pathway for pulmonary edema.[29] There has been

Table 2

Alveolar Protein Concentration and Lung Liquid Clearance in Sheep With Ligation of Inflow and Outflow Pulmonary Blood Vessels

Experimental condition	n	Total protein concentration in alveolar fluid (g/100 mL)		Lung liquid clearance, (% instilled)
		Initial	Final	
No ligation of pulmonary vessels	6	6.0±0.5	7.9±1.1	19±5
Ligation of pulmonary vessels	3	6.7±0.2	8.4±1.2	0±6*

Data are means ± SD; no. of sheep. *P<0.05 versus sheep without ligation of pulmonary vessels. Reproduced from Reference 14.

some interest in a possible role of the mediastinum as an overflow pathway, but no quantitative data are available.[29]

Edema Clearance in Pathological State

Although, as discussed above, there is a substantial amount of data to support the concept that lung liquid clearance is mediated by active Na^+ transport, it is only recently that investigations into the modulation of lung liquid clearance in pathological conditions were undertaken. Some studies have evaluated the impact of lung injury on the integrity and function of the alveolar epithelium. Interestingly, the results indicate that the alveolar and distal airway epithelium are remarkably resistant to injury, particularly compared to the adjacent lung endothelium (Table 3). Even when mild to moderate alveolar epithelial injury occurs, the capacity of the alveolar epithelium to transport salt and water is often preserved. In addition, several mechanisms may result in upregulation of the fluid transport capacity of the distal pulmonary epithelium, even after moderate to severe epithelial injury. Even when lung endothelial injury occurs, the alveolar epithelial barrier may remain normally impermeable to protein and retain its normal fluid transport capacity (Table 3). For example, intravenous endotoxin or bacteria were used to produce lung endothelial injury in sheep[38] and rats,[39] but permeability to protein across the lung epithelial barrier was not increased. When septic shock was induced in rats, there was a marked increase in plasma epinephrine levels. Even though endothelial injury and mild interstitial pulmonary edema occurred, alveolar ep-

Table 3

Effect of Pathological Conditions on Alveolar Epithelial Fluid Clearance in Several Species

Pathological Condition	Species	Severity of Lung Injury			Alveolar Epithelial Fluid Clearance
		Endothelium	Epithelium		
No pulmonary blood flow	Sheep	None	None		Normal
Endotoxin, intravenous	Sheep	Mild	None		Normal
Endotoxin, alveolar	Sheep	None	None		Normal
	Rat	None	None		Increased
Exotoxin, alveolar	Rat	None	None		Increased
Bacteria, intravenous	Sheep	Moderate/Severe	Mild/Severe		Increased/Decreased
	Rat	Mild	None		Increased
	Rabbit	Mild	None		Normal
Bacteria, alveolar	Sheep	Mild	Mild		Normal
	Rabbit	Mild	Moderate/severe		Normal/decreased
Oleic acid, intravenous	Sheep	Moderate	Moderate		Normal
Acid aspiration	Rabbit	Severe	Severe		Decreased
Salt water aspiration	Rabbit	Mild	Mild		Normal

For intravenous and alveolar bacteria, the extent of injury to the epithelial and endothelial barriers is dependent on the dose and virulence of bacteria that are administered. For intravenous oleic acid, initially the injury after intravenous oleic acid is severe, but the alveolar epithelium recovers sufficiently after 4 h to remove some of the excess edema fluid. Reproduced from Reference 21.

ithelial fluid transport was increased by 32% in septic rats. This enhanced liquid clearance was inhibited by instillation of amiloride (10^{-4} mol/L) or propranolol (10^{-4} mol/L) into the distal airspaces, demonstrating that stimulated clearance depended on β-agonist stimulation of alveolar epithelial sodium transport. When more severe septic shock was produced in sheep, the alveolar epithelial barrier was resistant to injury in the majority of animals, with confinement of edema to the pulmonary interstitium.[40] In some sheep, however, more severe systemic and pulmonary endothelial injuries were associated with alveolar flooding, a marked increase in epithelial permeability to protein, and the inability to transport fluid from the airspaces of the lung.[40] The inability to remove excess fluid from the airspaces in these sheep was probably related more to a marked increase in paracellular permeability from injury to the epithelial tight junctions than to a loss of salt and water transport capacities of alveolar epithelial cells.[40]

Although these studies suggest that active Na^+ transport could be modulated in lung injury, a question remains to be answered: is there intrinsic activation of active Na^+ transport during the development of pulmonary edema in vivo? Different groups of investigators have tried to answer this question. Most of the information was obtained in the hyperoxic lung injury model. Two different models of hyperoxic lung injury have been studied; one of them is subacute, where the animals are exposed to 85% O_2 for 7 days, and the second is acute, where animals are exposed to 100% O_2 for 60 hours.[41] In the acute model of hyperoxic lung injury, Nici et al[42] demonstrated increased expression of Na^+-K^+-ATPase mRNA and protein in exposed animals compared to the controls. The same group has shown that this adaptive response of Na^+-K^+-ATPase in alveolar type II cells is associated with enhanced active Na^+ transport in vivo.[43] However, recent work by Olivera et al[44] has demonstrated a decrease in active Na^+ transport at the end of hyperoxic exposure but an increase at 7 days postexposure. In the subacute model of hyperoxia (85% O_2 × 7 days), Sznajder et al[45] were able to show an increase in active Na^+ transport and lung liquid clearance at the end of the exposure period. Furthermore, this group of investigators has reported that enhanced Na^+ transport is associated with an increased Na^+-K^+-ATPase activity in the alveolar type II cells of these animals at the end of hyperoxic exposure.[46] More recently, Yue et al[47] observed an increased expression and activity of sodium channels in alveolar type II cells of rats exposed to 85% O_2 for 7 days. Although collectively these results suggest that there is activation of Na^+ transport mechanisms during pulmonary edema induced by hyperoxia, which would indicate that active Na^+ transport is important in the resolution of pulmonary edema, these two models of pulmonary edema are associated with structural changes that may influence interpretation of the data. A proliferative response of alveolar type II cells has been observed in the subacute hyperoxic lung injury model.[41] In the acute hyperoxic lung injury model, there is no proliferation of alveolar type II cells but the number of inflammatory cells in the interstitial space is increased.[41] Thus, it is unclear whether the increase in mRNA,[42] protein expression,[42] or enhanced enzyme activity[46] seen in these models represents a cellular reaction to edema or simply to the proliferation of alveolar type II cells or inflammatory cells present in the lung. The results of Carter et al[43] also suggest that this response can be secondary to hyperoxia itself, since they observed an increase of alveolar type II cell expression of Na^+-K^+-ATPase following hyperoxic exposure.

Because no previous studies have evaluated lung Na^+-K^+-ATPase activity during the resolution of pulmonary edema in models not associated with significant cell proliferation of the alveolar epithelium or interstitial compartment, or in models of edema not associated with hyperoxic exposure, Zuege and colleagues examined the changes in this parameter during recovery from thiourea-induced lung edema, a model of lung injury with no significant cell proliferation [48]. They measured Na^+-K^+-ATPase activity as a major endpoint, since Na^+-K^+-ATPase is the only mechanism for basolateral extrusion of sodium once it is absorbed from the apical membrane.[49] Thus, the activity of the enzyme should be a reasonable index of active sodium transport in the lung.[12,13,50] Zuege et al demonstrated that lung Na^+-K^+-ATPase activity was increased during recovery from thiourea-induced pulmonary edema. The activity of the enzyme started to increase 4 hours after the induction of edema, with maximal activation at 12 hours (Figure 4).[51] This increased activity was also associated with an elevated quantity of the enzyme in the lung at 12 hours.[51] Its stimulation during the resolution of lung edema provides evidence that the active sodium transport mechanism is upregulated during this process, suggesting that active sodium transport could be involved in recovery from thiourea-induced pulmonary edema. However, even if an increase of Na^+-K^+-ATPase activity and quantity in the whole lung is seen during recovery from edema, it does not necessarily follow that this enhanced activity is localized in alveolar epithelial cells, which are most likely to be involved in the resolution of alveolar flooding. To address this question, Zuege et al evaluated the quantity of Na^+-K^+-ATPase in alveolar type II cells isolated 12 hours after treatment, the time at which they could demonstrate an increased quantity of Na^+-K^+-ATPase in the whole lung. They showed that there was a significant increment of enzyme quantity in alveolar type II cells at that time, which suggests that alveolar type II cells may contribute to active lung sodium transport during edema recovery (Figure 5).[51] In summary, they have demonstrated that lung Na^+-K^+-ATPase is activated during

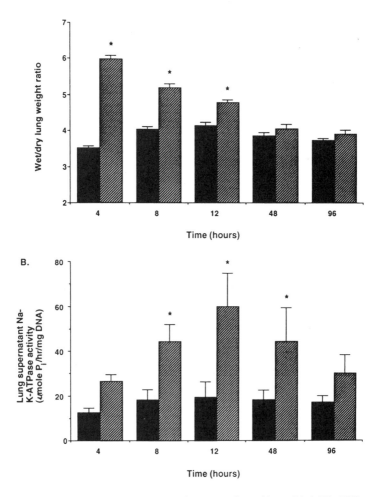

Figure 4. Wet/dry lung weigh ratios (top panel) and lung Na+-K+-ATPase activity (bottom Panel) over 96 hours after treatment with either thiourea (hatched bars) or saline (solid bars). There were significant increases over time in both wet/dry ratio and Na+-K+-ATPase activity in the thiourea group compared to the saline group. Values are means ± SEM. *Statistically different ($P<0.05$) from saline values at the same time point. Data from Reference 51.

recovery from pulmonary edema, indicating that active sodium transport mechanisms are upregulated during this process.

Even if active Na+ transport is involved in the resolution of pulmonary edema, can it become a therapeutic or prognostic tool clinically? In one study, 40% of patients were able to reabsorb some of the alveolar edema fluid within 12 hours of intubation and acute lung injury.[3] These patients recovered more rapidly from respiratory failure

KDa

alpha 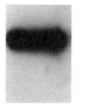 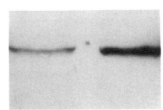 **-97**

Na-K   NS   TU

Figure 5. Quantity of Na^+-K^+-ATPase α_1-subunit in the alveolar type II cells of saline (NS) and thiourea-treated rats (TU). Alveolar type II cells were isolated 12 hours after treatment with either saline or thiourea and identical amounts of protein from the cell lysates were loaded on the gel from the two groups. Western blot was done with the MCK_1 monoclonal antibody against the Na^+-K^+-ATPase α_1-subunit. There is a greater amount of the α_1-subunit in the thiourea-treated rats. Data from Reference 51.

and had lower mortality. In contrast, patients who did not reabsorb any alveolar edema fluid in the first 12 hours after acute lung injury had protracted respiratory failure and a higher mortality.[3] Based on clinical studies, the ability of the alveolar epithelial barrier to reabsorb alveolar edema fluid from acute lung injury within the first 12 hours after acute lung injury is preserved in 30% to 40% of patients.[3] The results suggest that pharmacological manipulation of the alveolar epithelium can possibly accelerate the resolution of pulmonary edema in zones where the alveolar epithelium is intact. In other areas of the lung where significant injury to the alveolar epithelium has occurred, the reconstitution of the alveolar epitheliumis necessary before this process can be modulated.

Conclusions

Over the past two decades we have come a long way in understanding the mechanisms involved in edema clearance. The challenge in the future will be to identify the specific cellular mechanism involved in Na^+ transport and to develop pharmacological tools that will be useful to enhance lung liquid clearance and the resolution of pulmonary edema in patients.

References

1. Montaner JSG, Tsang J, Evans KG, et al. Alveolar epithelial damage. *J Clin Invest* 1986;77:1786–1796.
2. O'Brodovich HM. The role of active Na+ transport by lung epithelium in the clearance of airspace fluid. *New Horiz* 1995;3:240–247.
3. Matthay MA, Wiener-Kronish JP. Intact epithelial barrier function is critical for the resolution of alveolar edema in humans. *Am Rev Respir Dis* 1990;142:1250–1257.
4. Taylor AE, Gaar KA. Estimation of equivalent pore radii of pulmonary capillary and alveolar membranes. *Am J Physiol* 1970;218(4):1133–1140.
5. Matthay MA, Landolt CC, Staub NC. Differential liquid and protein clearance from the alveoli of anesthetized sheep. *J Appl Physiol* 1982;53(1):96–104.
6. Berthiaume Y, Staub NC, Matthay MA. Beta-adrenergic agonists increase lung liquid clearance in anaesthetized sheep. *J Clin Invest* 1987;79:335–343.
7. Matthay MA, Berthiaume Y, Staub NC. Long-term clearance of liquid and protein from the lungs of unanesthetized sheep. *J Appl Physiol* 1985;59(3):928–934.
8. Berthiaume Y, Broaddus VC, Gropper MA, Tanita T, Matthay MA. Alveolar liquid and protein clearance from normal dog lungs. *J Appl Physiol* 1988;65(2):585–593.
9. Jayr C, Garat C, Meignan M, Pittet JF, Zelter M, Matthay MA. Alveolar liquid and protein clearance in anesthetized ventilated rats. *J Appl Physiol* 1994;76:2636–2642.
10. Smedira N, Gates L, Hastings R, et al. Alveolar and lung liquid clearance in anasthetised rabbits. *J Appl Physiol* 1991;74(4):1827–1835.
11. Sakuma T, Okaniwa G, Nakada T, Nishimura T, Fujimura S, Matthay MA. Alveolar fluid clearance in the resected human lung. *Am J Respir Crit Care Med* 1994;150:305–310.
12. Goodman BE, Kim K-J, Crandall ED. Evidence for active sodium transport across alveolar epithelium of isolated rat lung. *J Appl Physiol* 1987;62(2):2460–2466.
13. Basset G, Crone C, Saumon G. Significance of active ion transport in transalveolar water absorption: A study on isolated rat lung. *J Physiol* 1987;384:311–324.
14. Sakuma T, Pittet JF, Jayr C, Matthay MA. Alveolar liquid and protein clearance in the absence of blood flow or ventilation in sheep. *J Appl Physiol* 1993;74(1):176–185.
15. Serikov VB, Grady M, Matthay MA. Effect of temperature on alveolar liquid and protein clearance in an in situ perfused goat lung. *J Appl Physiol* 1993;75(2):940–947.
16. Matalon S. Mechanisms and regulation of ion transport in adult mammalian alveolar type II pneumocytes. *Am J Physiol* 1991;261:C727–C738.
17. Matthay MA. Resolution of Pulmonary Edema. *Clin Chest Med* 1985;6(3):521–545.
18. Basset G, Crone C, Saumon G. Fluid absorption by rat lung in situ: Pathways for sodium entry in the luminal membrane of alveolar epithelium. *J Physiol* 1987;384:325–345.
19. O'Brodovich H. Epithelial ion transport in the fetal and perinatal lung. *Am J Physiol* 1991;261:C555–C564.

20. Saumon G, Basset G, Bouchonnet F, Crone C. cAMP and beta-adrenergic stimulation of rat alveolar epithelium. *Pflügers Arch* 1987;410:464–470.
21. Matthay MA, Folkesson HG, Verkman AS. Salt and water transport across alveolar and distal airway epithelia in the adult lung. *Am J Physiol* 1996; 270:L487–L503.
22. Hasegawa H, Zhang R, Dohrman A, Verkman AS. Tissue-specific expression of mRNA encoding rat kidney water channel CHIP28k by in situ hybridization. *Am J Physiol* 1993;264:C237–C245.
23. Folkesson HG, Matthay MA, Hasegawa H, Kheradmand F, Verkman AS. Transcellular water transport in lung alveolar epithelium through mercury-sensitive water channels. *Proc Natl Acad Sci U S A* 1994;91:4970–4974.
24. O'Brodovich H, Canessa C, Ueda J, Rafil B, Rossier BC, Edelson J. Expression of the epithelial Na+ channel in the developing rat lung. *Am J Physiol* 1993;265:C491–C496.
25. Effros RM. Osmotic extraction of hypotonic fluid from the lungs. *J Clin Invest* 1974;5:935–947.
26. Meyer EC, Ottaviano R, Higgins JJ. Albumin clearance from alveoli: Tissue permeation vs. airway displacement. *J Appl Physiol* 1977;43(3): 487–497.
27. Berthiaume Y, Albertine KH, Grady M, Fick G, Matthay MA. Protein clearance from the air spaces and lungs of unanesthetized sheep over 144 h. *J Appl Physiol* 1989;67(5):1887–1897.
28. Schultz AL, Grismer JT, Wado S, Grande F. Absorption of albumin from alveoli of perfused dog lung. *Am J Physiol* 1964;207(6):1300–1304.
29. Matthay MA, Berthiaume Y, Jayr C, Hasting RH. Alveolar liquid and protein clearance: In vivo studies. In: Effros RM, Chang HK (eds): *Fluid and Solute Transport in the Airspaces of the Lungs.* New York: Marcel Dekker Inc.; 1994;249–279.
30. Hastings RH, Grady M, Sakuma T, Matthay MA. Clearance of different-sized proteins from the alveolar space in humans and rabbits. *J Appl Physiol* 1992;73(4):1310–1316.
31. Bensch KG, Dominguez E, Liebow AA. Absorption of intact protein molecules across the pulmonary air-tissue barrier. *Science* 1967;157(3793): 1204–1206.
32. Williams MC. Endocytosis in alveolar type II cells: Effect of charge and size of tracers. *Proc Natl Acad Sci U S A* 1984;81:6054–6058.
33. Kim KJ, Lebon TR, Shinbane JS, Crandall ED. Asymmetric [14C] albumin transport across bullfrog alveolar epithelium. *J Appl Physiol* 1985;59(4): 1290–1297.
34. Hastings RH, Wright JR, Albertine KH, Ciriales R, Matthay MA. Effect of endocytosis inhibitors on alveolar clearance of albumin, immunoglobulin G, and SP-A in rabbits. *Am J Physiol* 1994;266(LCMP 10):L544–L552.
35. Effros RM, Mason GR. Measurements of pulmonary epithelial permeability in vivo. *Am Rev Respir Dis* 1983;127(5):S59–S65.
36. Folkesson HG, Westrom BR, Karlsson B. Permeability of the respiratory tract to different-sized macromolecules after intratracheal instillation in young and adult rats. *Acta Physiol Scand* 1990;139:347–354.
37. Jayr C, Matthay MA. Alveolar and lung liquid clearance in the absence of pulmonary blood flow in sheep. *J Appl Physiol* 1991;71:1679–1687.
38. Wiener-Kronish JP, Albertine KH, Matthay MA. Differential responses of the endothelial and epithelial barriers of the lung in sheep to escherichia coli endotoxin. *J Clin Invest* 1991;88:864–875.

39. Pittet JF, Wiener-Kronish JP, McElroy MC, Folkesson HG, Matthay MA. Stimulation of lung epithelial liquid clearance by endogenous release of catecholamines in septic shock in anesthetized rats. *J Clin Invest* 1994;94: 663–671.

40. Pittet JF, Wiener-Kronish JP, Serikov V, Matthay MA. Resistance of the alveolar epithelium to injury from septic shock in sheep. *Am J Respir Crit Care Med* 1995;151:1093–1100.

41. Crapo JD, Barry BE, Foscue HA, Shelburne J. Structural and biochemical changes in rat lungs occurring during exposures to lethal and adaptive doses of oxygen. *Am Rev Respir Dis* 1980;122:123–143.

42. Nici L, Dowin R, Gilmore-Hebert M, Jamieson JD, Ingbar DH. Upregulation of rat lung Na-K-ATPase during hyperoxic injury. *Am J Physiol* 1991;261(LCMP 5):L307–L314.

43. Carter EP, Duvick SE, Wendt CH, et al. Hyperoxia increases active alveolar Na^+ resorption in vivo and type II cell Na,K,ATPase in vitro. *Chest* 1994;105(suppl 3):75S–78S.

44. Olivera WG, Ridge KM, Sznajder JI. Lung liquid clearance and Na,K-ATPase during acute hyperoxia and recovery in rats. *Am J Respir Crit Care Med* 1995;152:1229–1234.

45. Sznajder JI, Olivera WG, Ridge KM, Rutschman DH. Mechanisms of lung liquid clearance during hyperoxia in isolated rat lungs. *Am J Respir Crit Care Med* 1995;151:1519–1525.

46. Olivera W, Ridge K, Wood Ld, Sznajder JI. Active sodium transport and alveolar epithelial Na-K-ATPase increase during subacute hyperoxia in rats. *Am J Physiol* 1994;26:L577–L584.

47. Yue G, Russell WJ, Benos DJ, Jackson RM, Olman MA, Matalon S. Increased expression and activity of sodium channels in alveolar type II cells of hyperoxic rats. *Proc Natl Acad Sci U S A* 1995;92:8418–8422.

48. Cunningham A, Hurley J. Alpha-napthyl-thiourea induced pulmonary edema in the rat: A topographical and electron-microscope study. *J Pathol* 1972;106:25–35.

49. Schultz SG, Hudson RL. How do sodium-absorbing cells do their job and survive? *NIPS* 1986;1:185–189.

50. Cheek JM, Kim K-J, Crandall ED. Tight monolayers of rat alveolar epithelial cells: Bioelectric properties and active sodium transport. *Am J Physiol* 1989;256:C688–C693.

51. Zuege D, Suzuki S, Berthiaume Y. Increase of lung sodium-potassium-ATPase activity during recovery from high-permeability pulmonary edema. *Am J Physiol* 1996;271:L896–L909.

Chapter 7

Role of Active Sodium Transport in Reabsorption of Pulmonary Edema

Richard L. Lubman, MD and
Edward D. Crandall, PhD, MD

Alveolar water and solute homeostasis is an important determinant of the lung's ability to participate in gas exchange in health and in disease. The recognition that the alveolar epithelium has an active role in maintaining lung fluid balance has been a major advance in the understanding of the pathophysiology of disease states that are characterized by respiratory failure due to alveolar edema such as congestive heart failure (CHF) and the adult respiratory distress syndrome (ARDS). This chapter discusses the role of active transepithelial sodium transport by the alveolar epithelium in the maintenance of alveolar fluid balance. In particular, current evidence demonstrating the central role of intercellular junctions (tight junctions),sodium channels, and sodium pumps are reviewed (Figure 1).

Alveolar Epithelial Cells: Type I Versus Type II

The distal airways terminate in approximately 3×10^8 alveolar air sacs in the adult human lung.[1] The alveolar epithelium that lines the surfaces of these alveolar air sacs is the interface between the mostly

This work was supported in part by the American Lung Association, the American Heart Association-Greater Los Angeles Affiliate, National Heart, Lung, and Blood Institute Research Grants HL38578, HL38621, and HL51928, and the Hastings Foundation.

From: Weir EK, Reeves JT (eds). *Pulmonary Edema*. Armonk, NY: Futura Publishing Company, Inc.; ©1998.

Alveolar Epithelium:
Salt and water transport

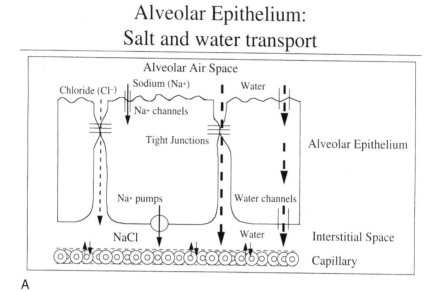

A

Alveolar Epithelial Injury:
Alveolar Edema

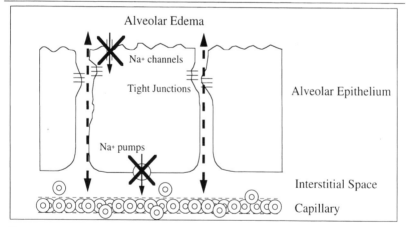

B

gaseous alveolar space and an aqueous internal milieu. Composed of alveolar type I and type II cells, it forms a continuous barrier that is one cell thick. Although the amount of type I cells in adult mammalian lungs is about half that of type II cells, type I pneumocytes cover more than 95% of the alveolar surface.[2,3] Type II pneumocytes are usually situated at the "corners" of alveolar air spaces, are cuboidal in shape, have numerous microvilli on their apical surfaces, and contain storage sites for pulmonary surfactant (lamellar bodies). Type II pneumocytes are progenitor cells for type I cells following injury to the adult alveolar epithelium,[4,5] and appear to play a similar role in the normal alveolar epithelial cell turnover.[6-9] The availability of purified type II cell populations for in vitro study has made feasible the investigation of the metabolic functions[10] and transport properties[11-14] of type II cells. Type I alveolar epithelial cells exhibit protruding nuclei with thin and widely spread cytoplasmic extensions. Little is known about the functional properties of type I cells, which have been isolated with only limited success.[15-18]

Alveolar Epithelial Permeability: Role of Tight Junctions

The relatively fluid-free condition of the alveolar space, historically viewed as resulting from the equilibrium of passive Starling forces, is now recognized to be affected by the transport properties of the alveolar epithelium. The alveolar epithelium provides the major re-

---

Figure 1. Alveolar fluid and solute homeostasis. A. Alveolar epithelial salt and water transport mechanisms. Mechanisms contributing to salt and water transport across the alveolar epithelium are illustrated diagrammatically. The alveolar surface is covered by a thin layer of fluid, the alveolar lining fluid (not shown), from which Na^+ enters the cells via apically situated sodium channels. Na^+ is extruded at the basolateral surface of the cells by active transport via the Na^+, K^+-ATPase (sodium pump). Cl^- follows passively to maintain electoneutrality via an unknown pathway, possibly via the intercellular junctions. Water follows passively due to the osmotic gradient thereby created, through intercellular junctions or transcellularly, possibly across one or more types of water channels (aquaporins). Alternate sodium and chlorine transport pathways have been omitted for clarity. B. Alveolar epithelial injury and edema formation. Effects of alveolar epithelial injury on transepithelial sodium transport and alveolar fluid homeostasis are shown diagrammatically. Loss of tissue integrity caused by damage to tight junctions and/or cell death makes vectorial salt and water transport impossible. Development of alveolar edema is inevitable. Many types of lung injury also cause direct impairment of sodium channel and/or pump activity, although specific effects of injury on water channels and other transport pathways are unknown.

sistance to the passage of water and solutes (eg, ions, small nonelectrolytes, and macromolecules) compared to other barriers present in the lung (eg, airway, interstitial, and endothelial). The alveolar epithelium is at least one order of magnitude less permeable to small solutes than the pulmonary endothelium is,[19,20] consistent with its major role in the regulation of fluid and solute movement across the alveolar-capillary wall.

Current experimental evidence supports the concept that the alveolar epithelium is a "tight" epithelial barrier that is capable of markedly restricting the flow of solutes and water. While measurement of the transepithelial resistance (TER) across the intact mammalian alveolar epithelium is made difficult by the complex anatomy of the lung,[21] measurements made in cultured alveolar epithelial cell monolayers[22] are consistent with TER on the order of several thousand $\Omega \cdot cm^2$. The resistance of this epithelial barrier, whose low paracellular permeability is of similar magnitude to other tight epithelia (eg, toad urinary bladder[23]), may be partly due to the large surface area covered by each alveolar type I cell and resultant minimum density of cell-to-cell contacts. The major factor that contributes to the resistance of the alveolar epithelial barrier, however, is the integrity of the intercellular contacts between alveolar epithelial cells, which in turn is determined by the properties of the junctional complexes that link the cells. The tight junctions (*zonulae occludentes*), whose structure and characteristics are presently the subject of active investigation,[24] appear to be primarily responsible for the maintenance and regulation of paracellular permeability of the alveolar epithelial barrier.

Salt and Water Transport by the Alveolar Epithelium

The alveolar epithelium functions as more than a passive barrier with respect to water and solute homeostasis in the lung. Evidence that the alveolar epithelium plays a major role in transepithelial transport in the lung has come from in vivo studies and from data obtained from many different experimental models. Fluid instilled into mammalian lungs is absorbed gradually over time, with the lung showing a surprisingly large capacity for fluid absorption.[25,26] Recent studies have estimated rates of lung liquid clearance using precise methods. Matthay et al[27] used ^{125}I-albumin as an airspace fluid marker in the lungs of anesthetized sheep, and showed that it was concentrated by 48% after 4 hours. The initial rate of liquid clearance estimated by this method was increased by agonists (eg, terbutaline), although species differences have since been observed in the degree of stimulation by these agents as well as in the baseline resorption rate of liquid.[28] Effros et al[29] measured lung liquid clearance in isolated rat lungs filled with an airspace marker (T1824-albumin) and found that ~100 nL/s of fluid was absorbed in control lungs. The rate of loss of airspace fluid increased to 200 nL/s when terbutaline (5×10^{-5} mol/L) was included in the airspaces and perfusate, whereas the sodium transport inhibitor, amiloride (10^{-4} mol/L), reduced fluid transport from the airspaces. Basset et al[30] and Saumon et al[31] reported similar rates of fluid movement out of the airspaces using ^{125}I-albumin as an alveolar fluid marker in rat lungs. These investigators also reported that cAMP and β-agonists (ie, isoproterenol, terbutaline) increased the fluid resorption rate. Berg et al[32] observed that terbutaline stimulated water resorption from 167 nL/s (baseline) to 305 nL/s in studies using radiolabeled dextran as an airspace marker in isolated perfused rat lungs. Passive permeability properties of the rat alveolar epithelial barrier (as measured by [^{14}C]sucrose and [^{14}C]glycerol fluxes) were not affected by the β-agonist. These and other studies[33–36] indicate that the adult mammalian lung is capable of reabsorbing excess fluid from the airspace in a regulable fashion, and suggest that fluid resorption occurs by mechanisms at least partially dependent on movement of ions (ie, Na^+) across the alveolar epithelium.

Numerous in situ studies using perfused lung preparations,[31,32,37–42] and both animal and human studies in vivo,[27,43–45] have established an important role for active transepithelial sodium transport in the modulation of alveolar fluid balance. Active sodium transport in situ was demonstrated by Crandall et al[37] and Goodman et al[40] with use of an isolated perfused rat lung model. In these studies, the authors measured unidirectional fluxes of ^{22}Na and [^{14}C]sucrose (as a passive transport marker) from airspace to blood across fluid-filled rat lungs and found that terbutaline increased ^{22}Na flux by 28%. The sodium pump inhibitor, ouabain, decreased ^{22}Na flux (by 20%), as did amiloride (by 35%), whereas [^{14}C]sucrose fluxes did not change with any of these agents. Confirmatory findings have been reported by other groups using similar approaches.[38,39] Taken together, these lung liquid clearance studies and solute flux measurements made in situ are consistent with a model of alveolar fluid homeostasis in which water resorption is driven by the local osmotic gradient established by active vectorial sodium transport from airspace to blood.

Although fluid and solute movement across pathways other than the alveolar epithelial barrier may account in part for some of these findings observed in situ, numerous in vitro studies have shown the capacity of alveolar epithelial cells for active transepithelial ion transport. Active transport by alveolar epithelial cells was first demonstrated in vitro in 1982.[46,47] In these studies, alveolar type II cell monolayers grown on plastic dishes were observed to form "domes," or fluid-filled blisters, whose production could be reduced by treatment with metabolic inhibitors. This evidence for active transepithelial transport was confirmed in many subsequent studies[48–50] and was shown more directly in studies in which alveolar epithelial cells were grown in monolayer culture on permeable filters. Cheek et al[22] first described formation of high electrical resistance (ie, "tight") monolayers of rat alveolar epithelial cells grown on tissue culture-treated polycarbonate filters. These monolayers exhibit a TER >2000 $\Omega \cdot cm^2$, consistent with a tight epithelial barrier in vivo, and develop a short-circuit current (ISC) of ≥ 4 $\mu A/cm^2$ that has been directly shown to reflect active transport of Na^+ in the apical-to-basolateral direction. Monolayers grown in this fashion have also been used to define the polarized distribution of acid/base transport mechanisms across the alveolar epithelium[51,52] and are well suited for study of vectorial transport of other substrates (eg, peptides).[53]

Alveolar Epithelial Polarity: Apical Sodium Channels and Basolateral Sodium Pumps

The alveolar epithelium, like all epithelial tissues, has luminal (apical) and serosal (basolateral) aspects, functionally compartmentalized by cell-to-cell junctions.[54] This "polarity" is the structural and functional hallmark of epithelia, and makes vectorial transport across the alveolar epithelium possible. Within each cell surface membrane domain, enzymes, lipids, receptors, and transport proteins are distributed in a polarized fashion. The mechanisms by which these molecules reach the appropriate cell membrane differ among different epithelia.[55] Interactions between the actin cytoskeleton and the surface membrane, and the presence of tight junctions, maintain the polarized localization of the molecular constituents of the membrane.[56]

Amiloride-sensitive sodium channels are the principal entry pathway for sodium at the apical membrane of alveolar epithelial cells,[22,57–59] although other sodium-coupled transport systems may be present. Sodium is actively extruded from the cells by Na^+, K^+-ATPase (Na pump), which most evidence indicates is present exclusively on the basolateral membrane of the cells.[22,60] Sodium channel and pump activities must remain equal at steady state in order for transepithelial transport to occur without a net change in intracellular [Na^+], volume, or osmolarity, indicating the need for precise regulation of these processes. The mechanisms that maintain this relationship, which are likely to be sensitive to derangement when the alveolar epithelium is injured,[61] are poorly understood at present. In contrast to the adult airway[62] or fetal lung epithelium,[63] adult rat alveolar epithelial cell monolayers do not actively secrete chloride under any experimental conditions.[64]

Some controversy remains concerning the properties and molecular identity of lung sodium channels. There is general agreement that sodium enters alveolar epithelial cells primarily via apically situated channels that are different from the voltage-gated sodium channels of neurons and other excitable cells. However, two different types of sodium channels,[59] as well as nonselective cation channels,[65] have been putatively identified in alveolar epithelial cells by use of immunochemical,[66] pharmacological,[67] and molecular biological[68] techniques. Senyk et al[69] purified sodium channels from adult mammalian lung and reconstituted them into lipid bilayers, which then displayed sodium conductances with low affinity for the sodium channel blocker, amiloride. Patch-clamp and pharmacological data from Yue et al[70] also showed evidence for low amiloride-affinity channels in alveolar epithelial cells in culture for 24 to 96 hours. However, data obtained from alveolar epithelial cells cultured on plastic,[57] and more recent data on alveolar epithelial cell monolayers grown on filters,[71] are more consistent with high amiloride-affinity channels (Figure 2). Voilley et al[58] and McDonald et al[72] recently cloned such high amiloride-affinity sodium channels from rat and human lung, respectively, which are essentially identical to those described in colon and kidney (αrENaC) by Canessa et al.[73] It is now recognized that these epithelial sodium channels are composed of at least three different subunits (α, β, and γ) that are regulated independently.[74,75] An inherited defect in the β-subunit of the sodium channel has recently been shown to be responsible for abnormal sodium transport in the kidney and for the resulting systemic hypertension present in individuals with Liddle's syndrome.[76] The α-subunit is developmentally regulated in fetal rat lung,[68] and its absence in an αENaC-deficient mouse has been shown to result in death within 40 hours of birth, due to defective neonatal lung liquid clearance.[77] The authors[77a] have also found 3.7, 2.2, and 3.2 kb transcripts in alveolar epithelial cell monolayers, corresponding to the data published for α-, β-, and γ-subunits, respectively, in rat kidneys. These results, along with pharmacological data, provide further evidence for the presence of high amiloride-affinity channels in the adult alveolar epithelium.

Epithelial sodium channel activity and expression can be regulated by hormones, by phosphorylation, by intracellular Ca^{++}, Na^+, and pH, by cytoskeletal elements (eg, actin filaments), and by G-proteins in epithelia.[78-84] Alveolar epithelial sodium channel activity can be regulated at the transcriptional and/or translational levels (ie, total number of channels), via intracellular trafficking and membrane targeting (ie, density of channels in the apical membrane), and/or at the level of activity of individual channels (ie, conductance and open-time probabil-

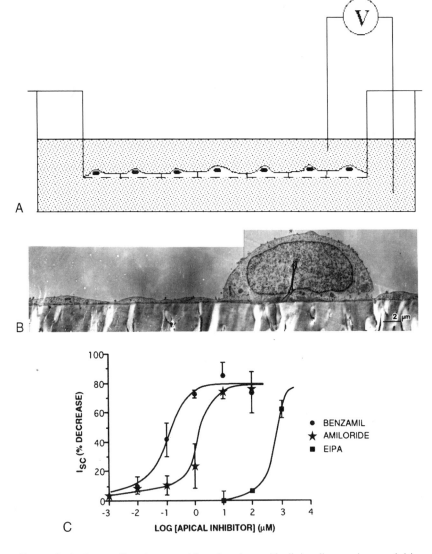

Figure 2. Active sodium transport by alveolar epithelial cell monolayers: inhibition by sodium channel blockade. A. Schematic representation of alveolar epithelial cell monolayers grown on permeable supports. Alveolar type II cells grown in primary culture form confluent electrically resistive monolayers by 3 to 4 days in culture (see References 22 and 71). Transepithelial resistance (TER) and spontaneous potential difference (SPD) are measured directly, and short-circuit current (ISC), an index of active transepithelial sodium transport, is calculated using Ohm's law. B. Representative transmission electron micrograph of alveolar epithelial cells grown on tissue culture-treated polycarbonate filter, day 5. Note protruding nucleus with closely pinched borders and thin cytoplasmic extensions, consistent with transition toward type I cell-like ap-

ity). Although it is known, for example, that expression of epithelial sodium channels is sensitive to thyroid-releasing hormone (TRH) and dexamethasone in the developing rat lung,[68] relatively few studies have been published concerning regulation of these channels in the adult lung. With the very recent availability of immunologic and molecular probes for these channels, and the further application of patch-clamp techniques, new information should become available shortly.

The sodium pump (Na^+, K^+-ATPase) is a heterodimeric protein consisting of an α- and a β- subunit. The α-catalytic subunit is responsible for extrusion of three Na^+ ions in exchange for two K^+ ions at the expense of cellular energy in the form of ATP. The function of the β-subunit, a glycoprotein, is currently unknown, but may include effects on subunit assembly, intracellular transport, and functional expression of sodium pumps, and effects on K^+ affinity of the enzyme.[85] Both subunits occur in one of several distinct isoforms that have different tissue distributions and, in some cases, different pharmacological properties.[86–88] Sodium pumps provide the driving force for transepithelial ion transport across alveolar epithelial cells, and probably constitute the major exit pathway at the basolateral surface of the cells. Current evidence is most consistent with predominant expression of the $α_1$- and $β_1$-subunit isoforms in the lung, and in the alveolar epithelium in particular.[89–92]

Several questions remain concerning the expression of sodium pumps in the alveolar epithelium. Ridge et al[93] published preliminary data suggesting that cultured alveolar epithelial cells express the $α_2$ isoform to a greater extent than the $α_1$ with time in culture, and that both alveolar type I and type II cells express the $α_2$ isoform by immunohistochemistry in situ. These data differ from another report that indicates relatively constant expression of $α_1$ isoform by cultured alveolar ep-

---

pearance. Micrograph is cropped to emphasize detail (6600×). Reprinted with permission from Reference 116. C. Effects of inhibitors of sodium transport on ISC. In the presence of epidermal growth factor (EGF), which upregulates active transepithelial sodium transport across alveolar epithelial cell monolayers, ISC is decreased at 10 minutes by apical (but not basolateral) sodium transport inhibitor. Here, ISC was decreased by the sodium channel blocker, amiloride, and by two analogues with augmented (benzamil) or decreased (5-[*N*-ethyl-*N*-isopropyl] amiloride [EIPA]) specificity for sodium channels. ISC was inhibited by benzamil > amiloride > EIPA (mean inhibitory concentration ~100 nmol/L, 1 µmol/L, and 200 µmol/L, respectively). Similar sensitivity to these inhibitors is seen in the absence of EGF. Each point represents average ± SE. These results are most consistent with the role of sodium channels having high affinity for amiloride as the principal sodium entry pathway for transepithelial sodium transport across alveolar epithelial cell monolayers. Reprinted with permission from Reference 71.

ithelial cells over time in culture,[94] and earlier studies[89,90] that found predominant expression of α_1 mRNA in adult lung, with minimal expression of other (ie, α_2 and α_3) isoforms. Several investigators have attempted to define the distribution of sodium pumps in situ in alveolar epithelium by immunochemical methods.[60,95] Although the basolateral surface of type II cells was labeled by antisera to the α-subunit of the sodium pump in these studies, the investigators were unable to detect any antigenic sodium pump in type I cells. Considering the low probability that these cells uniquely fail to express sodium pumps, however, the inability to detect Na^+, K^+-ATPase in situ probably reflects a problem of methodological resolution.

Regulation of sodium pump activity in alveolar epithelial cells may also occur at several different levels. Sodium pump regulation can occur over relatively short intervals (within hours) by mechanisms that include recruitment of sodium pumps from intracellular pools to the plasma membrane, phosphorylation of sodium pump subunits, or increased sodium pump kinetics due to elevations in intracellular $[Na^+]$.[96] As noted previously, the β-agonist, terbutaline, stimulates active transport of sodium in both cultured cells and whole lung,[22,37] prompting some to propose its therapeutic use in CHF and ARDS. These effects are thought to be mediated via cAMP-dependent signal-transduction pathways that are activated rapidly, and probably do not require changes in gene expression.

Longer-term regulation of active sodium transport is likely to require changes in the expression of sodium channels, sodium pumps, or both. Growth factors (ie, epidermal growth factor),[71,97] hyper- and hypoxia,[98–100] and terbutaline[94,101] have been reported to cause up- or downregulation of sodium transport by the alveolar epithelium via chronic effects on sodium pump expression. The molecular pathways by which sodium pump expression is regulated in alveolar epithelium are currently unknown. Recent developments, including characterization of the Na^+, K^+-ATPase α_1-subunit isoform promoter region,[102] should facilitate elucidation of these mechanisms.

Some of the reported effects of extracellular factors on sodium transport by alveolar epithelium, most notably those of hyperoxia, appear to vary considerably as a function of experimental model and condition. Olivera et al[42] found that exposure of rats to 85% O_2 for 7 days resulted in increased active Na^+ flux in isolated perfused lungs, increased Na^+, K^+-ATPase activity in isolated alveolar type II cells, and increases in type II cell α_1- and β_1-subunit by immunocytochemistry. Nici et al[95] similarly reported that exposure of rat lungs to 95% O_2 for 48 hours upregulated sodium pump gene and protein expression in alveolar endothelial cells (AECs). In contrast, a preliminary report from Harris et al[103] indicates that exposure of rats to hyperbaric oxygen (100% O_2 at 2.5 atm) results in an initial increase (1 to 3 hours' exposure), followed by a decrease (4 to 8 hours' exposure), in sodium pump message, basolateral membrane pumps, and Na^+, K^+-ATPase activity. In other preliminary reports, Carter et al[104] found that exposure of rats to 100% O_2 for 60 hours resulted in a transient reduction in lung Na^+, K^+-ATPase activity that lasted for several days postexposure, and Zheng and Goodman[105] found no effect on active sodium transport in lungs isolated from rats exposed to 95% O_2 for 48 hours or 60 hours.

Paracellular Versus Transcellular Water Movement: Role of Tight Junctions and Water Channels

Alveolar epithelial tight junctions (TJs) have been described as junctions that form a network of three to five interconnected strands that are similar in both alveolar type I and type II cells on freeze-fracture electron micrographs.[106] The junctional complex is associated with development and maintenance of epithelial polarity, and with regulation of paracellular permeability in epithelia. It has proven exceptionally difficult to characterize at the molecular level until very recently. Several TJ-associated proteins, including ZO-1 (*zonula occludens*-1), ZO-2, cingulin, and occludin, have recently been cloned and/or partially characterized with respect to their roles in TJ formation and regulation.[24] While the biology of TJs is complex and remains incompletely understood, the requirement of these proteins for TJ formation and regulation has become increasingly apparent. Preliminary data from the Will Rogers Institute Pulmonary Research Center indicate that the stimuli that modulate sodium channel and pump expression also affect cell-to-cell junctions and paracellular permeability across alveolar epithelial cell monolayers.[71,98,99] The development of electrically resistive alveolar epithelial cell monolayers coupled with the availability of cDNA and antibody probes for these proteins now makes it possible to investigate the relationship between alveolar epithelial permeability and the expression of TJ-associated proteins.

Tight junctions may also help to regulate movement of water across the cell-to-cell junction in alveolar epithelium. Water movement across the lipid bilayers of the cell membrane occurs by simple diffusion and is very slow. While there is substantial evidence that water traverses intact epithelia by the paracellular pathway, especially in "leaky" epithelia, transepithelial tissue conductance and hydraulic conductance do not always correlate well.[23] This apparent discrepancy led several investigators to infer the existence of water channels or pores in some epithelia. Such water channels, now known as aquaporins, were first demonstrated in 1992.[107] Aquaporin-1 (AQP-l), a 28 kd channel-forming integral membrane protein of human red blood cells (originally referred to as CHIP28), was the first of a family of related mercurial-sensitive proteins now shown to exist in many epithelial and nonepithelial tissues.[108] AQP-l, as well as a more recently cloned 32 kd mercurial-insensitive water channel (MIWC),[109–111] can be detected in alveolar epithelial cells. Of particular note, aquaporin-5 (AQP-5), a recently described mercury-sensitive water channel present in salivary lacrimal, and respiratory tissues,[112,113] is expressed in alveolar type I, but not type II, cells.[114] Preliminary evidence suggests that these and other[115] lung water channels contribute to alveolar fluid homeostasis, although their relative importance remains to be defined.

Summary and Overview

Current evidence strongly supports the concept that the alveolar epithelium contributes to alveolar fluid and solute homeostasis in the adult lung because of both its barrier or permeability properties and its ability to actively transport sodium in a vectorial fashion. Sodium enters the cells at the apical membrane passively via sodium channels, and is actively extruded at the basolateral membrane by sodium pumps. Water follows passively due to the osmotic gradient thus created, moving across intercellular junctions, water channels, or both (Figure 1).

The recent data discussed above are consistent with the notion that alveolar epithelial transport processes are influenced, and can be regulated, by a variety of extracellular factors. Lung injury increases paracellular permeability, either by impairing alveolar epithelial tissue integrity or tight junction integrity, thus resulting in alveolar flooding. Various forms of lung injury may also directly affect epithelial transport mechanisms (ie, sodium channels and pumps) directly, thereby causing alterations in lung fluid balance even in the absence of demonstrable pathological injury.

The morbidity and mortality of the ARDS and CHF are due in large measure to the development of alveolar edema. Although considerable information is now available concerning the role of the alveolar epithelium in the development of and recovery from alveolar edema, therapeutic advances based on this knowledge have not yet become a reality. Further research efforts will be directed toward finding safe and effective ways of modulating alveolar epithelial barrier and transport processes in humans via pharmacological, and in all likelihood, gene therapeutic approaches in the coming years.

Acknowledgments We are grateful to Drs. Zea Borok, Spencer I. Danto, and Kwang-Jin Kim for their important contributions to this work and for many helpful discussions.

References

1. Weibel ER. *The Pathway for Oxygen: Structure and Function in the Mammalian Respiratory System.* Cambridge: Harvard University Press; 1984: 211–230.
2. Haies DM, Gil J, Weibel ER. Morphometric study of rat lung cells. I. Numerical and dimensional characteristics of parenchymal cell population. *Am Rev Respir Dis* 1981;123:533–541.
3. Weibel ER, Gehr P, Haies D, et al. The cell population of the normal lung. In: Bouhuys A (ed): *Lung Cells in Disease.* Amsterdam: North-Holland; 1976;3–16.
4. Adamson IYR, Bowden DH. The type 2 cell as progenitor of alveolar epithelial regeneration. *Lab Invest* 1974;30:35–42.
5. Evans MJ, Cabral LJ, Stephens RJ, et al. Transformation of alveolar type 2 cells to type 1 cells following exposure to NO_2. *Exp Mol Pathol* 1975;22: 142–150.
6. Joyce-Brady MF, Brody JS. Ontogeny of alveolar epithelial markers of differentiation. *Dev Biol* 1990;137:331–348.
7. Williams MC, Dobbs LG. Expression of cell-specific markers for alveolar epithelium in the fetal rat lung. *Am J Respir Cell Mol Biol* 1990;2:533–542.
8. Brody JS, Williams MC. Pulmonary alveolar epithelial cell differentiation. *Annu Rev Physiol* 1992;54:351–371.
9. Danto SI, Zabski SM, Crandall ED. Late appearance of a type I alveolar epithelial cell marker during fetal rat lung development. *Histochemistry* 1994;102:297–304.
10. Dobbs LG, Geppert EF, Williams MC, et al. Metabolic properties and ultrastructure of alveolar type II cells isolated with elastase. *Biochim Biophys Acta* 1980;618:510–523.
11. Matalon S. Mechanisms and regulation of ion transport in adult mammalian alveolar type II pneumocytes. *Am J Physiol* 1991;261:C727–C738.
12. Lubman RL, Crandall ED. Regulation of intracellular pH in alveolar epithelial cells. *Am J Physiol* 1992;262:Ll–L14.
13. Cott GR. Active transport of Na^+ across epithelial monolayers. In: Effros RM, Chang HK (eds): *Fluid and Solute Transport in the Airspaces of the Lungs.* New York: Marcel Dekker; 1994;101–122.
14. Kim K-J, Crandall ED. Specialized alveolar epithelial transport processes. In: Effros RM, Chang HK (eds): *Fluid and Solute Transport in the Airspaces of the Lungs.* New York: Marcel Dekker; 1994;219–248.
15. Picciano P, Rosenbaum RM. The type I alveolar lining cells of the mammalian lung: I. Isolation and enrichment from dissociated rabbit lung. *Am J Pathol* 1978;90:99–122.
16. Weller NK, Karnovsky MJ. Isolation of pulmonary alveolar type I cells from adult rats. *Am J Pathol* 1986;122:448–456.
17. Dobbs LG, Williams MC, Gonzalez R. Monoclonal antibodies specific to apical surfaces of rat alveolar type I cells bind to surfaces of cultured, but not freshly isolated, type II cells. *Biochim Biophys Acta* 1988;970:146–156.
18. Banks MA, Porter DW, Pailes WH, Schwegler-Berry D, Martin WG, Cas-

tranova V. Taurine content of isolated rat alveolar type I cells. *Comp Biochem Physiol* 1991;100B:795–799.

19. Taylor AE, Gaar KA. Estimation of equivalent pore radii of pulmonary capillary and alveolar membranes. *Am J Physiol* 1970;218:1133–1140.

20. Normand ICS, Olver RE, Reynolds EOR, et al. Permeability of lung capillaries and alveoli to non-electrolytes in the foetal lamb. *J Physiol* 1971; 219:303–330.

21. Ballard ST, Gatzy JT. Alveolar transepithelial potential difference and ion transport in the adult rat lung. *J Appl Physiol* 1991;70:63–69.

22. Cheek JM, Kim K-J, Crandall ED. Tight monolayers of rat alveolar epithelial cells: Bioelectric properties and active sodium transport. *Am J Physiol* 1989;256:C688–C693.

23. Reuss L. Tight junction permeability to ions and water. In: Cereijido M (ed): *Tight Junctions*. Boca Raton, FL: CRC Press; 1992:49–66.

24. Anderson JM, Van Itallie CM. Tight junctions and the molecular basis for regulation of paracellular permeability. *Am J Physiol* 1995;269:G467–G475.

25. Courtice FC, Simmonds WJ. Absorption from the lung. *J Physiol* 1949; 109:103–116.

26. Kylstra JA. Lavage of the lung. *Acta Physiol Pharmacol Neerl* 1958;7: 163–221.

27. Matthay MA, Landolt CC, Staub NC. Differential liquid and protein clearance from the alveoli of anesthetized sheep. *J Appl Physiol* 1982;53:96–104.

28. Goodman BE, Waltz WF. Species differences in regulation of sodium transport. In: Effros RM, Chang HK (eds): *Fluid and Solute Transport in the Airspaces of the Lungs*. New York: Marcel Dekker; 1994;489–504.

29. Effros RM, Mason GR, Sietsema K, et al. Fluid reabsorption and glucose consumption in edematous rat lungs. *Circ Res* 1987;60:708–719.

30. Basset G, Crone C, Saumon G. Fluid absorption by rat lung in situ: Pathways for sodium entry in the luminal membrane of alveolar epithelium. *J Physiol* 1987;384:325–345.

31. Saumon G, Basset G, Bouchonnet F, et al. cAMP and β-adrenergic stimulation of rat alveolar epithelium. *Pflügers Arch* 1987;410:464–470.

32. Berg MM, Kim K-J, Lubman RL, et al. Hydrophilic solute transport across rat alveolar epithelium. *J Appl Physiol* 1989;66:2320–2327.

33. Jayr C, Matthay MA. Alveolar and lung liquid clearance in the absence of pulmonary blood flow in sheep. *J Appl Physiol* 1991;71:1679–1687.

34. Rutschman DH, Olivera A, Sznajder JI. Active and passive liquid movement in isolated perfused rat lungs. *J Appl Physiol* 1993;75:1574–1580.

35. Sakuma T, Pittet JF, Jayr C, et al. Alveolar liquid and protein clearance in the absence of blood flow or ventilation in the sheep. *J Appl Physiol* 1993;74:176–185.

36. Sakuma T, Okaniwa G, Nakada T, et al. Alveolar fluid clearance in the resected human lung. *Am J Respir Crit Care Med* 1994;150:305–310.

37. Crandall ED, Heming TA, Palombo RL, et al. Effects of terbutaline on sodium transport in isolated perfused rat lung. *J Appl Physiol* 1986;60: 289–294.

38. Basset G, Crone C, Saumon G. Significance of active ion transport in transalveolar water absorption: A study on isolated rat lung. *J Physiol* 1987;384:311–324.

39. Effros RM, Mason GR, Hukkanen J, et al. New evidence for active sodium transport from fluid-filled rat lungs. *J Appl Physiol* 1989;66:906–919.

40. Goodman BE, Kim K-J, Crandall ED. Evidence for active sodium transport

across alveolar epithelium of isolated rat lung. *J Appl Physiol* 1987;62: 2460–2466.

41. McLaughlin GE, Kim K-J, Berg MM, Agoris P, Lubman RL, Crandall ED. Measurement of solute fluxes in isolated rat lungs. *Respir Physiol* 1993; 91:321–334.

42. Olivera W, Ridge K, Wood LDH, Sznajder JI. Active sodium transport and alveolar epithelial Na-K-ATPase increase during subacute hyperoxia in rats. *Am J Physiol* 1994;266:L577–L584.

43. Matthay MA, Berthiaume Y, Staub NC. Long-term clearance of liquid and protein from the lungs of unanesthetized sheep. *J Appl Physiol* 1985;59: 928–934.

44. Berthiaume Y, Broaddus VC, Gropper MA, Tanita T, Matthay MA. Alveolar liquid and protein clearance from normal dog lungs. *J Appl Physiol* 1988;65:585–593.

45. Berthiaume Y, Staub NC, Matthay MA. Beta-adrenergic agonists increase lung liquid clearance in anesthetized sheep. *J Clin Invest* 1987;79:335–343.

46. Goodman BE, Crandall ED. Dome formation in primary cultured monolayers of alveolar epithelial cells. *Am J Physiol* 1982;243:C96–C100.

47. Mason RJ, Williams MC, Widdicombe JH, Sanders MJ, Misfeldt DS, Berry LC Jr. Transepithelial transport by pulmonary alveolar type II cells in primary culture. *Proc Natl Acad Sci U S A* 1982;79:6033–6037.

48. Goodman BE, Fleischer RS, Crandall ED. Evidence for active Na^+ transport by cultured monolayers of pulmonary alveolar epithelial cells. *Am J Physiol* 1983;245:C78–C83.

49. Goodman BE, Brown SES, Crandall ED. Regulation of transport across pulmonary alveolar epithelial cell monolayers. *J Appl Physiol* 1984;57: 703–710.

50. Cott GR, Sugahara K, Mason RJ. Stimulation of net active ion transport across alveolar type II cell monolayers. *Am J Physiol* 1988;250:C222–C227.

51. Lubman RL, Crandall ED. Polarized distribution of Na^+-H^+ antiport activity in rat alveolar epithelial cells. *Am J Physiol* 1994;266:L138–L147.

52. Lubman RL, Danto SI, Chao DC, Fricks CE, Crandall ED. Cl^--HCO_3^- exchanger isoform AE2 is restricted to the basolateral surface of alveolar epithelial cell monolayers. *Am J Respir Cell Mol Biol* 1995;12:211–219.

53. Kim K-J, Cheek JM, Crandall ED. ^{14}C-albumin transport across rat alveolar epithelial monolayers. *Am Rev Respir Dis* 1989;139:A477.

54. Schneeberger EE, Lynch RD. Structure, function, and regulation of cellular tight junctions. *Am J Physiol* 1992;262:L647–L661.

55. Matter K, Mellman I. Mechanisms of cell polarity in epithelial cells. *Curr Opin Cell Biol* 1994;6:545–554.

56. Rabito CA. Tight junction and apical/basolateral polarity. In: Cereijido M (ed): *Tight Junctions.* Boca Raton, FL: CRC Press; 1992;203–214.

57. Russo R, Lubman RL, Crandall ED. Evidence for amiloride-sensitive sodium channels in alveolar epithelial cells. *Am J Physiol* 1992;262:L405–L411.

58. Voilley N, Lingueglia E, Champigny G, et al. The lung amiloride-sensitive Na^+ channel: Biophysical properties, pharmacology, ontogenesis, and molecular cloning. *Proc Natl Acad Sci U S A* 1994;91:247–251.

59. Matalon S, Benos DJ, Jackson RM. Biophysical and molecular properties of amiloride-inhibitable Na^+ channels in alveolar epithelial cells. *Am J Physiol* 1996;271:Ll–L23.

60. Schneeberger EE, McCarthy KM. Cytochemical localization of Na^+, K^+-ATPase in rat type II pneumocytes. *J Appl Physiol* 1986;60:1584–1589.

61. Fish EM, Molitoris BA. Mechanisms of disease: Alterations in epithelial polarity and the pathogenesis of disease states. *N Engl J Med* 1994;330: 1580–1588.
62. Smith JJ, Welsh MJ. Fluid and electrolyte transport by cultured human airway epithelia. *J Clin Invest* 1993;91:1590–1597.
63. O'Brodovich H. Epithelial ion transport in the fetal and perinatal lung. *Am J Physiol* 1991;261:C555–C564.
64. Kim K-J, Cheek JM, Crandall ED. Contribution of active Na^+ and Cl^- transport to net ion transport by alveolar epithelium. *Respir Physiol* 1991; 85:245–256.
65. Feng Z-P, Clark RB, Berthiaume Y. Identification of nonselective cation channels in cultured adult rat alveolar type II cells. *Am J Respir Cell Mol Biol* 1993;9:248–254.
66. Yue G, Hu P, Oh Y, et al. Culture-induced alterations in alveolar type II cell Na^+ conductance. *Am J Physiol* 1993;265:C630–C640.
67. Matalon S, Bauer ML, Benos DJ, et al. Fetal lung epithelial cell contain two populations of amiloride-sensitive Na^+ channels. *Am J Physiol* 1993;264: L357–L364.
68. O'Brodovich H, Canessa C, Ueda J, et al. Expression of the epithelial Na^+ channel in the developing rat lung. *Am J Physiol* 1993;265:C491–C496.
69. Senyk O, Matalon S, Bradford. Reconstitution of immunopurified alveolar type II cell Na^+ channel protein into planar lipid bilayers. *Am J Physiol* 1995;268:Cl148–Cl156.
70. Yue G, Shoemaker RL, Matalon S. Regulation of low amiloride-affinity sodium channels in alveolar type II cells. *Am J Physiol* 1994;267:L94–L100.
71. Borok Z, Hami A, Danto SI, et al. Effects of EGF on alveolar epithelial junctional permeability and active sodium transport. *Am J Physiol* 1996; 270:L559–L565.
72. McDonald FJ, Snyder PM, McCray PB Jr, et al. Cloning, expression, and tissue distribution of a human amiloride-sensitive Na^+ channel. *Am J Physiol* 1994;266:L728–L734.
73. Canessa CM, Horisberger JD, Rossier BC. Epithelial sodium channel related to proteins involved in neurodegeneration. *Nature* 1993;361:467–470.
74. Canessa CM, Schild L, Buell G, et al. Amiloride-sensitive epithelial Na^+ channel is made of three homologous subunits. *Nature* 1994;367: 463–467.
75. Duc C, Farman N, Canessa CM, et al. Cell-specific expression of epithelial sodium channel α, β, and γ subunits in aldosterone-responsive epithelia from the rat: Localization by in situ hybridization and immunocytochemistry. *J Cell Biol* 1994;127:907–1921.
76. Shimkets RA, Warnock DG, Bositis CM, et al. Liddle's syndrome: Heritable human hypertension caused by mutations in the beta subunit of the epithelial sodium channel. *Cell* 1994;79:407–414.
77. Hummer E, Barker B, Gatzy J, et al. Early death due to defective neonatal lung liquid clearance in αENaC-deficient mice. *Nat Genet* 1996;12:325–328.
77a. Borok Z, Danto SI, Dimen LL, Zhang X-L, Lubman RL. NA^+, K^+-ATPase expression in alveolar epithelial cells: Upregulation of active ion transport by keratinocyte growth factor. *Am J Physiol* in press.
78. Berdiev BK, Prat AG, Cantiello HF, et al. Regulation of epithelial sodium channels by short actin filaments. *J Biol Chem* 1996;271:17704–17711.
79. Turnheim K. Intrinsic regulation of apical sodium entry in epithelia. *Physiol Rev* 1991;71:421–445.

80. Matsumoto PS, Ohara A, Duchatelle P, et al. Tyrosine kinase regulates epithelial sodium transport in A6 cells. *Am J Physiol* 1993;264:C246–C250.
81. Bubien JK, Jope RS, Warnock DG. G-proteins modulate amiloride-sensitive sodium channels. *J Biol Chem* 1994;269:17780–17783.
82. Lingueglia E, Renard S, Waldmann R, et al. Different homologous subunits of the amiloride- sensitive Na^+ channel are differently regulated by aldosterone. *J Biol Chem* 1994;269:13736–13739.
83. MacGregor GG, Olver RE, Kemp PJ. Amiloride-sensitive Na^+ channels in fetal type II pneumocytes are regulated by G proteins. *Am J Physiol* 1994;267:L1–L9.
84. Benos DJ, Awayda MS, Berdiev BK, et al. Diversity and regulation of amiloride-sensitive Na^+ channels. *Kidney Int* 1996;49:1632–1637.
85. McDonough AA, Geering K, Farley RA. The sodium pump needs its β-subunit. *FASEB J* 1990;4:1589–1605.
86. Shull GE, Greeb J, Lingrel JB. Molecular cloning of three distinct forms of the Na^+, K^+-ATPase α-subunit from rat brain. *Biochemistry* 1986;25: 8125–8132.
87. Sweadner KJ. Isozymes of the Na^+/K^+-ATPase. *Biochim Biophys Acta* 1989;988:185–220.
88. Lingrel JB. Na, K-ATPase: Isoform structure, function, and expression. *J Bioenerg Biomembr* 1992;24:263–270.
89. Young RM, Lingrel JB. Tissue distribution of mRNAs encoding the alpha isoforms and beta subunit of rat Na^+, K^+-ATPase. *Biochem Biophys Res Comm* 1987;145:52–58.
90. Orlowski J, Lingrel JB. Tissue-specific and developmental regulation of rat Na, K-ATPase catalytic α isoform and β subunit mRNAs. *J Biol Chem* 1988;263:10436–10442.
91. Shyjan AW, Levenson R. Antisera specific for $α_1$, $α_2$, $α_3$, and β subunits of the Na, K-ATPase: Differential expression of α and β subunits in rat tissue membranes. *Biochemistry* 1989;28:4531–4535.
92. O'Brodovich H, Staub O, Rossier B, et al. Ontogeny of $α_1$ and $β_1$-isoforms of Na^+, K^+-ATPase in fetal distal lung epithelium. *Am J Physiol* 1993; 264:Cl137–Cl143.
93. Ridge K, Factor P, Horowitz S, et al. Differential expression of Na, K-ATPase in rat alveolar epithelial cells. *Am J Respir Crit Care Med* 1994;149:A588.
94. Suzuki S, Zuege D, Berthiaume Y. Sodium-independent modulation of Na^+-K^+-ATPase activity by beta-adrenergic agonist in alveolar type II cells. *Am J Physiol* 1995;268:L983–L990.
95. Nici L, Dowin R, Gilmore-Hebert M, et al. Upregulation of rat lung Na, K-ATPase during hyperoxic injury. *Am J Physiol* 1991;261:L307–L314.
96. Bertorello AM, Katz AI. Regulation of Na^+, K^+-ATPase activity: Pathways between receptors and effectors. *NIPS* 1995;10:253–260.
97. Danto SI, Zabski SM, Borok Z, et al. Regulation of Na^+, K^+-ATPase $α_1$- and β-subunit protein expression by epidermal growth factor. *Am J Respir Crit Care Med* 1995;151:A189.
98. Borok Z, Kim K-J, Patel P, et al. Effects of hyperoxia on alveolar epithelial cell barrier properties and expression of Na^+, K^+-ATPase. *Am J Respir Crit Care Med* 1995;151:A190.
99. Borok Z, Dimen LL, Kim K-J, et al. Effects of hypoxia on alveolar epithelial cell ion transport and Na^+, K^+-ATPase gene and protein expression. *J Invest Med* 1995;43:275A.
100. Planès C, Friedlander G, Loiseau A, et al. Inhibition of Na-K-ATPase after

prolonged hypoxia in an alveolar epithelial cell line. *Am J Physiol* 1996;271: L70–L79.

101. Patel P, Borok Z, Kim K-J, et al. Phosphatase-mediated effects of terbutaline on active transport by alveolar epithelial cell monolayers. *Am Rev Respir Crit Care Med* 1995;151:A182.

102. Kawakami K, Masuda K, Nagano K, et al. Characterization of the core promoter of the Na^+ /K^+-ATPase α_1 subunit gene. Elements required for transcription by RNA polymerase II and RNA polymerase III in vitro. *Eur J Biochem* 1996;237:440–446.

103. Harris ZL, Ridge K, Sznajder JI. Modulation of alveolar Na, K-ATPase by hyperbaric oxygen in rats. *Am J Respir Crit Care Med* 1994;149:A59.

104. Carter EP, Duvick SE, Wangensteen OD, et al. Rat lung Na, K-ATPase activity is decreased following 60 hr of hyperoxia. *Am J Respir Crit Care Med* 1994;149:A588.

105. Zheng LP, Goodman BE. Effects of hyperoxia on sodium fluxes across the blood-gas barrier in rat lungs. *Am Rev Respir Dis* 1992;145:A366.

106. Schneeberger EE, Lynch RD. Tight junctions in the lung. In: Cereijido M (ed): *Tight Junctions*. Boca Raton, FL: CRC Press; 1992;337–352.

107. Preston GM, Carroll TP, Guggino WB, et al. Appearance of water channels in Xenopus oocytes expressing red cell CHIP28 protein. *Science* 1992;256:385–387.

108. Sabolic I, Brown D. Water channels in renal and nonrenal tissues. *NIPS* 1995;10:12–17. 109. Folkesson HG, Matthay MA, Hasegawa H, et al. Transcellular water transport through mercurial-sensitive water channels. *Proc Natl Acad Sci U S A* 1994;91:4970–4974.

110. Hasegawa H, Lian S-C, Finkbeiner WE, et al. Extrarenal tissue distribution of CHIP28 water channels by in situ hybridization and antibody staining. *Am J Physiol* 1994;266:C893–C903.

111. Hasegawa H, Ma T, Skach W, et al. Molecular cloning of a mercurial-insensitive water channel expressed in selected water-transporting tissues. *J Biol Chem* 1994;269:5407–5500.

112. Gropper MA, Frigeri A, Verkman AS. Localization of MIWC and GLIP water channel homologs in rat trachea and lung. *Am Rev Respir Crit Care Med* 1995;151:A179.

113. Raina S, Preston GM, Guggino WB, et al. Molecular cloning and characterization of an aquaporin cDNA from salivary, lacrimal, and respiratory tissues. *J Biol Chem* 1995;270:1908–1912.

114. Lee MD, Bhakta KY, Raina S, et al. The human Aquaporin-5 gene. Molecular characterization and chromosomal localization. *J Biol Chem* 1996; 271:8599–8604.

115. Zhang XL, Borok Z, Lubman RL, et al. Expression of aquaporin-5 (AQP5) in alveolar epithelial cells. *Am Rev Respir Crit Care Med* 1996;153:A508.

116. Cheek JM, Evans MJ, Crandall ED. Type I cell-like morphology in tight alveolar epithelial monolayers. *Exp Cell Res* 1989;184:375–387.

Chapter 8

Surfactant-Edema Interactions

Alan H. Jobe, MD, PhD

Introduction

Pulmonary surfactant is a complex lipoprotein structure that has as a primary physiological function the maintenance of low and variable surface tensions in alveoli and small airways. The low surface tensions stabilize the lung at low transpulmonary pressures and decrease the work of tidal breathing. Surfactant was identified by Clements and Pattle[1] as an anti-edema factor because agents that injured the lungs, such as toxic gases, caused severe edema. The surfactant film is the last barrier to the maintenance of the dry alveolus and it is essential for the prevention of atelectasis. Nevertheless, surfactant is not often discussed in the context of mechanical ventilation or edema. The text, *Edema* (1984), by Staub and Taylor contains no index entries for surfactant, and surfactant is minimally discussed in the otherwise complete text, *Principles and Practice of Mechanical Ventilation* (1994), by Tobin. The low surface tensions in the alveoli and small airways contribute to maintenance of a dry alveolus and factors that increase surface tensions promote edema formation. This chapter focuses on the interactions of edema fluid and the various components of edema fluid that affect the function of surfactant. The thesis of this chapter is that there is a reciprocal relationship between alveolar edema and surfactant. An intact surfactant system in the normal lung protects against edema accumulation; however, edema formation degrades surfactant function and promotes more edema accumulation. Several recent reviews[2,3] of surfactant inactivation have been published.

This work was supported by Grant HD-12714 from NIH—Child Health and Development.

From: Weir EK, Reeves JT (eds). *Pulmonary Edema.* Armonk, NY: Futura Publishing Company, Inc.; ©1998.

Surfactant and Edema Formation

Respiratory Distress Syndrome

The prototypic disease process associated with surfactant deficiency, edema, and lung injury is the respiratory distress syndrome (RDS) in the preterm infant.[4] In this disease atelectasis and alveolar edema are present soon after preterm delivery. The relationships between the surfactant deficiency and edema formation are complex and are the subject of much of this chapter. At a superficial level, infants with RDS have small surfactant pool sizes relative to term infants, but the preterm infant with RDS has pool sizes of about 5 mg/kg, similar to those of the healthy adult lung. The epithelial and endothelial barriers of the fetal lung prevent proteins and other large molecular weight substances from entering fetal lung fluid. However, with preterm birth and ventilation, interstitial and alveolar edema quickly develop.[5] The reasons for the increased permeability to plasma proteins are a combination of abnormal fluid clearance from the airspaces (a function of the immaturity of ion pumps), the immaturity of epithelial and endothelial barriers, stretch of distal lung structures that are susceptible to "volutrauma" with positive pressure ventilation, and perhaps other abnormalities of neonatal cardiopulmonary adaptation that injure epithelial and endothelial barriers. Samples of airspace fluid from infants with RDS or preterm lambs have very high minimum surface tensions, suggesting the presence of inadequate surfactant. However, the airspace fluid can be centrifuged to recover surfactant, and that surfactant has good surface tension-lowering characteristics.[6] Therefore, surfactant pool sizes similar to those of the healthy adult are not adequate because the edema fluid interferes with the function of the surfactant. Resolution of RDS is accompanied by improvements in minimum surface tensions, increased surfactant pool sizes, and decreased alveolar edema.

Effects of Surfactant on Edema Formation in the Preterm Lung

In several studies,[5,7] surfactant treatment of the preterm lung before the initiation of ventilation decreased the bidirectional flux of albumin from the vasculature to the airspace and from the airspace to the vasculature.[5] This effect of surfactant was more apparent at early gestational ages when surfactant deficiency and edema were more severe. The effect of the surfactant treatment was the preservation of the balance of transvascular fluid and protein movement into the lung that is characteristic of the fetal lamb during the early hours after preterm delivery and ventilation.[7] In the absence of surfactant treatment, lung lymph flow increased more than threefold and lymph and pleural space protein drainage more than doubled (Figure 1). No changes were noted in lymph or protein flows from fetal values in lambs treated with surfactant. The net effect at 8 hours of age was a 24% decrease in extravascular lung water in surfactant-treated lungs relative to control lungs. The mechanisms by which surfactant decreased edema formation in the preterm lung were probably a combination of the decreased surface tensions that facilitate alveolar expansion and fluid clearance, the promotion of more uniform alveolar expansion at lower transpulmonary pressures, which minimizes volutrauma, and a decrease in recruitment of white blood cells and/or the release of inflammatory mediators from the lung. Explanations other than improvements in surface tensions alone are needed to account for the decreased vascular permeability.

Surfactant, Edema, and Mechanical Ventilation

Ventilation of the normal lung can result in injury and edema if the lung is overstretched by either very large tidal volumes or more normal tidal volumes superimposed on a high functional residual capacity

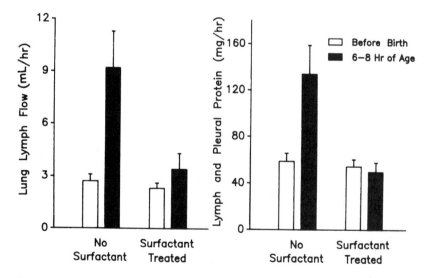

Figure 1. Effect of surfactant treatment on lung lymph and protein flow following delivery of preterm lambs. Preterm fetal sheep were instrumented for lung lymph measurements and baseline measurements were made before preterm delivery (open bars = before birth). The preterm lambs were delivered at 128 days' gestation and ventilated without surfactant treatment or after surfactant treatment; values for lymph flow and lymph and pleural protein were measured at 6 hours to 8 hours of age (solid bars). Data from Reference 7.

(FRC) such that maximal lung volumes are approached or exceeded.[8] This volutrauma occurs at the top end of the pressure-volume curve that is not dependent on surfactant function under normal circumstances.[9] With nonuniform lung injury, ventilation at high transpulmonary pressures tends to overdistend the compliant and more normal lung regions, resulting in injury to the lung that may be less involved with the primary injury process. In this situation, more normal surfactant function may facilitate injury to the overdistended lung regions, resulting in volutrauma injury and edema.

Surfactant treatment responses also depend on the strategy of mechanical ventilation selected and, in turn, may influence pulmonary edema development or progression. If the preterm or surfactant-deficient lung is ventilated at low FRC, white blood cells and edema accumulate. Ventilation of the preterm surfactant-deficient lung causes primarily bronchoepithelial disruption, rapid alveolar flooding with edema, and hyaline membrane formation.[10] The pathological lesions can be almost completely prevented by treatment of surfactant-deficient preterm animals with surfactant. This striking effect of surfactant treatment on lung edema is dependent on the composition of the surfactant and on the ventilation style. The surfactants that are used clinically to treat RDS are not equivalent to natural surfactant. When tested in preterm ventilated and surfactant-deficient rabbits, Exosurf® (Burroughs Wellcome, Research Triangle Park, NC), a synthetic surfactant that contains no surfactant-specific protein, does not improve compliance. However, it does decrease the leak of intravascular albumin into lung tissue and airspaces if the preterm rabbits are ventilated using 3 cm H_2O positive end-expiratory pressure (PEEP).[11] Survanta® (Ross Labs, Columbus, OH), a surfactant made from cow lung that contains the surfactant proteins SP-C and SP-B, has minimal effects on compliance in the absence of PEEP, but decreases lung edema. The addition of PEEP to the ventilation strategy improves compliance and further decreases lung edema. Natural sheep surfactant both improves compliance and decreases lung edema, independent of PEEP. These effects of the interaction of type of surfactant and PEEP on edema formation are, in part, explained by the surfactant protein content of the surfactant used for treatment. Rider et al[12] and Ogawa et al[13] reconstructed surfactant by adding native surfactant proteins to lipids and found that each of the surfactant proteins, SP-A, SP-B, and SP-C, enhanced the performance of surfactant lipids. The proteins complemented each other to achieve treatment responses similar to those of natural surfactant. The addition of each surfactant protein to lipids decreased edema accumulation (Figure 2). The more natural or complete the surfactant, the less PEEP needed to optimize FRC and decrease edema formation.

These observations, made with use of the preterm lung, are consistent with results for lung injury models with adult lungs. Kobayashi et

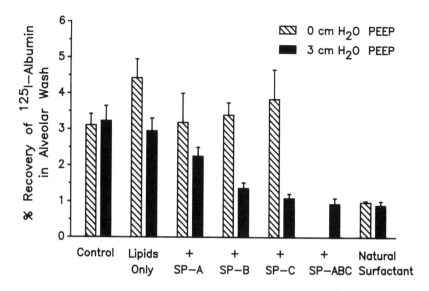

Figure 2. Effects of surfactant proteins and PEEP on the recovery of ^{125}I-albumin in alveolar washes 30 minutes after intravascular injection of ventilated preterm rabbits. The addition of each surfactant protein to the surfactant lipids decreased the recovery of radiolabeled albumin only if the preterm rabbits were ventilated with 3 cm H_2O PEEP. Natural surfactant decreased albumin recoveries from control values independently of PEEP. Data from Reference 12.

al[14] demonstrated in 1984 that surfactant treatment and conventional ventilation of saline-lavaged rabbits was ineffective unless PEEP was used. PEEP alone also was ineffective. As in the experiments in animals not treated with surfactant, ventilation at low lung volumes after surfactant treatment (no PEEP) resulted in severe lung injury, edema, and an irreversible loss of lung volume. PEEP was also necessary for surfactant treatments to decrease pulmonary edema in an acid aspiration model.[15]

Following saline lavage, adult rabbits had severe respiratory failure and died with conventional ventilation. The conventional ventilation strategy using 6 cm H_2O PEEP was associated with rapid accumulation of white blood cells in the lungs, and systemic granulocyte depletion prevented most of the lavage-induced respiratory failure.[16] The granulocytes were activated and the resulting inflammation damaged the conventionally ventilated and surfactant-deficient lung. A high-frequency ventilation strategy resulted in restoration of the partial pressure of oxygen (PO_2) to prelavage values and prevented white blood cell accumulation and the development of alveolar edema.[17] But what do these observations have to do with surfactant?

Other observations have provided some insight into why these effects were observed. Argiras et al[18] found that the injury resulting from conventional mechanical ventilation of surfactant-depleted lungs was minimized by using a PEEP above the inflection point for opening of the lung as determined by an inflation pressure-volume curve. McCulloch and colleagues[19] made the parallel observation that after saline lavage, oscillatory ventilation with a mean lung volume 23 mL/kg above FRC maintained normal PO_2 values. Pressure-volume curves after several hours of oscillation demonstrated no loss of lung volume. In contrast, oscillation at a mean lung volume approximately 8 mL/kg above FRC or conventional ventilation at a mean lung volume 4 mL/kg above FRC resulted in hypoxia and permanent volume loss at the end of the ventilation period. Low-volume strategies, using either conventional or oscillatory ventilation, resulted in bronchiolar epithelial injury, edema, and hyaline membranes. The beneficial effects of oscillation strategies are apparent only if oscillation occurs at lung volumes well above a normal FRC. Therefore, ventilation strategies interact with surfactant to determine, in part, the sequence of lung injury and edema formation.

Substances that Interfere with Surfactant Function

Alveolar Metabolism of Surfactant

In order to understand why multiple substances can interfere with surfactant function, it is necessary to evaluate each substance in terms of how it interacts with surfactant in the alveolar environment. The flow diagram in Figure 3 is used to organize this discussion.[20] As presently understood, the lipid components of surfactant (primarily saturated phosphatidylcholines, monounsaturated phosphatidylcholines, the acidic phospholipids phosphotidylglycerol and phosphatidylinositol, and small amounts of neutral lipids) are secreted by type II cells together with the two small hydrophobic proteins SP-B and SP-C as condensed lipid-protein structures called lamellar bodies. The lamellar arrays then unfold into tubular myelin or loose lipid protein arrays within the hypophase (the thin film of fluid covering the alveolus and the fluid pools in the corners of alveoli). Tubular myelin contains all surfactant components plus a higher SP-A content than the lamellar bodies because de novo synthesized SP-A is secreted independently of lamellar bodies by type II cells. SP-A seems to form the corner anchors for tubular myelin. This structure is highly surface active in that it adsorbs to an air-water interface, spreads rapidly, and will achieve very low surface tensions on surface area compression. However, most of the surfactant in the hypophase is in a loose lipid array that is less structured than tubular myelin. Transgenic mice lacking SP-A have no tubular myelin and have essentially normal surfactant function.[21] The con-

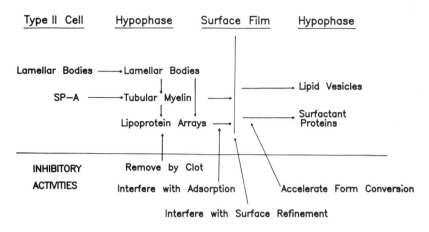

Figure 3. Summary of alveolar forms of surfactant and inhibitory activities that interfere with surfactant function.

version of lamellar bodies to tubular myelin or to loose lipid arrays is probably a spontaneous process that occurs following secretion and is not influenced by inhibiting substances.

The biophysical process of film formation by surface adsorption requires lipids with a high saturated phosphatidylcholine content and the hydrophobic proteins SP-B and SP-C for optimal absorption rates. The "surface film" is itself a complex structure, thought to be a monolayer of primarily phospholipid with multilayers just below the monolayer that contain lipids and proteins that provide substrate for film formation. The monolayer is refined by the loss of surfactant proteins and lipids other than saturated phosphatidylcholine by surface area compression. Lipids are lost from the surface film by collapse into small vesicles that contain very little surfactant protein. The process of surface film maintenance and lipid form conversion from tubular myelin and loose lipid arrays to vesicles is facilitated by a serine protease that may be an integral component of the surfactant complex.[22] This enzymatic activity, referred to as convertase, requires surface film formation and surface area changes for activity. The mechanisms for loss of surfactant proteins from the surface film are not understood, but condensed aggregates of SP-B have been recovered from alveolar washes.[23]

The clearance and catabolism of surfactant lipids and proteins is done by macrophages and type II cells. Both cell types can take up all surfactant components and degrade them. Type II cells also take up phospholipids and surfactant proteins and recycle them, intact, back into lamellar bodies for resecretion. The process of recycling alveolar saturated phosphatidylcholine is approximately 50% efficient in adult animals, and the surfactant proteins are recycled at somewhat lower efficiencies. In the adult rabbit, approximately 20% to 30% of the saturated phosphatidylcholine from surfactant is catabolized by macrophages.

Lavage fluid from the airspaces of normal animals and humans contains approximately 50% of the lipids in tubular myelin plus loose lipid arrays, and approximately 50% of the lipids in small vesicles that have very poor surface-active properties. Therefore, only about 50% of the alveolar pool is in a biophysically active form. Recent estimates of surfactant pool sizes in humans are on the order of approximately 4 mg/kg,[24] of which perhaps 2 mg/kg is capable of surface film formation. Estimates of alveolar fluid volume range from 15 mL to 70 mL in humans.[25] With use of a value of 40 mL for a 70 kg man, the total surfactant concentration is on the order of approximately 7 mg/mL hypophase fluid.

Inhibition by Proteins

In 1965, Tierney and Johnson[26] reported that blood or serum could elevate the minimum surface tension of surfactant. Subsequently, multiple interactions between surfactant and the protein components of plasma have been described and some of the mechanisms of inactivation have been explored (Table 1).[2,3] Albumin, γ-globulin, and fibrinogen, when mixed with natural surfactant (containing all lipid and protein components), will interfere with surface adsorption.[27,28] The plasma-derived proteins also prevent the development of low surface tensions on surface area compression.[29] These effects of proteins are extremely dependent on both the relative concentration and the absolute concentration of the plasma proteins and surfactant. Plasma protein components at low concentrations are very inhibitory when mixed with concentrations of surfactant that are just sufficient to form stable films. However, if surfactant concentration is high, little interference with adsorption and the surface tension behavior of surfactant occurs.[30] This nonlinear concentration-dependent behavior is thought to result from a competition for the air-liquid interface between proteins and surfactant.[29] The proteins also interfere with the development of low surface tensions by interfering with surface enrichment for saturated phosphatidylcholine.[28]

The effects of most proteins on surfactant function are not the result of direct molecular interactions because surfactant can be separated from albumin or protein mixtures by centrifugation, and surface properties are restored.[29,30] The interference with the surface biophysical behavior of surfactant also is path-dependent in vitro. A preformed surface film of albumin, hemoglobin, or fibrinogen will inhibit the ad-

Table 1

Substances That Inhibit Surfactant

Protein Inhibitors

Edema fluid	Globulins	Laminin
Plasma	Fibrinogen	Elastin
Serum	Fibrinogen degradation products	Hemoglobin
Albumin	110-kDa protein	C-reactive protein

Lipid inhibitors

Lyso-Phosphatidylcholine	Red cell membranes
Cholesterol	Oleic acid

Other inactivators

Amino acids	Proteases
Meconium	Lipases
Oxidizing agents	Bilirubin

Table abstracted from Reference 2.

sorption of a surfactant suspension that would not be affected if the proteins were mixed with surfactant and absorption allowed to occur.[29] The reciprocal effect is that a surfactant film preformed from a dilute surfactant suspension will not be inactivated by proteins added in high concentration to the hypophase. These concentration-dependent and path-dependent effects may be important to understanding surfactant inactivation in lung injury. Surfactant concentration in the alveolar hypophase is high because the hypophase volume is very low; it is perhaps 30 mL in humans.[25] A modest amount of regional alveolar edema can dilute the surfactant several fold, permitting surfactant inactivation by protein components of the edema fluid.

Most of the studies of surfactant inactivation by proteins have not explored the mechanism of inactivation. Plasma and serum components, such as albumin, globulins, hemoglobin, and a 110 kd inhibitory protein found in the plasma and airspaces of preterms with RDS, probably interfere with surfactant function nonspecifically as described above.[29] Fibrinogen and fibrinogen split products resulting from clot formation are very potent inhibitors of surfactant in vitro.[31] There have not been studies of the mechanism of inactivation. C-reactive protein is a potent inhibitor of surfactant adsorption, and this inhibition can be prevented by phosphocholine.[32] Therefore, C-reactive protein seems to interfere with the adsorption of surfactant by binding to the phosphocholine head groups of phosphatidylcholine.

Sensitivity of Different Surfactants to Proteins

A uniform observation is that natural surfactant is much more resistant to inactivation by any of the plasma components than is a less complete surfactant.[33] Lipid-only surfactants made from either the lipids from natural surfactant or from synthetic lipids are extremely sensitive to inactivation by protein. Addition of SP-C or SP-B increases resistance to inactivation and inclusion of both proteins in general further protects the surfactant from inactivation.[3] These observations also apply to synthetic sequences of SP-C and SP-B as well as to synthetic peptides designed to enhance the function of lipid mixtures.[34] The hydrophobic surfactant proteins organize the lipids in the hypophase and in the surface film, and this structure presumably results in less effective competition by other proteins for the surface. SP-A also increases the resistance of surfactant to inhibition by proteins,[35] and an antibody to SP-A increases sensitivity of surfactant to inactivation by fibrinogen in vivo.[36]

Lipid Inhibitors of Surfactant

The lipid composition of surfactant is conserved across mammalian species, although changes in composition (substitution of phosphatidylglycerol by phosphatidylinositol) in native surfactant or changes in the ratios of lipids in synthetic surfactant do not significantly alter function in vivo. Nevertheless, certain lipids do inactivate surfactant, presumably by mixing with the lipid-protein structures and interfering with adsorption and surface film refinement. High concentrations of cholesterol can interfere with surfactant function. Lysophosphatidylcholine can injure the lungs and cause pulmonary edema, and it can interfere with surfactant function by sensitizing surfactant to inactivation by proteins.[37,38] Although the first enzymatic step in the normal catabolism of phosphatidylcholine by type II cells and by macrophages is the production of lysophosphatidylcholine by phospholipase A_2, this reaction is intracellular and is carefully regulated.[20] Release of phospholipases into the alveolus (pancreatitis or inflammation) can generate lysophosphatidylcholine from surfactant and result in a sequence of lung injury and surfactant inactivation. Oleic acid can also directly interfere with surfactant by mixing with surfactant lipids to disrupt structures or by generating lung injury, edema, and subsequent surfactant inactivation.[39] Another source of abnormal lipids in the airspace is pulmonary hemorrhage. The lipids from red cell membranes are not very surface active and they can interfere with surfactant function by mixing with surfactant lipids to change biophysical properties. As with protein inactivation, lipid inactivation of incomplete (lacking one or more of the surfactant proteins) surfactants or of lipid-only surfactants is more potent than is the effect of these lipids on natural surfactant.

Other Inactivators of Surfactant

Surfactant also is susceptible to inactivation by other substances that are likely to be in the airspace with lung injury. Infants who aspirate meconium can have severe respiratory failure. Meconium can directly inhibit the function of surfactant, and surfactant treatment can improve lung function in both experimental models and in infants.[40] With lung injury, the free amino acid content of alveolar fluid can increase several fold and the cationic amino acids, lysine, arginine, and ornithine, inhibit the minimum surface tension of surfactant in a dose-dependent fashion in the presence of Ca^{+}[41] SP-A makes the surfactant less susceptible to inactivation by amino acids. Cationic polyamino acids can inhibit surfactant function as well. Bilirubin associates with surfactant and disrupts its function. It also can sensitize surfactant to further inactivation by serum proteins, again demonstrating interactions between different classes of inactivators that further disrupt surfactant function.

Oxidation can inactivate surfactant. Although the primary surface-active phospholipid class, saturated phosphatidylcholine, is quite resistant to oxidation, unsaturated lipids are important for surface adsorption. Activated macrophages produce both nitric oxide and superoxide, and the injured lung is often exposed to high oxygen concentrations. Haddad et al[42] and Gilliard et al[43] demonstrated lipid peroxidation of the unsaturated phospholipids of surfactant with degradation of surface biophysical properties. The hydrophobic surfactant proteins SP-B and SP-C can be damaged by oxidants as well. Nitration of SP-A resulted in fragmentation and polymerization and in decreased ability to aggregate lipids.[44] Surfactant from lambs exposed to 80 ppm or 200 ppm NO had abnormal surface properties and damaged SP-A.[45] Interactions between oxidized surfactants and protein inactivators have not been evaluated. Illustrative of the reciprocal relationships between surfactant and edema, surfactant can inhibit the respiratory burst of neutrophils and macrophages and thus suppress the inflammatory response that may release oxidants and other inhibitory substances.[46]

Proteases and Surfactant Form Conversion

The normal process of form conversion from lamellar bodies and loose lipid arrays via the surface film to vesicles and residual surfactant protein aggregates is also susceptible to interference by components of edema (Figure 3). In the normal lung the form changes of surfactant catalyzed by a serine protease (convertase) presumably maintain the balance of substrate in the hypophase for film formation and postfilm forms for recycling and catabolism.[22] When plasma or proteases are mixed with surfactant in vitro and surface area is cycled at 37°C according to the procedure of Gross and Schultz,[22] there is an increased rate of form conversion from surface active to inactive forms.[47] The process is inhibited by α_1-antitrypsin and by SP-A. In experimental models of lung injury, the inactive forms increase relative to the active surfactant fractions and lung function deteriorates proportionately to the increase in inactive surfactant forms.[48] It is of interest that this change in ratio of active to inactive surfactant forms is one of the earliest indicators of lung injury in a septic lung injury model.[49] Lavage samples from patients with adult respiratory distress syndrome (ARDS) have increased amounts of the inactive surfactant forms relative to the active forms.[50] Furthermore, surfactant from lung injury models and patients also contain less SP-A. The net result is a situation that promotes depletion of functional surfactant pools because edema fluid and inflammation products increase proteases and injury depletes SP-A. Proteases in edema fluid can also degrade the surfactant proteins directly and alter surfactant function.

Clotting in the Alveoli and Resolution

The above discussion emphasizes that soluble proteins such as fibrinogen can reversibly inactivate surfactant and that nonspecific proteases can increase the rate of form conversion of surfactant. The complex relationships between surfactant, clotting, and fibrinolysis further complicate the intra-alveolar behavior of surfactant in lung injury. Hyaline membranes in both RDS and ARDS are, in essence, coagulums of fibrin and debris resulting from the edema-injury-inflammation sequence. In 1966, Taylor and Abrams[51] proposed that surfactant was a thromboplastin and that it might interfere with fibrinolysis. Balis et al[52] reported in 1971 that not only was surfactant a potent thromboplastin, but that the subsequent clot removed surfactant from plasma-surfactant suspensions, resulting in a "coagulation type of surfactant depletion." Subsequent experiments demonstrated that clot formation yielding 0.3 mg/mL fibrin trap about 50% of surfactant within the clot, and higher fibrin concentrations remove essentially all the surfactant from suspension.[53] Surfactant does not bind to preformed clots; therefore, the surfactant depletion is an integral part of clot formation. Fibrin monomers and fibrinogen split products generated during clotting are potent reversible inhibitors of surfactant. Thrombin and other proteases that degrade clots and lung ground substances during fibrinolysis also generate fragments that will reversibly inhibit the surface properties of surfactant.[54] Fragments of molecular weight >30 kd are more inhibitory than are smaller fragments.[55] Therefore, surfactant dysfunction can persist during the resolution phase of lung injury. In complex injuries associated with ARDS, both clot formation and fibrinolysis no doubt occur simultaneously in different lung regions, and both processes may interfere with surfactant function. As a further twist to the interactions of surfactant with the clotting pathways, surfactants containing the hydrophobic proteins inhibit the cleavage of fibrinogen by plasmin and can contribute to delayed clearance of fibrin from alveoli.[56]

Models and Clinical Correlates of Surfactant Inactivation

Assessment of the importance of surfactant inactivation by the mechanisms discussed above are complicated by other factors that contribute to lung injury. Inactivation phenomena probably seldom occur in isolation from cardiopulmonary abnormalities, inflammation, and other mechanisms of lung injury. Soon after birth, the infant destined to develop severe RDS will often transiently oxygenate well. Airway samples collected at the time of intubation for progressive respiratory failure have high minimum surface tensions that are explained by plasma proteins.[2] Preterm lambs with RDS respond to exogenous surfactant treatment with an acute improvement in surface tensions, and recurrent respiratory failure correlates with subsequent increases in surface tensions[6] (Figure 4). In these experiments performed on preterm lambs, the surfactant used for treatment was recovered by alveolar lavage and its surface properties were intact once the soluble proteins were removed. Therefore, in the early phases of RDS, surfactant inactivation by soluble proteins seems to contribute to the respiratory failure. Kobayashi et al[57] directly evaluated the effects of proteins from edema fluid recovered from oxidant-injured rabbits by mixing the proteins with surfactant and then treating surfactant-deficient preterm rabbits with mixtures containing different ratios of edema protein to surfactant lipid. Protein-to-lipid ratios >4.5 (mg/mg) caused severe inhibition of surface properties in vitro. Ratios higher than 11 were required for interference with in vivo treatment responses in the preterm

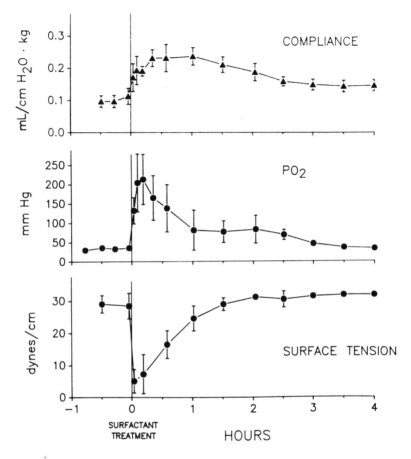

Figure 4. Compliance, arterial PO_2, and minimum surface tension for preterm lambs treated with surfactant. After delivery and ventilation for a short period, the lambs were treated at zero time with 100 mg/kg natural sheep surfactant. The treatment resulted in improved PO_2 and compliance values that correlated with low minimum surface tensions measured for samples of lung fluid collected by suction of the large airways. The subsequent deterioration in lung function correlated with increased surface tensions. Data abstracted from Reference 6.

rabbits. In similar experiments, Yukitake et al[58] reported that plasma added to natural surfactant had little effect on treatment responses in preterm rabbits, but plasma interfered with treatment responses for a surfactant that lacked SP-A. Addition of SP-A restored function even in the presence of plasma. This experiment demonstrated in vivo the general observation from in vitro studies of surface properties that natural surfactant is much more resistant to plasma inactivation than are surfactants lacking SP-A or synthetic surfactants.

Surfactant treatment responses in lung injury models and in term infants that are not surfactant deficient also are consistent with inhibition of function in the mature lung. Infants with severe pulmonary hemorrhage will respond to surfactant treatments, demonstrating what may be a pure response to severe inhibition.[59] Similarly, rabbits with acute edema caused by bilateral vagotomy will respond to surfactant treatments.[5] More complex acute injuries that are associated with severe edema, such as smoke inhalation, will also respond to exogenous surfactant, as will animals with viral pneumonia.[60] Nevertheless, some severe injuries, such as oleic acid-induced edema/hemorrhage, and more chronic injuries caused by agents such as N-nitroso-N-methyl urethane do not respond consistently to surfactant treatments. These mixed results suggest that more complex injuries and/or more severe inactivation phenomena make treatments designed to restore surfactant function less successful.

In lavage samples from ARDS patients plasma proteins, fibrinogen split products, free amino acids, and proteolytic enzyme levels are elevated.[48,61] Surfactant with abnormal in vitro surface properties and increased amounts of small vesicle forms is recovered. This surfactant also contains less SP-A and may have decreased amounts of SP-B. Therefore, the potential for inactivation includes most of the mechanisms described in this chapter.

Summary

Surfactant interfaces with alveolar edema at multiple levels that have been primarily characterized by in vitro studies. The low and variable surface tensions of surfactant balance interstitial pressures to prevent alveolar flooding in the normal lung. Once edema is present, surfactant concentration falls and inhibition of surfactant can occur by soluble proteins, lipids, or other substances. Surfactant is a thromboplastin-causing fibrinogen that enters the airspace to clot. The clotting process interferes with surfactant by two mechanisms: (1) by removal of surfactant in the clot and (2) by generation of fibrinogen breakdown products that are extremely inactivating. Edema and inflammatory fluid also contain enzymes that deplete the functional surfactant pool by conversion of surfactant to forms that are biophysically inactive. Further damage to lipids and proteins may result from oxidants. The amount and mechanisms of damage to the surfactant system in an injury that includes alveolar edema depends on the characteristics of the injury. However, the contribution of surfactant inactivation to lung dysfunction cannot be quantified at this time. The inactivation phenomena are likely to be influenced by clinical management decisions that include fluid administration, ventilation strategies, and oxidant exposure.

References

1. Clements JA. Surface tension of lung extracts. *Proc Soc Exp Biol Med* 1957;95:170–172.
2. Ikegami M. Surfactant inactivation. In: Boynton BR, Carlo WA, Jobe AH (eds): *New Therapies for Neonatal Respiratory Failure*. New York: Cambridge University; 1994;36–48.
3. Gunther A, Seeger W. Resistance to surfactant inactivation. In: Robertson B, Taeusch HW (eds): *Surfactant Therapy for Lung Disease*. New York: Marcel Dekker, Inc.; 1995;269–292.
4. Jobe AH. Pulmonary surfactant therapy. *N Engl J Med* 1993;328:861–868.
5. Jobe AH, Ikegami M. Protein permeability abormalities in the preterm lung. In: Effros RM, Chang HK (eds): *Fluid and Solute Transport in the Airspaces of the Lungs*. New York: Marcel Dekker; 1994;335–355.
6. Ikegami M, Jobe AH, Glatz T. Surface activity following natural surfactant treatment in preterm lambs. *J Appl Physiol* 1981;51:306–312.
7. Carlton DP, Cho SC, Davis P, et al. Surfactant treatment at birth reduces lung vascular injury and edema in preterm lambs. *Pediatr Res* 1995;37:265–270.
8. Dreyfuss D, Saumon G. Ventilator-induced injury. In: Tobin MJ (ed): *Principles and Practice of Mechanical Ventilation*. New York: McGraw-Hill; 1994;793–811.
9. Goerke J. Prediction of mechanical responses to surfactant therapy. In: Robertson B, Taeusch HW (eds): *Surfactant Therapy for Lung Disease*. New York: Marcel Dekker; 1995;349–369.
10. Robertson B. Animal models of neonatal surfactant dysfunction. In: Robert B, Van Golde LMG, Batenburg JJ (eds): *Pulmonary Surfactant: From Molecular Biology to Clinical Practice*. Amsterdam: Elsevier; 1992;459–484.
11. Rider ED, Jobe AH, Ikegami M, et al. Different ventilation strategies alter surfactant responses in preterm rabbits. *J Appl Physiol* 1992;73:2089–2096.
12. Rider ED, Ikegami M, Whitsett JA, et al. Treatment responses to surfactant containing natural surfactant proteins in preterm rabbits. *Am Rev Respir Dis* 1993;147:669–676.
13. Ogawa A, Brown CL, Schlueter MA, et al. Lung function, surfactant apoprotein content, and level of PEEP in prematurely delivered rabbits. *J Appl Physiol* 1994;77:1840–1849.
14. Kobayashi T, Kataoka H, Ueda T, et al. Effects of surfactant supplement and end-expiratory pressure in lung-lavaged rabbits. *J Appl Physiol* 1984;57:995–1001.
15. Zucker AR, Holm BA, Crawford GP, et al. PEEP is necessary for exogenous surfactant to reduce pulmonary edema in canine aspiration pneumonitis. *J Appl Physiol* 1992;73:679–686.
16. Kawano T, Mori S, Cybulsky M, et al. Effect of granulocyte depletion in a ventilated surfactant-depleted lung. *J Appl Physiol* 1987;62:27–33.
17. Froese AB, McCulloch PR, Sugiura M, et al. Optimizing alveolar expansion prolongs the effectiveness of exogenous surfactant therapy in the adult rabbit. *Am Rev Respir Dis* 1993;148:569–577.
18. Argiras EP, Blakeley CR, Dunnill MS, et al. High PEEP decreases hyaline membrane formation in surfactant deficient lungs. *Br J Anaesth* 1987;59:1278–1285.
19. McCulloch PR, Forkert PG, Froese AB. Lung volume maintenance prevents lung injury during high frequency oscillatory ventilation in surfactant-deficient rabbits. *Am Rev Respir Dis* 1988;137:1185–1192.

20. Jobe AH, Rider ED. Catabolism and recycling of surfactant. In: Robertson B, Van Golde LMG, Batenburg JJ (eds): *Pulmonary Surfactant: From Molecular Biology to Clinical Practice.* Amsterdam: Elsevier; 1992;313–337.
21. Korfhagen TR, Bruno MD, Ross GF, et al. Preservation of lung function and deficiency of tubular myelin in SP-A gene targeted mice. *Proc Natl Acad Sci U S A* 1996;93:9594–9599.
22. Gross NJ, Shultz RM. Requirements for extracellular metabolism of pulmonary surfactant: Tentative identification of serine protease. *Am J Physiol* 1992;262:446–453.
23. Baritussio A, Alberti D, Quaglino D, et al. SP-A, SP-B, and SP-C in surfactant subtypes around birth: Reexamination of alveolar life cycle of surfactant. *Am J Physiol* 1994;266:436–447.
24. Rebello CM, Jobe AH, Eisele J, Ikegami M. Alveolar and tissue surfactant pool sizes in humans. *Am J Res Crit Care Med* 1996;154:625–628.
25. Rennard SI, Basset G, Lecossier D, et al. Estimation of volume of epithelial lining fluid recovered by lavage using urea as marker of dilution. *J Appl Physiol* 1986;60(2):532–538.
26. Tierney DF, Johnson RP. Altered surface tension of lung extracts and lung mechanics. *J Appl Physiol* 1965;20:1253–1260.
27. Holm BA, Notter RH, Finkelstein JN. Surface property changes from interactions of albumin with natural lung surfactant and extracted lung lupids. *Chem Phys Lipids* 1985;38:287–298.
28. Keough KMW, Parsons CS, Tweeddale MG. Interactions between plasma proteins and pulmonary surfactant: Pulsating bubble studies. *Can J Physiol Pharmacol* 1989;67:663–668.
29. Holm BA, Enhorning G, Notter RH. A biophysical mechanism by which plasma proteins inhibit lung surfactant activity. *Chem Phys Lipids* 1988;49: 49–55.
30. Ikegami M, Jacobs H, Jobe AH. Surfactant function in the respiratory distress syndrome. *J Pediatr* 1983;102:443–447.
31. Seeger W, Stöhr G, Wolf HRD, et al. Alteration of surfactant function due to protein leakage: Special interaction with fibrin monomer. *J Appl Physiol* 1985;58:326–338.
32. McEachren TM, Keough KMW. Phosphocholin reverses inhibition of pulmonary surfactant adsorption caused by C-reactive protein. *Am J Physiol* 1995;13:492–497.
33. Seeger W, Günther A, Thede C. Differential sensitivity to fibrinogen inhibition of SP-C vs SP-B based surfactants. *Am J Physiol* 1992;5:286–291.
34. Amirkhanian JD, Bruni R, Waring AJ, et al. Inhibition of mixtures of surfactant lipids and synthetic sequences of surfactant proteins SP-B and SP-C. *Biochem Biophys Acta* 1991;1096:355–360.
35. Cockshutt AM, Weitz J, Possmayer F. Pulmonary surfactant-associated protein A enhances the surface activity of lipid extract surfactant and reverses inhibition by blood proteins in vitro. *Biochemistry* 1990;29:8424–8429.
36. Strayer DS, Herting E, Sun B, et al. Antibody to surfactant protein A increases sensitivity of pulmonary surfactant to inactivation by fibrinogen in vivo. *Am J Respir Crit Care Med* 1996;153:1116–1122.
37. Holm BA, Keicher L, Liu M, et al. Inhibition of pulmonary surfactant function by phospholipases. *J Appl Physiol* 1991;71:317–321.
38. Cockshutt AM, Possmayer F. Lysophosphatidylcholine sensitizes lipid extracts of pulmonary surfactant to inhibition by serum proteins. *Biochem Biophys Acta* 1991;1086:63–71.

39. Hall SB, Lu RZ, Venkitaraman R, et al. Inhibition of pulmonary surfactant by oleic acid: Mechanisms and characteristics. *J Appl Physiol* 1992;72: 1708–1716.
40. Findlay RD, Taeusch HW, Walther FJ. Surfactant replacement therapy for meconium aspiration syndrome. *Pediatrics* 1996;97:48–52.
41. Hallman M, Merritt TA, Akino T, et al. Surfactant protein A, phosphatidylcholine, and surfactant inhibitors in epithelial lining fluid. *Am Rev Respir Dis* 1991;144:1376–1384.
42. Haddad IY, Zhu S, Ischiropoulos H, et al. Nitration of surfactant protein A results in decreased ability to aggregate lipids. *Am J Physiol* 1996;14: 281–288.
43. Gilliard N, Heldt GP, Loredo J, et al. Exposure of the hydrophobic components of porcine lung surfactant to oxidate stress alters surface tension properties. *J Clin Invest* 1994;93:2608–2615.
44. Haddad IY, Ischiropoulos H, Holm BA, et al. Mechanisms of peroxynitrite-induced injury to pulmonary surfactants. *Am J Physiol* 1993;265: 555–564.
45. Matalon S, DeMarco V, Haddad IY, et al. Inhaled nitric oxide injures the pulmonary surfactant system of lambs in vivo. *Am J Physiol* 1996; 270:273–280.
46. Ahuja A, Oh N, Chao W, et al. Inhibition of the human neutrophil respiratory burst by native and synthetic surfactant. *Am J Respir Cell Mol Biol* 1996;14:496–503.
47. Ueda T, Ikegami M, Jobe AH. Surfactant subtypes: In vivo function, and effects of serum proteins. *Am J Respir Crit Care Med* 1994;149:1254–1259.
48. Veldhuizen RAW, Marcou J, Yao L-J, et al. Alveolar surfactant aggregate conversion in ventilated normal and injured rabbits. *Am J Physiol* 1996;14: 152–158.
49. Lewis JF, Veldhuizen R, Possmayer F, et al. Altered alveolar surfactant is an early marker of acute lung injury in septic adult sheep. *Am J Respir Crit Care Med* 1994;150:123–130.
50. Veldhuizen RAW, McCaig LA, Akino T, et al. Pulmonary surfactant subfractions in patients with the acute repiratory distress syndrome. *Am J Respir Crit Care Med* 1995;152:1867–1871.
51. Taylor FB Jr, Abrams ME. Effect of surface active lipoprotein on clotting and fibrinolysis, and of fibrinogen on surface tension of surface active lipoprotein. *Am J Med* 1966;40:346–350.
52. Balis JU, Shelley SA, McCue MJ, et al. Mechanisms of damage to the lung surfactant system ultrastructure and quantitation of normal and in vitro inactivated lung surfactant. *Exp Mol Pathol* 1971;14:243–262.
53. Seeger W, Elssner A, Günther A, Krämer H-J, et al. Lung surfactant phospholipids associate with polymerizing fibrin: Loss of surface activity. *Am J Respir Cell Mol Biol* 1993;9:213–220.
54. O'Brodovich HM, Weitz JI, Possmayer F. Effect of fibrinogen degradation products and lung ground substance on surfactant function. *Biol Neonate* 1990;57:325–333.
55. Seeger W, Grube C, Günther A. Proteolytic cleavage of fibrinogen: Amplification of its surfactant inhibitory capacity. *Am J Respir Cell Mol Biol* 1993;9:239–247.
56. Günther A, Bleyl H, Seeger W. Apoprotein-based synthetic surfactants inhibit plasmic cleavage of fibrinogen in vitro. *Am J Physiol* 1993;265: 186–192.

57. Kobayashi T, Nitta K, Ganzuka M, et al. Inactivation of exogenous surfactant by pulmonary edema fluid. *Pediatr Res* 1991;29:353–356.
58. Yukitake K, Brown CL, Schlueteer MA, et al. Surfactant apoprotein A modifies the inhibitory effect of plasma proteins on surfactant activity in vivo. *Pediatr Res* 1995;37:21–25.
59. Pandit PB, Dunn MS, Colucci EA. Surfactant therapy in neonates with respiratory deterioration due to pulmonary hemorrhage. *Pediatrics* 1995;95: 32–36.
60. Nieman GH, Paskanik AM, Fluck RR, et al. Comparison of exogenous surfactant in the treatment of wood smoke inhalation. *Am J Respir Crit Care Med* 1995;152:597–602.
61. Günther A, Siebert C, Schmidt R, et al. Surfactant alterations in severe pneumonia, acute respiratory distress syndrome, and cardiogenic lung edema. *Am J Respir Crit Care Med* 1996;153:176–184.

Section II

Filtration Pressures and Pulmonary Edema

Chapter 9

Interstitial Mechanics and Fluid Flow

Stephen J. Lai-Fook, PhD

Introduction

The pulmonary interstitium, the route by which the microvascular filtrate is cleared from the lung, is not a single homogeneous compartment. The work of Staub and coworkers[1] identifies three interstitial compartments in the lung, which can be categorized on the basis of the surface forces acting on their boundaries: the interstitium around capillaries, the (perivascular) interstitium around large (extra-alveolar) blood vessels and bronchi, and the alveolar airspaces.

The perivascular interstitium is extremely thin under normal conditions, occupying a volume that is only 1% to 3% of the vascular volume. However, with edema formation the interstitium can expand almost 100-fold, equaling the size of the vessel.[2] The focus of this chapter is to describe the flow-resistive properties of this loose connective interstitium that contributes to this remarkable storage capacity.

Interstitial Cuff Growth

The filling of the perivascular interstitium occurs by bulk flow driven by differences in interstitial (hydrostatic) pressure. The rate of filling depends on the interstitial compliance and flow resistance of the interstitium. Implied in this description is the absence of diffusion driven

This research was supported by National Institute of Health Research Grants HL40362 and HL36552.

From: Weir EK, Reeves JT (eds). *Pulmonary Edema*. Armonk, NY: Futura Publishing Company, Inc.; ©1998.

by protein concentration gradients. Recent study results[3,4] indicate that this is only an approximation.

Interstitial Pressure and Compliance

Reviews of the aforementioned literature have recently appeared.[5,6] The fundamental tenet is that interstitial pressure in lung tissue is determined by forces acting on the interstitial boundaries. At the alveolar level, the alveolar air pressure acting on the flat alveolar walls is transmitted directly to the interstitium that surrounds the capillaries. At alveolar corners, interstitial pressure is below the alveolar air pressure because of the pressure drop across the air-liquid interface. Alveolar liquid pressure, measured in nonedematous rabbit lungs,[7] and in edematous dog lungs[8] by the micropuncture-servonulling technique, was slightly above the pleural pressure at all lung volumes. However in these studies alveolar liquid pressure always below the alveolar air pressure, the relevant reference pressure in the intact chest. Alveolar surface tension calculated from the interfacial pressure, the difference between alveolar air pressure and alveolar liquid pressure, showed a reduction in surface tension to ~2 dyne/cm at functional residual capacity with lung deflation, consistent with direct estimates.[9]

Perivascular interstitial pressure is determined by the force interaction between the lung parenchyma surrounding blood vessels and the vessel wall. When interstitial pressure was measured with use of wick catheters inserted in the perivascular interstitium between the main airway and artery at the hilum of isolated dog lungs, it was 2 to 4 cm H_2O below the pleural pressure (zero reference) at functional residual capacity (5 cm H_2O transpulmonary pressure), and it decreased with lung inflation.[10] At constant lung volume, perivascular interstitial pressure decreased with a reduction in vascular pressure. This behavior is similar to that of the surface pressure acting on the vessel wall due to the recoil of the surrounding lung parenchyma,[11] indicating an identity between interstitial fluid pressure and surface pressure.

Measurements in isolated dog lungs have indicated a longitudinal gradient in interstitial pressure between the alveolar liquid space and the perivenous interstitium at the lung hilum.[8,12] Alveolar liquid pressure is initially 5 cm H_2O above the perivenous interstitial pressure at the lung hilum. This fluid pressure gradient is reduced to zero as interstitial pressure increases with water accumulation.

In several studies, direct measurements of alveolar liquid pressure[13] and perivascular interstitial pressure[14] in isolated lung showed that interstitial pressure is fairly uniform at different heights in the lung at constant lung volume. Interstitial pressure is determined by parenchymal forces around large vessels, and alveolar liquid pressure is determined by alveolar surface forces. These forces are uniform with height in uniformly expanded lungs. The force due to gravity is compensated for by viscous forces due to the downward flow of interstitial liquid.

The increase in interstitial pressure with water accumulation is a measure of interstitial compliance defined as the change in interstitial volume (ΔVi) divided by the change in interstitial pressure (ΔPi). Because of the heterogeneity of pulmonary interstitium, definitive measurements of interstitial compliance have proved elusive.[5,6] A theoretical approach to the problem considered the perivascular interstitium surrounding blood vessels as a thin layer surrounded by two elastic structures: the lung parenchyma and the vessel wall.[19] Since these two structures are mechanically in series, interstitial compliance is the sum of the parenchymal and vessel wall compliances. From elasticity theory, parenchymal specific compliance ($\Delta D/D$)/ΔPi, the fractional change in diameter (D) divided by ΔPi, is $1/2G$ where G is the shear modulus of the parenchyma.[11] Parenchymal compliance is the major determinant of interstitial compliance because it is much larger than the vessel wall compliance. For small changes in cuff diameter, interstitial compliance in terms of ΔVi as a fraction of vascular volume (Vv) is:

$$(\Delta Vi/Vv)/\Delta Pi = (1/G) \qquad [1]$$

Using a G of $0.7 \times$ Ptp (transpulmonary pressure), measured by indentation tests in a variety of species,[16] interstitial compliance is reduced by a factor of 3 from 0.29 cm H_2O^{-1} at 5 cm H_2O Ptp to 0.10 cm H_2O^{-1} at 15 cm H_2O Ptp. This trend was verified by interstitial pressure measured in the hilar periarterial interstitium versus water accumulation in isolated dog lobes.[15] Compliance estimated from the maximum cuff area-to-vessel area ratio in liquid-inflated rabbit lungs showed a reduction from 0.25 cm H_2O^{-1} at 5 cm H_2O Ptp to 0.05 cm H_2O^{-1} at 15 cm H_2O Ptp.[17] Similar studies indicate that interstitial compliance varies among the dog, sheep, and rabbit lung, with measured values of 0.25, 0.13, and 0.045, respectively, at Ptp values of 14 to 19 cm H_2O (Table 1). These differences might be due to the nonlinear behavior of the lung parenchyma undergoing large deformations.[17]

From geometry, interstitial compliance (Ci) in terms of fractional change in interstitial volume is:

$$Ci = (\Delta Vi/Vi)/\Delta Pi = (1/G)/(2t/r) \qquad [2]$$

Here Vi/Vv is 2t/r, the interstitial cuff thickness-to-vessel radius ratio.

Table 1

Cuff Growth Parameters for Dog, Sheep, and Rabbit Lungs Inflated With 3 g/dL albumin solution

Vessel Diameter (mm)	Species[+]	Maximum (Ac/Av)	Compliance[∧] (cm H_2O^{-1})	Time constant[#] (min)	Resistance* (cm $H_2O \cdot$ min)
	Rabbit	0.91±0.47 (185)	0.06	30	2200
≤ 0.5	Sheep	2.6±1.4 (79)	0.14	6	800
	Dog	3.6±1.4 (116)	0.26	1.5	80
	Rabbit	0.45±0.21 (137)	0.03	30	4600
> 0.5	Sheep	2.3±1.2 (258)	0.12	12	1200
	Dog	3.4±1.5 (150)	0.24	3	160

[+]Inflation pressures were 15, 19, and 14 cm H_2O in rabbit, sheep, and dog lungs, respectively. [#]Time constant based on first-order kinetics, time at 0.63 of maximum Ac/Av. *Initial values (at t=0) used in the nonlinear solutions to model B that fit the data. Ac/Av: cuff-to-vessel area ratio. [∧]Maximum Ac/Av divided by inflation pressure.
Data from References 17–19.

Interstitial Resistance

Interstitial flow is assumed to obey Darcy's law for a permeable material. Darcy's law states that the hydrostatic pressure gradient, the driving pressure (ΔP) per unit length (L), is proportional to the fluid velocity:

$$\Delta P/L = \nu Q/(KA) \qquad [3]$$

Velocity is flow (Q) divided by interstitial cross-sectional area (A); ν is fluid viscosity; and K is the interstitial permeability constant. Interstitial resistance, $\nu L/(KA)$ (driving pressure divided by flow [$\Delta P/Q$]), varies inversely with cross-sectional area. This results in nonlinear equations defining the pressure-flow relationships.

Interstitial resistance was estimated from modeling studies of the growth of perivascular interstitial fluid cuffs in isolated dog, sheep, and rabbit lungs.[17-20] Isolated degassed lungs were inflated with liquid to a fixed inflation pressure and frozen in liquid N_2 at different times after inflation. Cuff and vessel cross-sectional areas were measured. The cuff-to-vessel area ratio (Ac/Av) increased to a maximum value that was species-dependent. The rate of cuff growth was measured by the time constant at 63% maximum Ac/Av. To interpret the experimental data, Conhaim and coworkers[17-20] used electrical analog models with in-series resistances and shunt compliances. Interstitial compliance was given by the maximum Ac/Av divided by ΔPi at equilibrium, the inflation pressure. From solutions of the pressure-flow equations that fit the data, estimated interstitial resistance was 60 cm $H_2O \cdot min \cdot cm^{-2}$.

Differences in Cuff Growth Among Dog, Sheep, and Rabbit Lungs

The growth rate of perivascular cuffs in liquid-filled lungs varied considerably among the dog, sheep, and rabbit lungs. Table 1 summarizes maximum Ac/Av, interstitial compliance, time constant for cuff growth, and the calculated interstitial resistance among the three species at comparable inflation pressures, 14 cm H_2O to 19 cm H_2O.[17–19] In general, cuff growth was slower and cuff size smaller in the rabbit than in the dog; the responses in the sheep were intermediate. Maximum Ac/Av was 3 to 7 times smaller in the rabbit than in the dog, indicating a much smaller perivascular interstitial capacity in the rabbit lung. The smaller maximum Ac/Av in the rabbit pointed to a proportional decrease in interstitial compliance compared to the dog. The time constant for cuff growth in the rabbit was 10- to 20-fold greater than in the dog, indicating a much slower rate of cuff growth. The longer time constant and smaller interstitial compliance indicated a much larger (30-fold) interstitial resistance in rabbit lung compared to the dog lung.

Effect of Lung Inflation Pressure on Cuff Growth Reponse

To determine whether the high inflation pressure used in the experiments was responsible for differences in cuff growth between rabbit and dog lungs, cuff growth was compared in liquid-filled rabbit lungs at 5 cm H_2O and 15 cm H_2O inflation pressure.[17,20] The time constant for cuff growth was twofold greater at the lower inflation pressure. Interstitial compliance based on maximum cuff size was smaller at the higher inflation pressure, reflecting the increased shear modulus of lung parenchyma at higher transpulmonary pressures.

Direct Measurements of Interstitial Resistance

The foregoing analysis of cuff growth was an indirect way to arrive at interstitial resistance. Accordingly, the following experiment was developed to measure interstitial resistance directly.[21] The airways and blood vessels of degassed rabbit lungs were filled with silicon rubber (Microfil). After the rubber set, the caudal lobes were cut into 1 cm thick slabs. Two compartments were bonded to the sides of a slab to enclose a vessel 2 mm to 3 mm in diameter. The compartments were filled with normal saline and the driving pressure varied across the interstitium to measure its pressure-flow behavior.

To determine interstitial resistance and interstitial thickness, driving pressure was kept constant at 5 cm H_2O and the mean interstitial pressure was varied. Flow decreased as mean interstitial pressure was reduced and reached a small but finite limiting value at a mean interstitial pressure of -7 cm H_2O. The pressure-flow behavior was analyzed by considering flow through a permeable material surrounded by elastic walls. Interstitial resistance estimated from the analysis of the pressure-flow curves averaged 78 ± 60 (SD) cm $H_2O \cdot min \cdot cm^{-2}$, comparable to that estimated from the analysis of cuff growth, but two to three orders of magnitude smaller than that estimated for the subcutaneous interstitium.[22]

This interstitial model was used to study the effect of albumin and electric charge on interstitial permeability. For these experiments, the flow of a solution, such as albumin, relative to that of saline at a constant driving pressure was measured. This allowed for the comparison of experiments in which the flow magnitude might vary greatly. For each lung slab A, L, and ΔP were held constant so that flow was proportional to permeability divided by fluid viscosity: $Q \propto K/v$. If permeability were constant, flow of any solution (eg, albumin) relative to that of saline must be equal to the inverse ratio of their viscosities:

$$Q_a/Q_s = v_s/v_a \qquad [4]$$

where subscripts a and s refer to albumin and saline, respectively.

Effect of Albumin Concentration

The effects of albumin concentration on the flow through the pulmonary interstitium were studied.[23] The flow of saline, followed by albumin solutions of either 3 g/dL, 5.5 g/dL, 8 g/dL, or 15 g/dL concentration was measured. The driving pressure was constant at 15 cm H_2O to 25 cm H_2O. This was followed by the flow of hyaluronidase, then followed by the flow of albumin. If the flow was entirely viscosity dependent, the flow ratio should have decreased with an increase in albumin concentration as the viscosity ratio was reduced. However, the measured albumin-to-saline flow ratio increased with albumin concentration, reaching a value of 1.5 at a concentration of 15 g/dL (Table 2), which indicates an increase in interstitial permeability. This might be due to a decrease in the volume of albumin excluded by in-

Table 2

Effect of Albumin, Cationic Protamine Sulfate,
Cationic Dextran, and Anionic Dextran
on Interstitial Conductivity in Hydrated Interstitium

	Flow Ratios*	Concentration (g/dL)	Viscosity Ratio#
Albumin			
Saline	1.5±0.36 (6)^	15	0.5
Dextran 72K			
Saline	0.64±0.30 (5)	5	0.44
Cationic Protamine			
Saline	2.3±0.92 (7)^	0.008	1
Cationic Dextran			
Saline	3.0±1.2 (6)^	0.1	0.95
Anionic Dextran			
Saline	0.72±0.28 (13)+	0.1	0.95
Hyaluronidase			
Saline	10±9.8 (33)^	0.02	1

*mean±SD. (n): No. of measurements. Driving pressure was 10, 15, 20, or 25 cm H_2O.
^Significant greater than viscosity ratio ($P<0.05$). +Significant less than viscosity ratio.
#Saline-to-solution viscosity ratio. Data from References 23 and 28.

terstitial molecules with the increase in albumin concentration.[24] The increased albumin-to-saline flow ratio was reduced after treatment by hyaluronidase, suggesting that the osmotic interaction between hyaluronan and albumin was partly responsible for the reduced albumin excluded volume.

Effect of Hyaluronidase

Because it was uncertain exactly where flow occurred through the lung slab, the flow of hyaluronidase (0.02 g/dL) was studied in every experiment. Hyaluronidase increased the flow on an average of 10-fold in studies with albumin and electrically charged solutions (Table 2). This is in agreement with the longstanding result found by Day.[25] Accordingly, hyaluronan, which accounts for only 0.01% of the interstitial weight,[26] was responsible for 90% of the interstitial resistance. The increased flow of hyaluronidase indicated that the flow was primarily through the interstitium and not through the vessel wall that does not respond to hyaluronidase.[27]

Effect of Electric Charge

For examination of the effect of electric charge on permeability of pulmonary interstitium (Table 2), the flow of polycationic protamine sulfate (0.08 mg/mL), cationic dextran (0.1 g/dL and 1.5 g/dL), and anionic dextran (0.1 g/dL and 1.5 g/dL) was measured.[28] All solutions were adjusted to a pH of 7.4. Driving pressure was constant between 10 cm H_2O and 25 cm H_2O. The flow of polycationic protamine and dextran increased two- to threefold relative to that of saline. By contrast, the flow of anionic dextan decreased relative to that of neutral dextran. Thus the pulmonary interstitium acts as a negatively charged barrier which by virtue of its molecular attraction for positively charged molecules enhances flow. This is consistent with the conclusions of Parker and coworkers.[29] To determine if hyaluronan, with its negatively charged sulfated groups, was responsible for the changes in resistance, the flow of the positively and negatively charged solutions after treatment with hyaluronidase was remeasured. The flows of polycationic protamine and cationic dextran were much reduced after hyaluonidase, suggesting a major role for hyaluronan in enhancing the flow of the positively charged solutions. Hyaluronidase, however, had no effect on the reduced flow of anionic dextran, indicating that other constituents were responsible for the reduced flow of anionic dextran.

Effect of Hydration

The increased permeability measured with albumin and positively charged solutions might have been a function of the hydration. Thus the studies were repeated at different degrees of hydration brought about by varying interstitial pressure.[30] For these experiments a constant driving pressure of 5 cm H_2O was used, and the mean interstitial pressure varied. Based on the shear modulus of silicon rubber (140 cm H_2O) and an initial cuff thickness-to-vessel radius ratio of 0.01, interstitial volume expansion was 40% per cm H_2O increase in mean interstitial pressure (Equation 2). Figure 1 shows that the flow of albumin relative to that of Ringer's solution increased with mean interstitial pressure attaining a value of 1.6 to 2 at a mean interstitial pressure of 15 cm H_2O. This increased permeability was absent for nonedematous conditions at interstitial pressures near to zero (ambient). A similar effect of hydration was observed with hyalurondase (Figure 1) and with positively charged protamine sulfate.[31] Thus, the increased permeability might be the result of an interaction between albumin and hyaluronan that is exposed with hydration. The functional significance of these

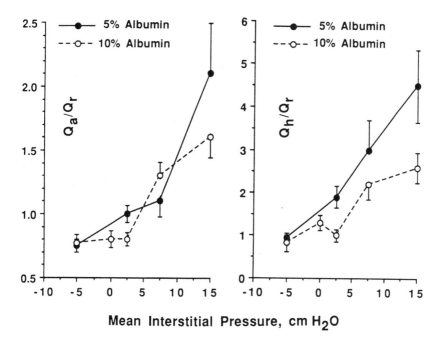

Mean Interstitial Pressure, cm H₂O

Figure 1. Effect of hydration on interstitial flow response to albumin and hyaluronidase. Left: Albumin-to-Ringer's solution flow ratio (Q_a/Q_r) versus mean interstitial pressure (Pm) with 5% and 10% albumin concentrations. Right: Hyaluronidase-to-Ringer's solution flow ratio (Q_h/Q_r) versus Pm. Hyaluronidase flow was measured after the flow of 5% and 10% albumin solutions. Hydration increased by 40% per cm H₂O increase in Pm. Reproduced from Reference 30.

findings is that during pulmonary edema formation caused by endothelial damage, interstitial conductivity increases to compensate for the reduced protein osmotic pressure gradients across the microvascular barrier.

Interstitial Pressure Response in Liquid-Filled Lungs

The response in cuff growth in lungs inflated with 3 g/dL albumin solution to 15 cm H₂O inflation pressure was similar to the interstitial pressure response measured at the lung hilum by micropuncture.[17] Thus, the interstitial pressure response could be used as a measure of the cuff growth response. This represented an enormous saving in effort. The response of hilar interstitial pressure to inflation was studied with different solutions: 3 g/dL albumin, 0.08 mg/mL polycationic protamine sulfate, albumin plus protamine, lactated Ringer's, and 1.5 g/dL anionic dextran sulfate.[17] The results indicated that albumin has the quickest response, followed by polycationic protamine, Ringer's solution, and anionic dextran sulfate (Figure 2). The flow of albumin and protamine relative to that of Ringer's solution verified the changes in permeability observed in the steady flow experiments. The flow of anionic dextran was reduced relative to that of saline, but only to the extent predicted from the increased viscosity.

Restriction of Protein by Pulmonary Interstitium

In the foregoing studies, an implicit assumption in the use of Darcy's law for the pressure-flow behavior of a permeable material was that the pulmonary interstitium does not restrict the passage of plasma proteins. The degree to which this is true was studied in experiments in which the flow of 2 g/dL albumin dyed with Evan's blue was measured across a 1 cm length of pulmonary interstitium.[4] The driving pressure was 5 cm H_2O and the mean interstitial pressure was varied. After 6 hours, the measured downstream-to-upstream albumin concentration ratio was 0.27 at a mean interstitial pressure of 5 cm H_2O and increased to 0.57 at a mean interstitial pressure of 25 cm H_2O. Thus, the interstitial concentration gradient was reduced from 1.7 g/dL/cm to 1.5 g/dL/cm as hydration increased from 1.5-fold to fivefold. These results indicated changes in albumin concentration of 0.017 g/dL over a 100 μm length of interstitium, the typical pathlength from filtration sites to lymphatic stomata in the peripheral lung tissue.[2] This estimate supports the assumption that lung lymph protein concentration is a reasonable estimate of microvascular filtrate.[2] However, during the formation of interstial cuffs where pathlengths might be on the order of several centimeters, significant spatial differences in protein concentration might be detectable. For example, studies in edematous lamb lungs have indicated a larger protein concentration in the hilar periarterial interstitium than in the perivenous interstitium.[3] Based on the measured gradients in albumin concentration, this can be explained by a microvascular filtrate from arterial blood vessels that flowed from periarterial sites to perivenular sites.

Summary

The starting point of the aforementioned studies was the elastic interaction between the lung parenchyma and blood vessels. This provided a prediction of perivascular interstitial pressure and compliance

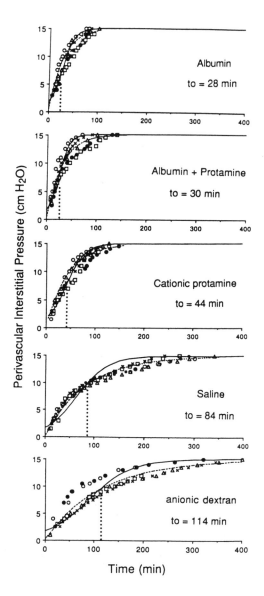

Figure 2. Perivascular (perivenous) interstitial pressure measured by micropuncture versus time in rabbit lungs inflated with 3 g/dL albumin solution, 0.008 g/dL polycationic protamine sulfate, albumin plus protamine, saline, and 1.5 g/dL anionic dextran solution. Full and dashed lines are solutions to nonlinear and linear one-compartment electric analogs, respectively. Time constants (to) were obtained from the linear system response. Reproduced from Reference 17.

that motivated the direct measurement of interstitial pressure by wick catheters and micropuncture. The micropuncture technique also allowed the direct measurements of alveolar liquid pressure. The studies of interstitial cuff growth in liquid-filled lungs was an independent series of studies done in parallel with the interstitial pressure studies. The measurements of cuff growth provided an estimate of interstitial resistance through mathematical modeling with electrical analogs. These indirect estimates of interstitial resistance motivated the direct measurement of interstitial resistance using steady flow through interstitial segments of rubber-filled lungs. The latter method was used to determine the effects of albumin, electrically charged solutions, and hyaluronidase on interstitial conductivity. The increased interstitial permeability to the flow of albumin and positively charged solutions was dependent on the presence of hyaluronan and edema. In nonedematous interstitium, flow was viscosity dependent. Only the bulk flow of interstitial fluid caused by fluid pressure gradients was considered. The effects of diffusion, which is likely to be more important under normal conditions, under which the effects of osmosis dominate the effects of bulk flow, must be studied.

References

1. Staub NC, Nagano H, Pearce ML. Pulmonary edema in dogs, especially the sequence of fluid accumulation in lungs. *J Appl Physiol* 1967;22:227–240.
2. Staub NC. Pulmonary edema. *Physiol Rev* 1974;54:678–811.
3. Raj JU, Anderson J. Regional differences in interstitial fluid albumin concentration in edematous lamb lungs. *J Appl Physiol* 1992;72:699–705.
4. Saini R, Brown LV, Lai-Fook SJ. Effect of hydration on albumin concentration gradient in pulmonary interstitium. (Abstract) *FASEB J* 1996;10:A351.
5. Lai-Fook SJ. Mechanical factors in lung liquid distribution. *Ann Rev Physiol* 1993;55:155–179.
6. Taylor AE, Parker JC. Pulmonary interstitial spaces and lymphatics. In: *Handbook of Physiology. The Respiratory System. Circulation and Nonrespiratory Functions. Section 3*. Bethesda: American Physiological Society. 1985; 167–230.
7. Ganesan S, Lai-Fook SJ, Schurch S. Alveolar liquid pressures in nonedematous and kerosene-washed rabbit lung by micropuncture. *Respir Physiol* 1989;78:281–296.
8. Lai-Fook SJ, Beck KC. Alveolar liquid pressure measured by micropipets in isolated dog lung. *J Appl Physiol* 1982;53:737–743.
9. Schurch S, Goerke J, Clements JA. Direct determination of surface tension in the lung. *Proc Natl Acad Sci U S A* 1976;73:4698–4702.
10. Goshy M, Lai-Fook SJ, Hyatt RE. Perivascular pressure measurements by the wick catheter technique in isolated dog lobes. *J Appl Physiol* 1979;46:1003–1010.
11. Lai-Fook SJ. A continuum mechanics analysis of pulmonary vascular interdependence in isolated dog lobes. *J Appl Physiol* 1979;46:419–429.

12. Lai-Fook SJ. Perivascular interstitial fluid pressure measured by micropipets in isolated dog lung. *J Appl Physiol* 1982;52:9–15.
13. Beck KC, Lai-Fook SJ. Effect of height on alveolar liquid pressure in isolated edematous dog lung. *J Appl Physiol* 1983;54:619–622.
14. Lai-Fook SJ, Kaplowitz MR. Perivascular interstitial pressure versus height in isolated saline filled sheep lungs. (Abstract) *Microvasc Res* 1984; 27:250.
15. Lai-Fook SJ, Toporoff B. Pressure-volume behavior of perivascular interstitium measured directly in isolated dog lung. *J Appl Physiol* 1980;48: 939–946.
16. Hajji MA, Wilson TA, Lai-Fook, SJ. Improved measurements of the shear modulus and pleural membrane tension of the lung. *J Appl Physiol* 1979;47: 175–181.
17. Liang J, Lai-Fook SJ. Effect of inflation on interstitial cuff and pressure in liquid-filled rabbit lung. *Respir Physiol* 1996;106:293–305.
18. Conhaim RL, Lai-Fook SJ, Staub NC. Sequence of perivascular liquid accumulation in liquid-inflated dog lung lobes. *J Appl Physiol* 1986;60: 513–520.
19. Conhaim RL, Lai-Fook SJ, Eaton A. Sequence of perivascular liquid accumulation in liquid inflated sheep lung lobes. *J Appl Physiol* 1989;66: 2659–2666.
20. Li J, Lai-Fook SJ, Conhaim RL. Effect of hyaluronidase on the growth of perivascular interstitial cuffs in liquid-filled rabbit lungs. *J Appl Physiol* 1992;72:1261–1269.
21. Lai-Fook SJ. Pressure-flow behavior of pulmonary interstitium. *J Appl Physiol* 1988;64:2372–2380.
22. Guyton AC, Scheel K, Murphree D. Interstitial fluid pressure. III. Its effect on resistance to interstitial tissue motility. *Circ Res* 1966;19:412–419.
23. Lai-Fook SJ, Rochester NL, Brown LV. Effects of albumin, dextran, and hyaluronidase on pulmonary interstitial conductivity. *J Appl Physiol* 1989; 67:606–613.
24. Wiederhielm CA, Black LL. Osmotic interaction of plasma proteins with interstitial macromolecules. *Am J Physiol* 1976;231:638–641.
25. Day TD. The permeability of interstitial connective tissue and the nature of the interfibrillary substance. *J Physiol (Lond)* 1952;117:1–8.
26. Horwitz AL, Crystal RG. Content and synthesis of glycosaminoglycans in the developing lung. *J Clin Invest* 1975;56:1312–1318.
27. Sunnergren KP, Fairman RP, DeBlois GG, et al. Effects of protamine, heparinase, and hyaluronidase on endothelial permeability and surface charge. *J Appl Physiol* 1987;63:1987–1992.
28. Lai-Fook SJ, Brown LV. Effect of electric charge on hydraulic conductivity of pulmonary interstitium. *J Appl Physiol* 1991;70:1928–1932.
29. Parker JC, Gilchrist S, Cartledge JT. Plasma-lymph exchange and interstitial distribution volume of charged molecules in the lung. *J Appl Physiol* 1980;59:1128–1136.
30. Tajadinni A, Brown LV, Lai-Fook SJ. Effect of hydration on lung interstitial permeability response to albumin and hyaluronidase. *J Appl Physiol* 1994;76:578–583.
31. Saini R, Brown LV, Lai-Fook SJ. Effect of interstitial pressure on lung interstitial permeability response to the flow of polycationic protamine sulfate. (Abstract) *FASEB J* 1994;8:A415.

Chapter 10

The Interstitial and Microvascular Unit of the Lung:
From the Neonate to the Adult

Giuseppe Miserocchi, MD

Introduction

During fetal life, potential airspaces are filled with liquid that is actively secreted.[1] After birth the lung quickly switches from a water-filled to an air-filled organ to assure alveolar gas exchange. Three major events occur at birth that have a direct or indirect impact on lung fluid balance: (1) the secretion of luminal liquid decreases towards the end of gestation[2,3] and right at birth, alveolar cells start absorbing luminal fluid, a process that is triggered by adrenaline release,[4] (2) with onset of breathing there is a sudden increase in pulmonary vascular perfusion, and (3) lung recoil pressure increases due to aeration of alveoli and to expansion of the chest wall. From the standpoint of water exchange, clearly, the whole process of maturation of lung fluid balance can be regarded as an example of recovery from alveolar and interstitial lung edema. Although it seems well established that most of alveolar fluid is drained in the first postnatal hours,[5,6] it is probable that a much longer time is required for lung fluid balance to attain the adult condition that is characterized by the very dehydrated state of the interstitial matrix.[7] A key variable to model the development of lung fluid balance is pulmonary interstitial pressure (P_{ip}), namely the hydraulic pressure of the free liquid phase that is present within the lung interstitium. A free liquid phase is normally present in all interstitial spaces. The hydraulic pressure of the free liquid phase reflects on one side the hydration state of the interstitium and on the other side, the tissue

From: Weir EK, Reeves JT (eds). *Pulmonary Edema*. Armonk, NY: Futura Publishing Company, Inc.; ©1998.

forces developing within the tissue itself. In the case of the lung, the latter forces relate to the parenchymal stresses that increase when lung volume increases due to the elastic component of the lung tissue matrix. P_{ip} is expected to become more positive when the interstitium is volume loaded, as in the case of luminal fluid reabsorption after birth. In fact, data in adult animals show that P_{ip} increases when lung interstitial edema develops.[8] However, with the onset of respiration, lung volume increases and this represents a condition that causes P_{ip} to decrease.[9] Therefore, the increase in interstitial volume and the increase in lung volume, both occurring in the postnatal hours, result in opposite effects on P_{ip}; in turn this should influence fluid balance, as P_{ip} is an important variable that appears in the well-known Starling equation, which describes water fluxes among compartments. The measurement of P_{ip}, and in general, the study of the lung microvascular unit, always posed a big challenge to scientists on experimental grounds due to the delicacy of the tissue that requires minimally invasive techniques. A major contribution was made by the development of the so-called "pleural window" technique, which allowed micropuncture of the lung interstitium and microvessels through the intact pleural space, thus preserving lung mechanics. The surgical procedure involves resection of the intercostal muscles and of the endothoracic fascia, leaving the parietal pleura intact.[7] The major advantage offered by the technique is that it is possible to study the lung while preserving the physiological pleural space mechanics and lung perfusion. The technique has, in fact, allowed us to study the pleuro-pulmonary compartments and to quantify pressure gradients and fluid and solute fluxes. Figure 1 shows, as an example, three microphotographs taken through the pleural window. The bottom and center panels refer to a mature adult lung and to a term newborn lung, respectively. The top image, taken from a preterm animal, shows the generation of immature airways of a saccular type, surrounded by a rather homogeneous atelectatic lung tissue. The experimental data base gathered in rabbits by micropuncturing intact in situ lungs through the "pleural window technique" is used in this chapter to describe the pattern of fluid exchanges in the pleuro-pulmonary compartments during development from birth to adulthood. To this aim, it is also useful to recall how the lung interstitial matrix behaves when the lung interstitium is volume loaded: this occurs, indeed, in the early postnatal life due to luminal liquid reabsorption and may occur in the adult when microvascular filtration increases and pulmonary edema develops.

Figure 1. Microphotographs of pleural surface as seen through the pleural window. Top: immature airways surrounded by atelectatic lung region in preterm rabbit. Center: aerated lung in newborn rabbit. Bottom: adult lung.

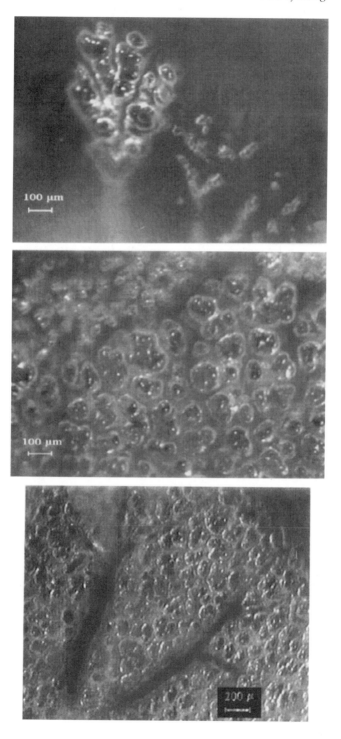

The Pulmonary Interstitial Compartment

The lungs are a compartment in series between the right and the left ventricle and their function is to act as a gas exchanger between alveolar air and blood. In the adult lung, diffusion processes are under very efficient physiological conditions, as the thickness of the alveolo-capillary membrane is only 0.5 μm and the overall alveolar surface area is as large as 70 m² in humans. The thinness of the alveolo-capillary membrane is assured by a minimum volume of interstitial tissue. The latter is limited by the capillary endothelial barrier, the visceral pleura, and the alveolar epithelial layer. Pulmonary interstitial tissue contains a macromolecular matrix and a free liquid phase; the matrix structure includes several molecules that constitute the fiber scaffold of the lung.[10] The matrix accomplishes two main functions: on the one hand, it provides support to alveolar cells and is responsible for the elastic recoil properties of the lung, on the other, its biochemical structure and mechanical properties contribute to the maintenance of a minimal interstitial volume of water. Recoil properties are mostly provided by elastin and by collagen that amounts to approximately 15% to 20% of the dry weight of the lung. Other important macromolecules such as proteoglycans and hyaluronan fill the fibrous network and, being highly hydrophilic, influence the water content of the interstitium.[11,12] Proteoglycans represent a minor component of dry lung weight but represent important molecules that provide attachments with other fibril components of the matrix and between cells. Proteoglycans have a core protein to which one or more glycosaminoglycan chains are attached by covalent bonds. Glycosaminoglycans are the main determinants of the physical properties of proteoglycans in that they allow them to resist compressive forces and to maintain the hydration state of the tissue. Proteoglycans also constitute a selective sieve of various size and charge density for molecules, in particular plasma proteins, escaping from the microvascular bed. Finally, heparan sulfate-containing proteoglycans are important components of basal membranes. Another important matrix molecule is hyaluronan, a glycosaminoglycan with gel-like properties that acts as an organizer of proteoglycans aggregates.[11,12] Interstitial water is either bound to hydrophilic molecules or is present as a free liquid phase dispersed in the spaces left free by the macromolecules; this latter form is in dynamic equilibrium with the microvascular district.

Interstitial spaces are drained by an extended network of lymphatics. The casting of lung lymphatics by the injection of resin either through the vascular system or through the airways (when damage of the epithelial wall is present)[13] made it possible to establish that lymphatics reach the alveolar septa. Initial lymphatics, at the boundary where lymphatics begin in the interstitial spaces, appear as thin, leaf-like, saccular forms.

The Law Governing Fluid Exchanges

A useful description of the microvascular fluid exchanges is given by the so-called Starling law:

$$J_v = K_f \cdot [(P_1 - P_2) - \sigma(\pi_1 - \pi_2)]$$

where J_v, the water flux between two compartments labeled 1 and 2, results from the balance of hydraulic (P) and colloid osmotic (π) pressures in the two compartments. K_f is the filtration coefficient defined as $K_f = L_p \cdot S$, where L_p is the hydraulic permeability coefficient and S is the surface available for fluid exchanges. σ, termed total protein reflection coefficient, varies between 0 and 1. For $\sigma = 1$, plasma proteins are too large to permeate the capillary endothelium, while for $\sigma = 0$ there is no restriction to protein movement across the capillary endothelium. For $0 < \sigma < 1$, a condition of partial restriction to plasma protein movement occurs. On experimental grounds it appears rather difficult to measure J_v directly, so that researchers aim to measure the variables and coefficients that appear in the above equation for the system under study. Alveoli, lung interstitium, and microvessels are three compartments in series, therefore, P_{ip} appears in the above equation defining flows between any two of the above compartments.

Fluid Balance in the Pleuro-Pulmonary Compartments in the Adult

The situation in the adult mammal is shown first, as it represents a useful reference framework.[14] No experimental data are available in humans, however physiological and pathophysiological considerations lead one to believe that the model is valid at least in mammals up to 30 kg.[15]

Figure 2 presents a summary of the balance of pressures in the pleuro-pulmonary compartments in rabbits at approximately 50% lung height (right atrium level). Pulmonary capillary pressure was obtained from experimental measurement of the microvascular pressure profile in intact in situ lungs.[16,17] Most of the information provided in Figure 2 is rather new and at variance with other data obtained in different experimental conditions. In fact, most of the previous micropuncture data were gathered in isolated perfused lungs expanded at positive alveolar pressure. In this condition the lungs tend to spontaneously develop

ADULT LUNG

NET PRESSURE GRADIENTS , cmH₂O

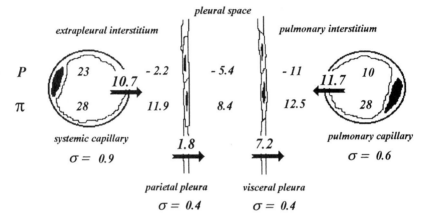

Figure 2. Starling balance of pressures in the pleuro-pulmonary compartments. Sigma for mesothelia and for systemic and pulmonary capillaries were taken from Reference 15. Adapted from Reference 15.

edema.[18] Furthermore, vascular pressures are set by the experimenter and, in particular, left atrial pressure is kept relatively high (higher than alveolar pressure) to allow capillary perfusion. The major difference between the two experimental preparations concerns P_{ip}: in fact, when the lung is expanded by positive alveolar pressure a compressive stress is applied to lung interstitium, consequently rendering P_{ip} more positive. On the contrary, when lungs are expanded by a subatmospheric pleural pressure (with zero alveolar pressure) a tensile stress is applied to lung interstitium and this renders P_{ip} subatmospheric. Therefore, use of P_{ip} data gathered with positive alveolar pressure to define the microvascular Starling pressure balance in the lung in physiological conditions (namely, with negative pleural pressure and zero alveolar pressure) is not appropriate. As it can be seen, net filtration occurs from pulmonary capillaries into lung interstitium; note that the same would occur even at venular level due to the rather subatmospheric pulmonary interstitial pressure. Since the pulmonary microvasculature provides net filtration into the surrounding lung parenchyma, a negative pulmonary interstitial pressure may only depend on a powerful draining action of interstitial lymphatics. The ability of the lymphatic system to balance net transmicrovascular fluid filtration under steady state conditions has been demonstrated for other interstitial compartments, as well; in

ADULT LUNG

FLUID TURNOVER , flows in mL/(kg·h)

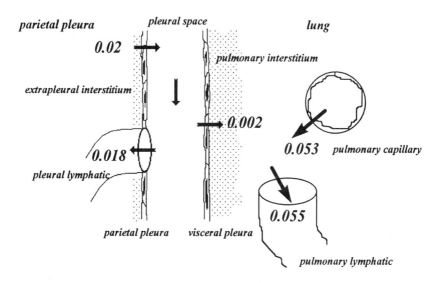

Figure 3. Estimated fluid fluxes among the pleuro-pulmonary compartments. Adapted from Reference 14.

fact, interstitial fluid reabsorption into capillaries may only occur as a transient phenomenon being self-limited by the increase in interstitial colloid osmotic pressure.[19,20] Note also in Figure 2 that a pressure gradient exists to drive fluid from pleural space into lung interstitium. Figure 3 shows the estimated fluid fluxes in the pleuro-pulmonary compartment. Note that the visceral transpleural flow is negligible due to the low hydraulic conductance of the visceral pleura, and that the major route for pleural liquid drainage is via lymphatics of the parietal pleura.[15,21,22] No pleural fluid can drain into pulmonary capillaries as hypothesized in 1927[23] and maintained until the 1980s.

Development of Fluid Balance in the Pleuro-Pulmonary Compartment

After birth, luminal fluid is absorbed into the lung interstitium from where it can be drained down the following pathways: (1) into pulmonary microcirculation, (2) via pulmonary lymphatics, and (3) in part through the visceral pleura. As result of this fluid clearance, total lung water decreases as a function of time, as shown by the decrease in wet-to-dry weight ratio (W/D) of the lung (Figure 4) from ≈ 7.5 in term (31 days of gestation) vaginally delivered rabbits at birth, to the physiological value of ≈ 5 found in the adult. In preterm animals the W/D ratios are significantly higher at any postnatal age. Based on the available information, this chapter attempts to estimate the quantitative relative roles of the three draining pathways of lung water removal as a function of time. Figure 5 shows that plasma and pleural liquid protein concentrations sharply decrease in the early postnatal phase; the former subsequently rises to attain the adult value, while the latter keeps decreasing to attain the final adult value of ≈ 1.5 g/dL. Figure 6 shows the time course of end-expiratory P_{ip} in the postnatal life.[24,25] In term animals (continuous line) P_{ip} increases from zero up to approximately 5 cm H_2O: in this phase more fluid is transferred from alveoli into the interstitium than is drained out of the interstitium.[5] Thereafter, P_{ip} decreases, indicating that interstitial fluid drainage is becoming predominant, until a steady state condition is reached around 60 days of life, at

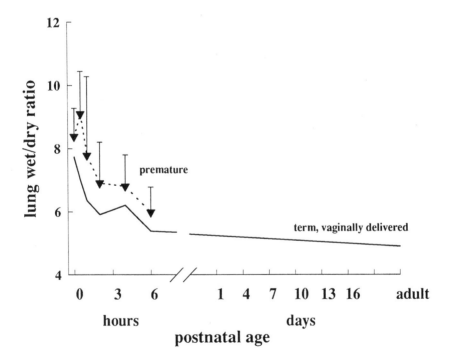

Figure 4. Wet/dry weight ratio of the lungs from birth to adulthood.

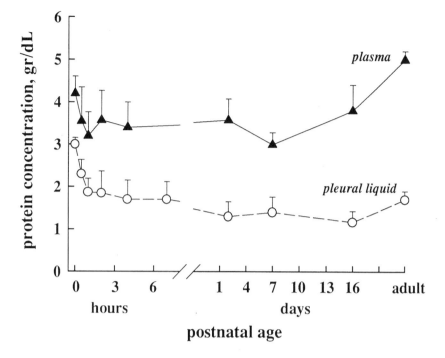

Figure 5. Plasma and pleural liquid protein concentration as a function of post-natal age.

which age P_{ip} has become equal to that found in the adult ≈ -10 cm H_2O). From day 1, the time course of P_{ip}, which is also valid for term cesarean delivered animals, can be described by the function: P_{ip} (cm H_2O) = 7.95 $e^{-0.049t} - 10$, where t is expressed as days of postnatal life. The knowledge of P_{ip} is a good hint to estimate, based on some assumptions, the Starling pressure balance acting across the microvascular barrier that is shown in Figure 7. Assumptions tend to underestimate the gradient, namely: (1) a pulmonary capillary pressure equal to that of the adult, (2) a protein reflection coefficient equal to 1, and (3) an interstitial colloid osmotic pressure corresponding to the lowest estimate of protein concentration in pulmonary lymph in newborn lambs (1.7 g/dL).[26] As data in Figure 7 suggest, interstitial fluid drains into microcirculation (indicated by a pressure gradient with a negative sign) in the first 3 hours of postnatal life, corresponding to a major decrease in W/D ratio and to a decrease in plasma protein concentration. After 3 hours, the W/D ratio continues to decrease, though to a much smaller extent, but the pressure gradient reverses in sign—namely filtration occurs from microcirculation into lung interstitium. Therefore, other

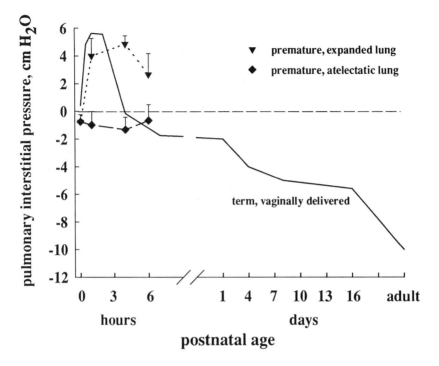

Figure 6. Time course of pulmonary interstitial pressure from birth to adulthood in term, vaginally delivered rabbits. Data are also shown for expanded and at-electatic lung regions of preterm rabbits.

mechanisms should be considered to bring lung interstitium to its final "dehydrated" adult state. Figure 8 shows that lung fluid can drain into the pleural space down a corresponding estimated Starling pressure gradient for up to 9 hours of postnatal life.[24] Despite such a relatively long time, the transpleural fluid flow is expected to be a minor share of interstitial fluid drainage as there is much less pleural surface than pulmonary capillary surface. The decrease in pleural liquid protein concentration (Figure 5) is in keeping with the existence of a transpleural flow of liquid.

As for the contribution of pulmonary lymphatics to postnatal fluid drainage, there is a discrepancy between the data of Humphreys et al,[6] who claim that pulmonary lymphatics account for up to 40% of fluid removal, and those of Bland et al[27] who estimate that they drain no more than 11%. There is little doubt that microvascular absorption is quantitatively more important than lymphatic drainage early after birth, due to the high surface area of pulmonary capillaries. Luminal fluid has been estimated at $\approx$ 6 mL/kg at birth.[27] Assuming that 90% of

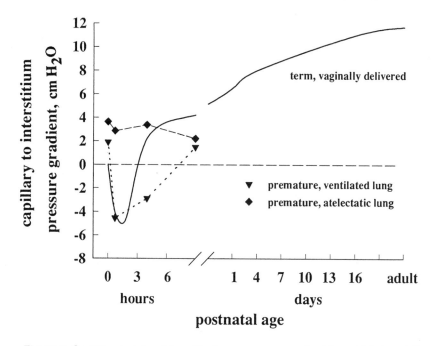

Figure 7. Capillary to interstitium Starling pressure gradient from birth to adulthood in term, vaginally delivered rabbits. Data are also shown for ventilated and atelectatic lung regions of preterm rabbits. Negative values indicate fluxes from interstitium to capillaries.

lung clearance has occurred in the first 6 hours of postnatal life,[5] the average clearance rate amounts to about 0.9 mL/(kg·h), most of it being due to capillary absorption. In Figure 9 Miserocchi and colleagues attempted to partition the role of capillary absorption (J_v), lymphatic drainage (J_l), and transpleural flow (J_{pl}) to the total rate of decrease in lung water in the postnatal life. The latter tends to zero approaching the adult state (60 days). J_v represents the major mechanism of lung water clearance early after birth, and drops to zero at 3 hours. J_{pl} provides a modest contribution that vanishes at about 6 hours. Finally, J_l also provides a modest contribution to the early postnatal lung water clearance but accounts for almost 100% of lung water clearance after 6 hours of life. Figure 10 presents the estimated absolute values of J_v, J_l, and J_{pl} during maturation. Microvascular absorption (J_v) turns to filtration at 3 hours and slowly rises to the steady state adult value; filtration is assured by J_{pl} up to 6 hours and by J_l to maturation. Data in Figures 9 and 10 are normalized to body weight on the basis of the growing rate of rabbits from birth to adulthood.

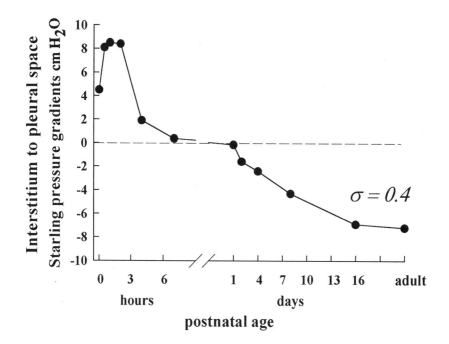

Figure 8. Pulmonary interstitium to pleural space Starling pressure gradient from birth to adulthood in term, vaginally delivered rabbits. It was assumed $\sigma = 0.4$ for the visceral pleura.[15] Adapted from Reference 24.

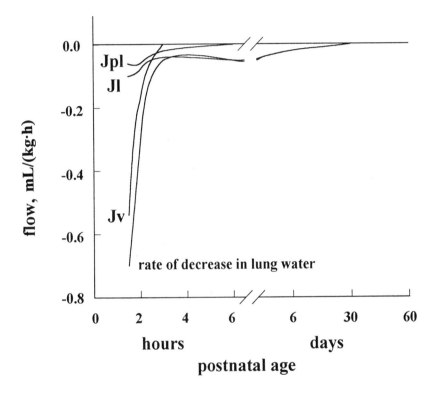

Figure 9. Estimated contribution of microvascular absorption (J_v), lymphatic flow (J_1), and transpleural flow (J_{pl}) to total rate of decrease of lung water in the postnatal life. The latter tends to zero as the steady state condition of turnover is attained.

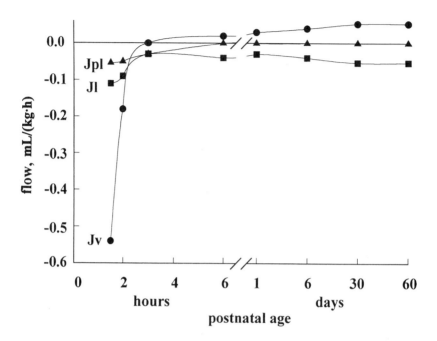

Figure 10. Estimated absolute values of J_v, J_1, and J_{pl} during lung maturation from birth to adulthood.

Age and Size Dependence of the Starling-Lymphatic Interaction

The steady state condition of interstitial fluid turnover reached at maturation represents a balance between Starling-dependent capillary filtration and lymphatic flows. In the adult, the pulmonary capillary filtration rate is about one order of magnitude lower (in absolute terms) than the average absorption rate occurring in the first 3 hours of life, yet the Starling pressure gradient (that is opposite in sign) is about threefold higher (see Figures 2 and 7). Thus, there is a suggestion that the permeability of the membranes to water and solutes decreases with increasing age. This indication is strengthened by observations gathered from the pleural compartment. In fact, it was found that the pleural liquid-to-plasma protein concentration ratio (Cliq/Cpl) decreases with increasing age, going from newborn to adult rabbits, from puppies to dogs, and from lambs to sheep (Figure 11). Yet, as can be appreciated from Figure 11, the decrease in Cliq/Cpl ratio seems to fit a general relationship by having body mass on the abscissa.[24,28] Other data from comparative studies show that pleural liquid pressure becomes more subatmospheric with increasing size, and furthermore, the protein con-

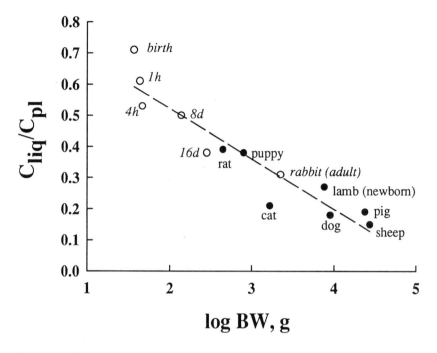

Figure 11. Pleural liquid to plasma protein concentration ratio as a function of body mass. Data gathered from References 28, 29, and 42. Redrawn from Reference 24.

centration of the pleural fluid also decreases with increasing size.[28,29] Correspondingly, the transpleural Starling pressure gradients increase with increasing size, though the corresponding flows decrease. As far as the lung is concerned, many reports indicate that lymph flow, normalized per unit body mass, decreases with increasing animal size.[30–33] Furthermore, Humphreys et al[6] found that pulmonary lymph flow may decrease by one order of magnitude from lambs to sheep. Based on these considerations, one may hypothesize that a steady state interstitial fluid balance develops through two parallel mechanisms: (1) a progressive decrease in conductance of the endothelial membranes that can be easily explained by an increased deposition of matrix macromolecules, and (2) a progressively increasing importance of the lymphatic pump to set the interstitial pressure. Lymphatics act as a draining system that has a relatively small capacity, but a high power to generate a subatmospheric pressure; the relatively dehydrated condition is maintained as long as the conductance of the endothelial membrane remains low. The ability of initial lymphatics to generate rather subatmospheric pressures has been demonstrated for lymphatics on the peritoneal surface of the diaphragm.[34]

Respiratory Mechanics

As previously stated, an increase in lung volume, as during tidal breathing, causes P_{ip} to decrease. In fact, in one study,[24] at 2 hours of postnatal age, end-inspiratory P_{ip} was found to be about 3 cm H_2O less positive compared to end expiration; the corresponding Starling gradient still favored absorption into pulmonary capillaries but was reduced by the same amount. In the adult, increasing parenchymal stresses, as during tidal breathing, causes a greater decrease in P_{ip},[9] likely due to a lower interstitial compliance. During the first 30 minutes of life, lung volume seems to be maintained by closure of upper airways as indicated by the finding that tracheal pressure equals lung recoil pressure.[24] Thereafter, the chest wall develops an outward recoil and therefore FRC is established by the opposing pressures generated by lung and chest wall, a condition that causes pleural pressure to become subatmospheric. Figure 12 shows the time course of end-expiratory lung re-

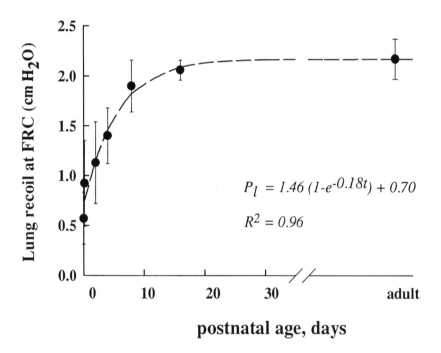

$$P_l = 1.46\,(1\text{-}e^{-0.18t}) + 0.70$$

$$R^2 = 0.96$$

postnatal age, days

Figure 12. Time course of lung recoil pressure at the end-expiratory volume of the respiratory system from birth to adulthood. Recoil pressure is shown relative to alveolar pressure. On the pleural side, the corresponding pressure (pleural surface pressure) would be equal in module but of negative sign. Redrawn from Reference 24.

coil in the postnatal age. The adult value would be reached at approximately 16 days of life. The absolute change in lung recoil pressure at end-expiratory volume from birth to adulthood is only ≈ 2 cm H_2O. Therefore, the impact of an increase in lung recoil on P_{ip} is relatively small and, in fact, the decrease in P_{ip} reflects more closely the process of progressive dehydration of the lung interstitium. To guarantee the coupling of lung and chest wall, a mechanism should be present at pleural level to drain pleural fluid and to maintain pleural pressure subatmospheric. Were this not the case, pleural fluid would eventually collect in the pleural space, leading to hydrothorax. From direct measurements it appears that pleural liquid pressure is already fairly subatmospheric at birth (approximately -2 cm H_2O)[24]; since the Starling pressure gradient at mesothelial level would favor filtration into the pleural space both at visceral and parietal side, it follows that pleural lymphatics play an important role in maintaining the pleural space at subatmospheric pressure. Given the features of the lymphatic drainage outlined in the preceding paragraph, it appears likely that the fluid flux from lung interstitium to pleural space occurring in the first postnatal hours is quantitatively not relevant. It is interesting to note that already at birth the pressure of the pleural liquid is more negative than pleural surface pressure, namely, the pressure exerted by the opposite recoil pressure of lungs and chest wall. Such dissociation is maintained in the adult life.[14]

Lung Fluid Balance in Preterm Animals

In the premature lung there may be deficiency in alveolar surfactant. Furthermore, the lung epithelium does not switch rapidly from alveolar secretion (Cl^- dependent) to alveolar absorption (Na^+ dependent).[35] As a result, the aeration of alveoli may be retarded and the respiratory distress syndrome, characterized by a condition of interstitial and alveolar edema ("leaky lungs") with protein-rich alveolar fluid forming hyaline membranes, may develop.[36] In preterm rabbits (27 days to 30 days of gestation) the pleural window technique allows us to see lung regions that are mostly aerated and others that appear mostly atelectatic.[25] In the ventilated areas P_{ip} can be followed up to 6 hours: P_{ip} increases (Figure 6), peaking at a value similar to that found in term animals, but fails to show a rapid decline. The corresponding Starling pressure gradient favoring absorption into pulmonary capillaries (Figure 7) lasts twice as long compared to term animals; this is in keeping with the fact that there is a greater amount of lung water to be drained. In the atelectatic lung regions P_{ip} remains substantially unchanged. A Starling balance of pressures based on the aforementioned assumption would indicate that, due to the lack of an increase in P_{ip}, the pressure gradient would favor filtration into the interstitial space. Although the microvascular conditions in these areas are rather undefined, this is in keeping with the reported "leaky lung" when respiratory distress syndrome develops. In one study,[37] pulmonary lymph flow and lymph protein concentration were both found to be higher in preterm compared to term animals, particularly in animals developing respiratory distress syndrome, suggesting a higher solute permeability and water permeability of capillary wall.

Pulmonary Interstitial Matrix in the Transition to Interstitial and Alveolar Lung Edema

In order to learn more about the mechanical behavior of the lung tissue matrix when lung interstitium is volume loaded, Miserocchi and colleagues[8,38] measured P_{ip} in the adult rabbit with a model of increased filtration rate induced by intravenous saline infusion at a very low rate (approximately 0.5 mL/[kg·min]). In the early phase of interstitial edema, they observed a marked increase in P_{ip} with a minimal change in W/D, indicating a very low compliance of the pulmonary interstitium estimated to be ≈ 0.5 mL·mm Hg^{-1}·100 g^{-1}, approximately 30-fold lower than other interstitial spaces. Therefore, in the adult mature lung there is a strong "tissue safety factor" against the development of edema. When severe edema develops in the adult lung,[38] P_{ip} tends to decrease toward zero, indicating a sudden increase in interstitial tissue compliance. This was interpreted as an overcoming of the mechanical tolerance of the interstitial matrix to volume loading with a loss of structural organization. In fact, a biochemical study of pulmonary interstitial tissue when severe edema develops, revealed loosening of chemical bonds of proteoglycans of the interstitial matrix and of the basal membranes (heparan sulfate-containing proteoglycans) of alveolar and capillary walls.[38] This information allows the investigators to comment on the time course of P_{ip} in newborn animals. Before luminal reabsorption starts, interstitial matrix is in an unstressed state. As luminal fluid reabsorption proceeds, this causes P_{ip} to increase in term animals, and peak value of P_{ip} found in term newborn animals during reabsorption of alveolar liquid is similar to that observed in the initial edematous state of the adult lung; this suggests a similar mechanical behavior of the pulmonary interstitial matrix. Although the lung is still developing in the postnatal age to achieve its final maturation,[39] the indication is that in the term newborn animal the structural organization of the lung matrix is fairly complete; indeed matrix deposition has been shown to increase exponentially in the late fetal life[11,40] to assure low interstitial compliance. This mechanical feature is important during luminal liquid reabsorption as it leads to an increase in P_{ip} that, in turn, generates a Starling gradient favoring microvascular absorption. One may further observe that the peak value of P_{ip} is set by the ability of the luminal pump to work against a hydraulic pressure gradient. In atelectatic regions of preterm animals, no increase in P_{ip} is observed. In immature lungs, matrix deposition is incomplete[41] and therefore interstitial tissue compliance is not low as it is in case of a mature matrix. Consequently, P_{ip} cannot rise when luminal fluid is reabsorbed. One should recall also that in premature animals there may be a less efficient alveolar liquid absorption[35]; the resulting situation, considering that these animals have a higher-than-normal W/D ratio, is rather unfavorable to fluid drainage, which depends critically on the increase in P_{ip}.

References

1. Olver RE, Strang LB. Ion fluxes across the pulmonary epithelium and the secretion of lung liquid in the fetal lamb. *J Physiol (Lond)* 1974;241:327–357.
2. Dickinson KA Maloney JE, Berger PJ. Decline in lung liquid volume before labor in fetal lambs. *J Appl Physiol* 1986;61:2266–2272.
3. Kitterman JA, Ballard PL, Clements JA, et al. Tracheal fluid in fetal lambs: Spontaneous decrease prior to birth. *J Appl Physiol* 1979;47:985–989.
4. Brown MJ, Olver RE, Ramsden CA, et al. Effects of adrenaline and of spontaneous labour on the secretion and absorption of lung liquid in the foetal lamb. *J Physiol (Lond)* 1983;344:137–152.
5. Aherne W, Dawkins MJR. The removal of fluid from the pulmonary airways after birth in the rabbit, and the effect on this of prematurity and prenatal hypoxia. *Biol Neonate* 1964;7:214–229.
6. Humphreys PW, Normand ICS, Reynolds EOR, et al. Pulmonary lymph flow and the uptake of liquid from the lungs of the lamb at the start of breathing. *J Physiol (Lond)* 1967;193:1–29.
7. Miserocchi G, Negrini D, Gonano C. Direct measurements of interstitial pulmonary pressure in in-situ lung with intact pleural space. *J Appl Physiol* 1990;69:2168–2174.
8. Miserocchi G, Negrini D, Del Fabbro M, et al. Pulmonary interstitial pressure in intact in situ lung: Transition to interstitial edema. *J Appl Physiol* 1993;74:1171–1177.
9. Miserocchi G, Negrini D, Gonano C. Parenchymal stress affects interstitial and pleural ressures in in situ lung. *J Appl Physiol* 1991;71:1967–1972.
10. Weibel ER, Bachofen H. The fiber scaffold of lung parenchyma. In: Crystal RG, West JB (eds): *The Lung: Scientific Foundations.* New York: Raven Press; 1991;787–794.
11. Juul SE, Wight TN, Hascall VC. Proteoglycans. In: Crystal RG, West JB (eds): *The Lung: Scientifc Foundations.* New York: Raven Press; 1991;413–420.
12. Laurent TC. Structure of the extracellular matrix and the biology of

hyaluronan. In: Reed RK, McHale NG, Bert JL, et al (eds): *Interstitium, Connective Tissue and Lymphatics*. London: Portland; 1995;1–12.

13. Hainis KD, Sznajder JI, Schraufnagel DE. Lung lymphatics cast from airspace. *Am J Physiol* 1994;267:L199–L205.
14. Miserocchi G. Pleural pressures and fluid transport. In: Crystal RG, West JB (eds): *The Lung: Scientific Foundations*. New York: Raven Press; 1991; 885–893.
15. Negrini D. Integration of capillary interstitial and lymphatic function in the pleural space. In: Reed RK, McHale NG, Bert JL, et al (eds): *Interstitium, Connective Tissue and Lymphatics*. London: Portland; 1995;283–299.
16. Negrini D, Gonano C, Miserocchi G. Microvascular pressure profile in intact in situ lung. *J Appl Physiol* 1992;72:332–339.
17. Negrini D. Pulmonary microvascular pressure profile during development of hydrostatic edema. *Microcirculation* 1995;2:173–180.
18. Bhattacharya J, Nakahara K, Staub NC. Effect of edema on pulmonary blood flow in the isolated perfused dog lung lobe. *J Appl Physiol* 1980;48: 444–449.
19. Curry FR. Mechanism and thermodynamics of transcapillary exchange. In: Renkin EM, Michel CC (eds): *Handbook of Physiology. The Cardiovascular System*. Microcirculation. Bethesda, MD: American Physiological Society; 1984;309–374.
20. Michel CC. Fluid movements through capillary walls. In: Renkin EM, Michel CC (eds): *Handbook of Physiology. The Cardiovascular System. Microcirculation*. Bethesda, MD: American Physiological Society; 1984;375–409.
21. Miserocchi G, Venturoli D, Negrini D, et al. Model of pleural fluid turnover. *J Appl Physiol* 1993;75:1798–1806.
22. Negrini D, Del Fabbro M, Venturoli D. Fluid exchanges across the parietal peritoneal and pleural mesothelium. *J Appl Physiol* 1993;74:1779–1784.
23. Neergard K. Zur Frage des Druckes in Pleuraspalt. *Beitr Klin Erfosch Tuberk Lungenkr* 1927;65:476–485.
24. Miserocchi G, Haxhiu Poskurica B, Del Fabbro M. Pulmonary interstitial pressure in anesthetized paralyzed newborn rabbits. *J Appl Physiol* 1994; 77:2260–2268.
25. Miserocchi G, Haxhiu Poskurica B, Del Fabbro M, et al. Pulmonary interstitial pressure in premature rabbits. *Respir Physiol* 1995;102:239–249.
26. Bland RD. Fetal lung liquid and its removal near birth. In: Crystal RG, West JB (eds): *The Lung: Scientific Foundations*. New York: Raven Press; 1991;1677–1685.
27. Bland RD, Hansen TN, Haberkern CM, et al. Lung fluid balance in lambs before and after birth. *J Appl Physiol* 1982;53:992–1004.
28. Miserocchi G, Negrini D, Mortola J. Comparative features of Starling-lymphatic interaction at the pleural level in mammals. *J Appl Physiol* 1984;56: 1151–1156.
29. Negrini D, Miserocchi G. Size related differences in parietal extrapleural and pleural liquid pressure distribution. *J Appl Physiol* 1989;67(5):1967–1972.
30. Parker JC, Crain M, Grimbert F. Total lung fluid flow and fluid compartmentation in edematous dog lungs. *J Appl Physiol* 1981;51:1269–1277.
31. Brace RA, Power GG. Thoracic duct lymph flow and protein flux dynamics: Response to intravascular saline. *Am J Physiol* 1981;240:R282–R288.
32. Havill AM, Gee MH. Role of the interstitium in clearance of alveolar fluid in normal and injured lungs. *J Appl Physiol* 1984;57:1–6.

33. Matthey MA, Landolt CC, Staub NC. Differential liquid and protein clearance from the alveoli of anesthetized sheep. *J Appl Physiol* 1982;53:96–104.
34. Miserocchi G, Negrini D, Mukenge S, et al. Liquid drainage through the peritoneal diaphragmatic surface. *J Appl Physiol* 1989;66:1579–1585.
35. Bland RD. Lung epithelial ion transport and fluid movement during perinatal period. *Am J Physiol* 1990;259:L30–L37.
36. Normand ICS, Reynolds EOR, Strang LB, et al. Flow and protein concentration of lymph from lungs of lambs developing hyaline membrane disease. *Arch Dis Child* 1968;43:334–339.
37. Bland RD, Carlton DP, Scheerer RG et al. Lung fluid balance in lambs before and after premature birth. *J Clin Invest* 1989;84:568–576.
38. Negrini D, Passi A, De Luca G, Miserocchi G. Pulmonary interstitial pressure and proteoglycans during development of pulmonary edema. *Am J Physiol* 1996;39:H2000–H2007.
39. Burn PH. Postnatal development of the lung. In: Crystal RG, West JB (eds): *The Lung: Scientifc Foundations*. New York: Raven Press; 1991;677–687.
40. Mecham RP, Prosser IW, Hascall VC. Elastic fibers. In: Crystal RG, West JB (eds): *The Lung: Scientifc Foundations*. New York: Raven Press; 1991; 389–398.
41. Gross I. Regulation of fetal lung maturation. *Am J Physiol* 1990;259: L337–L344.
42. Broaddus VC, Araya M, Carlton DP, et al. Developmental changes in pleural liquid protein concentration in sheep. *Ann Rev Respir Dis* 1991; 143:38–41.

Chapter 11

Strength, Failure, and Remodeling of the Pulmonary Blood-Gas Barrier

John B. West, MD, PhD, DSc, Ellen C. Breen, PhD, and Odile Mathieu-Costello, PhD

Structure of the Blood-Gas Barrier

In 1661 Marcello Malpighi of Bologna wrote to his friend, Alfonso Borelli, professor of mathematics at Pisa, about the appearances of frog lung under his new microscope and reported that he could see "an aggregate of very fine thin membranes [*levissimis et tenuissimis membranis*] which, stretched and folded, form an almost infinite number of orbicular bladders . . ."[1] This was the first observation of the pulmonary blood-gas barrier (BGB). Although some further progress was made as the light microscope was refined, the components of the BGB remained controversial until the introduction of the electron microscope. For example, as late as 1929 the French pathologist, Albert Policard[2] argued that the internal surface of the lung was "like the flesh of an open wound," with only the capillary endothelium intervening between the alveolar gas and capillary blood. However when Frank Low[3] made the first electron micrographs of the BGB, it immediately became clear that on the thin side, the barrier consisted of the alveolar epithelium, capillary endothelium, and the intervening interstitium composed of the fused basement membranes of the two cell layers. Modern electron micrographs show the ultrastructure of the barrier with great clarity.

From both anatomical and physiological points of view, it is use-

This work was supported by NHLBI grant R01 HL46910.

From: Weir EK, Reeves JT (eds). *Pulmonary Edema*. Armonk, NY: Futura Publishing Company, Inc.; ©1998.

ful to divide the BGB into two parts, the thick side and the thin side. The thick side contains several elements including cords of type I collagen and interstitial cells, and it may be 1 μm thick or more. The consequent diffusion resistance to gas exchange presumably means that the thick side participates principally in fluid exchange and, certainly, thickening of this region occurs in early pulmonary edema. By contrast, the thin side of the barrier is extremely efficient for diffusive gas exchange and, because of the sparse, tight interstitium, its role in fluid exchange is probably small. The thin part of the BGB occupies about half of the total area, that is some 25 m^2 to 50 m^2, of the human lung.

Strength of the Blood-Gas Barrier

Although the extreme thinness of the BGB was immediately recognized when the first electron micrographs became available, it has only been appreciated during the last 5 years that the barrier is also immensely strong. The main reason why this important feature was not appreciated previously was the persisting belief that the pressures in the pulmonary capillaries are low at rest and remain low during exercise. For example, in the early days of cardiac catheterization, some studies apparently showed that the mean pulmonary arterial pressure decreased as a result of exercise![4,5] We now know that both pulmonary arterial and venous pressures increase substantially with exercise.

Another misconception was that much of the pressure drop in the pulmonary circulation occurs in the arterioles, as is the case in the systemic circulation. However, direct measurements made by the insertion of tiny cannulas into small blood vessels show that pulmonary capillary pressure is about halfway between arterial and venous pressure and, in addition, much of the pressure drop in the pulmonary circulation occurs in the capillaries.[6,7]

Modern measurements on healthy humans exercising on a bicycle ergometer at an oxygen consumption of 80% to 90% of their maximal oxygen consumption show that the mean pulmonary arterial pressure increases from 13.2 mm Hg at rest to 37.2 mm Hg on exercise, while the mean pulmonary arterial wedge pressure increases from 3.4 mm Hg at rest to 21.1 mm Hg on exercise.[8] Other studies on normal subjects have produced similar results.[9,10] This means that the capillary pressure at the bottom of the upright human lung during near-maximal exercise is approximately 36 mm Hg.[11]

As a result of these high capillary pressures, the circumferential or hoop stress in the wall of the capillary becomes extremely high. It is important to understand what type of stress is being referred to here. This is not shear stress, which depends on rapid blood flow and has been studied extensively in large systemic blood vessels because of its possible importance in atherogenesis. Hoop stress is generated by the difference in pressure between the inside and the outside (transmural pressure) of a tube such as a capillary. An analogy is a garden hose, which may burst if someone blocks it by standing on it when the tap is turned on.

The hoop stress in a cylindrical tube is easily calculated from the Laplace relationship and, taking representative values for capillary radius and wall thickness, the hoop stress in the capillary wall of rabbit lung at a capillary transmural pressure of 36 mm Hg is approximately $5.1 \times 10^4 \, \text{N/m}^2$. This is an enormous stress comparable to that in the aorta, the wall of which is armored with large amounts of collagen and elastin. It is truly remarkable that the extremely thin BGB (Figure 1) can tolerate such an enormous stress. Incidentally, it is also remarkable that apparently no one made this simple calculation until approximately 5 years ago. Probably the reason is that people were misled by the small radius of the capillary which, others things being equal, reduces wall stress. What was overlooked was the extreme thinness of the wall.

What is responsible for the great strength of the thin part of the BGB? There is now strong evidence that the strength comes from the type IV collagen in the basement membranes of the alveolar epithelial

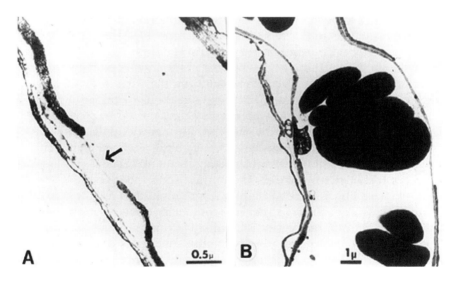

Figure 1. Ultrastructural changes in the blood-gas barrier when pulmonary capillaries are exposed to high transmural pressures (rabbit). In A, the endothelium is disrupted (arrow) but the alveolar epithelium and two basement membranes are continuous. In B, the alveolar epithelial layer (right) and the capillary endothelial layer (left) are disrupted. Note the platelet closely applied to the exposed endothelial basement membrane (left). From Reference 14.

and capillary endothelial cells. The type IV collagen molecules are about 400 nm long. Two join at the C terminal end, and four come together at the N terminal end to give a matrix configuration similar to that of chicken wire.[12,13] The resulting mesh structure apparently combines great strength with porosity. Few measurements of the ultimate tensile strength of basement membrane have been made, but they suggest that it approaches that of the enormously strong type I collagen, perhaps the strongest soft tissue in the body.[14–16] It is clear, however, that with the enormous stresses that are referred to here, the BGB is at some risk of failing during heavy exercise.

Failure of the Blood-Gas Barrier

In view of the high stresses in the capillary walls, it is not surprising that when capillary pressure is raised to abnormally high levels, ultrastructural changes are seen. These have been described in detail elsewhere[14,17–19] and are briefly reviewed here. Most of the results were obtained with use of anesthetized rabbit preparations where the pulmonary artery and left atrium were cannulated and the capillary pressure was increased to known levels by raising the pulmonary arterial and venous reservoirs.

Figure 1A shows an example of stress failure in the wall of a pulmonary capillary when the transmural pressure was 52.5 cm H_2O (39 mm Hg). It can be seen that there is disruption of the capillary endothelium but its basement membrane is continuous, as is the basement membrane of the alveolar epithelial layer and the epithelial layer itself. Figure 1B shows another example at the same capillary transmural pressure, where the alveolar epithelial layer is disrupted on the right side, while on the left the endothelium is broken and a platelet is closely applied to the exposed endothelial basement membrane. This membrane is electrically charged and highly reactive, and it is not surprising that it attracts platelets and red and white blood cells.

In the rabbit preparation, stress failure begins at a capillary transmural pressure of about 32.5 cm H_2O (24 mm Hg), but the pressure has to be raised to approximately 52.5 cm H_2O (39 mm Hg) before breaks are consistently seen. The number of breaks increases when the pressure is further raised.[17] Of course it cannot be assumed that the transmural pressure required for stress failure is the same in all species. Indeed we have evidence that the critical pressure increases with the aerobic capacity of the animal such that the dog is less vulnerable than the rabbit and the thoroughbred racehorse less vulnerable than the dog.[20–22] Species differences in the variables in the Laplace equation fit with the different pressures required for stress failure. The BGB is thinnest in the rabbit, intermediate in the dog, and thickest in the horse, whereas average capillary radius tends to be largest in the rabbit, intermediate in the dog, and smallest in the horse. The result is that calculated capillary wall stress for a given transmural pressure decreases from rabbit to dog to horse.[20]

Stress failure in mesenteric capillaries of the frog at high-capillary pressures has recently been reported.[23] It is remarkable that the findings in this very different structure in an amphibian are so similar to the authors' results in the rabbit lung. For example, the frog mesenteric capillaries begin to fail at a capillary pressure of about 30 cm H_2O, and as the pressure is raised more breaks are seen. Another similarity is that most of the breaks are rapidly reversible when the transmural pressure is decreased. This fits with the authors' studies on the rabbit lung, where about 70% of the breaks disappear within a few minutes of lowering the pressure.[24] Finally, painstaking three-dimensional reconstructions of the electron micrographs in the frog study show that over 80% of the breaks in the capillary endothelium are transcellular rather than intercellular. The authors of this chapter do not have data on this point for the capillary endothelial cells of rabbit lung, but studies of alveolar epithelial cells by scanning electron microscopy show that essentially all of the breaks there are transcellular.[18]

The structure of the frog mesentery and the rabbit lung are very different in that the mesenteric capillaries are surrounded by interstitial tissue but have no closely adjacent epithelium, while the thin side of the BGB has little interstitium but an alveolar epithelial layer. The fact that approximately the same transmural pressures are necessary for stress failure in both preparations is consistent with the fact that the strength of the capillary is attributable to the basement membrane and that the surrounding interstitial tissue in the mesentery, or the surrounding epithelial layer in the lung, confer little structural support.

Dilemma of the Blood-Gas Barrier

It is natural to ask why evolutionary processes have resulted in such a critical structure as the BGB being so close to mechanical failure during heavy exercise. Clearly, failure could be catastrophic for gas exchange if the alveoli fill with blood. The answer is that the barrier has to satisfy two conflicting requirements. On the one hand it has to be extremely thin for efficient gas exchange by diffusion. Indeed, some studies indicate that the barrier is not thin enough (or does not have a large enough surface area) for optimal diffusion rates during maximal exercise in some elite athletes. It is well documented that some human athletes develop arterial hypoxemia during heavy exercise as a result of diffusion limitation across the BGB.[8,25] Diffusion limitation is even more marked in the highly aerobic racehorse, which develops marked arterial hypoxemia during galloping.[26] Thus, there would be a clear advantage for aerobic performance in having a thinner BGB, and presumably there is continuous evolutionary pressure to maintain it as thin as possible.

However at the same time, the BGB must be maintained strong enough to prevent mechanical failure which, as indicated above, could be catastrophic for gas exchange. As we shall see shortly, failure of the barrier does occur in humans when the capillary pressure is raised to abnormally high levels, and remarkably, it occurs in *all* thoroughbred racehorses under the physiological conditions of galloping. Thus, the BGB faces a dilemma in that it has to be extremely thin for gas exchange but just strong enough to maintain its integrity when the capillary pressure rises maximally during exercise. This means that the capillaries are the most vulnerable vessels in the pulmonary circulation.

Physiological and Pathological Conditions Causing Failure of the Blood-Gas Barrier

The most dramatic example of stress failure of the BGB under *physiological* conditions is seen in thoroughbred racehorses. All of these bleed into their lungs during training as evidenced by the presence of hemosiderin-laden macrophages in tracheal washings.[27] The failure occurs because of the extremely high capillary pressures, which in turn are a consequence of enormously high left ventricular filling pressures. For example, the left atrial pressure measured directly with an indwelling catheter can be as high as 70 mm Hg and the mean pulmonary artery pressure can be 120 mm Hg.[28–30] Therefore, the pulmonary capillary pressure approaches 100 mm Hg. The high left ventricular filling pressures are necessary for the enormous cardiac outputs that allow the extraordinary aerobic performance of these animals, which have been selectively bred for more than 400 years.[31]

Hopkins and colleagues[32] wondered whether some elite human athletes might show changes in the permeability of their BGB with intense exercise and therefore studied six top-level cyclists with a history of hemoptysis or tasting blood following exercise, but who were otherwise healthy.[32] Bronchoalveolar lavage (BAL) using normal saline was carried out 1 hour following a 4 km uphill sprint at maximal effort, which was sufficient to give a mean heart rate of 177 beats·min^{-1}. The controls were normal sedentary subjects who did not exercise prior to BAL. The athletes showed significantly higher concentrations of red blood cells and total protein in their BAL fluid, which is evidence of an increased permeability of the BGB (Figure 2). There was also an increase in concentra-

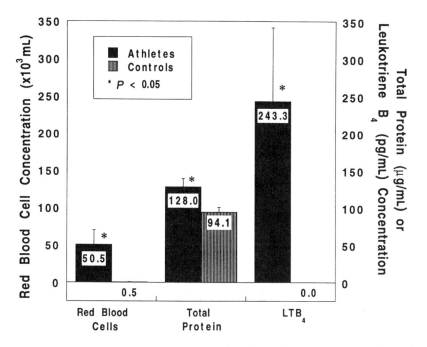

Figure 2. Increases in concentrations of red blood cells, total protein, and leukotriene B$_4$ in the BAL fluid of elite cyclists after 7 minutes of maximal exercise. From Reference 32.

tion of leukotriene B$_4$, a potent chemotactic mediator that has previously been shown to be raised in the BAL fluid of patients with high-altitude pulmonary edema (HAPE)[33] and also in the rabbit preparation of Tsukimoto et al[34] at high capillary pressures. A possible mechanism for the increased leukotriene B$_4$ is exposure of the basement membrane of alveolar epithelial cells (Figure 1B), which activate macrophages, or capillary endothelial cells (Figure 1A), which activate leukocytes.

Pathological conditions that result in stress failure of the BGB include HAPE, neurogenic pulmonary edema, severe left ventricular failure, and overinflation of the lung. The last is responsible for the increased capillary permeability seen in patients in the intensive care unit who are treated with high levels of positive end-expiratory pressure (PEEP). These conditions are discussed in detail elsewhere.[11]

Remodeling of the Pulmonary Blood-Gas Barrier

How is the enormous area of the thin side of the BGB (over 30 m^2 in the human lung) maintained so extremely thin (0.2 μm to 0.4 μm in the human lung) and yet just strong enough to withstand the largest normal physiological stresses? Presumably, capillary wall stress is being continually monitored, and the structure of the wall, especially the amount of type IV collagen, continually adjusted.

Remodeling in other parts of the pulmonary circulation has been extensively studied. For example, rats made hypoxic by exposure to air at half the normal barometric pressure, and thus increasing pulmonary artery pressure by hypoxic vasoconstriction, show rapid morphological changes in their pulmonary arteries, including increases in the amount of vascular smooth muscle and extracellular matrix.[35,36] The increase in smooth muscle can be detected histologically within 48 hours, and involution of both smooth muscle and extracellular matrix is rapid when the animals are returned to a normoxic environment.[37] The rapidity of remodeling has been demonstrated by stretching excised rings of pulmonary artery in Krebs-Ringer solution to simulate an increased wall tension equivalent to a transmural pressure of 50 mm Hg.[38] Within 4 hours there were increases in collagen synthesis, elastin synthesis, mRNA for pro-α1(I) collagen, and mRNA for proto-oncogene v-cis. The last may implicate platelet-derived growth factor or transforming growth factor β (TGF-β) as the mediator. The responses were endothelium-dependent because they did not occur when the endothelium was removed from the arterial rings.

What is the evolutionary advantage of this pulmonary artery remodeling? It is likely that it is to protect the vulnerable pulmonary capillaries because, in the adult lung, there is meager vascular smooth muscle in the pulmonary arteries, and this is unevenly distributed. The result is that when hypoxic pulmonary vasoconstriction occurs, those capillaries that are downstream from areas of the lung that lack arteriolar smooth muscle will be exposed to a high pressure, and consequently liable to stress failure. Indeed the authors of this chapter believe this is the mechanism of HAPE.[39] Remodeling of the pulmonary arteries allows the resistance of all vessels to be increased, thus protecting all the capillaries. It is of note that the result is the return of the structure of the pulmonary arteries to a state similar to that in the fetus where the capillaries must be protected from the high pulmonary artery pressure in utero.

A clinical feature of HAPE may throw light on this process. It is known that if a person goes to high altitude, HAPE will develop within 3 to 5 days or not at all. A reasonable explanation is that the pulmonary arterial remodeling progresses far enough to completely protect the capillaries at the end of this time. However, if someone who has been at high altitude for a period goes to sea level for several days and subsequently returns to high altitude, so-called "re-ascent" HAPE may develop, particularly in children. Possibly, the mechanism is that the involution of vascular smooth muscle and connective tissue that occurs in response to descent makes the capillaries vulnerable again.

By contrast, with the extensive information available on remodeling of pulmonary arteries, almost nothing is known about remodeling in pulmonary capillaries. It is known, however, to occur in patients with mitral stenosis and left ventricular failure.[40,41] Figure 3 shows an example with obvious thickening of the basement membrane in a patient with mitral stenosis. Presumably, this is in response to the increase in capillary wall stress, and the thickening will result in strengthening of the BGB.

Regulation of the thickness and strength of the BGB is central to the success of the mammalian lung as a gas exchanger, and it remarkable that it has been so little studied and that the mechanisms are essentially unknown. This is one of the central thrusts of the current research by the authors of this chapter. Recently, these authors increased capillary wall stress in one lung of anesthetized rabbits by separately cannulating the trachea and the left main bronchus and exposing one side to 8 cm H_2O PEEP while exposing the other side to only 1 cm H_2O PEEP. Control animals had both lungs exposed to low levels of PEEP. The authors have previously shown that high lung inflation increases capillary wall stress.[19] The results (Figure 4) show that high states of lung inflation cause increases in mRNA for pro-α1(III) collagen, fibronectin, and TGF-

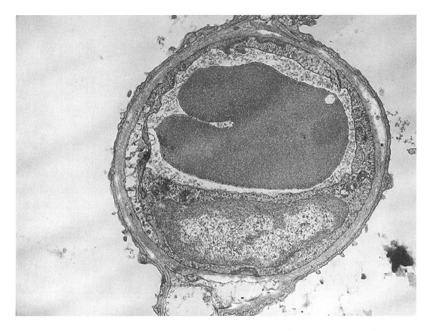

Figure 3. Electron micrograph of pulmonary capillary from a young patient with mitral stenosis. Note thickening of the basement membranes of the capillary endothelium and alveolar epithelium, particularly the former. Courtesy of S.G. Haworth.

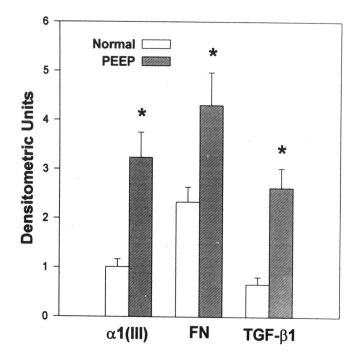

Figure 4. Increases in mRNA for α1(III) procollagen, fibronectin, and TGF-β1 from peripheral parenchyma of lungs at high states of inflation compared with other animals with normally inflated lungs. Modified from Reference 42.

β1 within 4 hours.[42] An unexpected finding was that the changes in gene expression are similar in both lungs in the animals where one lung is exposed to high inflation, indicating that information is being transferred from the high-inflation lung to the other side. Additional studies are being carried out in isolated rat lungs where preliminary results show increased gene expression for α2(IV) procollagen mRNA. Much further work is needed to understand this central dilemma of the mammalian lung, namely how to provide an extremely thin membrane of large area, while protecting it against large mechanical stresses.

Acknowledgments We acknowledge the collaboration of John Berg, Eric Birks, Michael Costello, Ann Elliott, Zhenxing Fu, James Jones, Sanli Kurdak, Yasuo Namba, John Pascoe, Renato Prediletto, Koichi Tsukimoto, and Walter Tyler.

References

1. Malpighi M. *Duae epistolae de pulmonibus*. Florence: 1661.
2. Policard A. Les nouvelles idées sur la disposition de la surface respiratoire pulmonaire. *Presse Med* 1929;37:1293–1295.

3. Low FN. Electron microscopy of the rat lung. *Anat Rec* 1952;113:437–443.
4. Riley RL, Himmelstein A, Motley HL, et al. Studies of the pulmonary circulation at rest and during exercise in normal individuals and in patients with chronic pulmonary disease. *Am J Physiol* 1948;152:372–382.
5. Donald KW, Bishop JM, Cumming G, et al. The effect of exercise on the cardiac output and circulatory dynamics of normal subjects. *Clin Sci* 1955;14:37–73.
6. Bhattacharya J, Staub NC. Direct measurement of microvascular pressures in the isolated perfused dog lung. *Science* 1980;210:327–328.
7. Bhattacharya J, Nanjo S, Staub NC. Micropuncture measurement of lung microvascular pressure during 5-HT infusion. *J Appl Physiol* 1982;52: 634–637.
8. Wagner PD, Gale GE, Moon RE, et al. Pulmonary gas exchange in humans exercising at sea level and simulated altitude. *J Appl Physiol* 1986;61: 260–270.
9. Groves BM, Reeves JT, Sutton JR, et al. Operation Everest II: Elevated high-altitude pulmonary resistance unresponsive to oxygen. *J Appl Physiol* 1987;63:521–530.
10. Reeves JT, Groves BM, Cymerman A, et al. Operation Everest II: Cardiac filling pressures during cycle exercise at sea level. *Respir Physiol* 1990; 80:147–154.
11. West JB, Mathieu-Costello O. Vulnerability of pulmonary capillaries in heart disease. *Circulation* 1995;92:622–631.
12. Timpl R, Wiedemann H, van Delden V, et al. A network model for the organization of type IV collagen molecules in basement membranes. *Eur J Biochem* 1981;120:203–211.
13. Yurchenco PD, Schittny JC. Molecular architecture of basement membranes. *FASEB J* 1990;4:1577–1590.
14. West JB, Tsukimoto K, Mathieu-Costello O, et al. Stress failure in pulmonary capillaries. *J Appl Physiol* 1991;70:1731–1742.
15. Welling LW, Grantham JJ. Physical properties of isolated perfused renal tubules and tubular basement membranes. *J Clin Invest* 1972;51:1063–1075.
16. Fisher RF, Wakely J. The elastic constants and ultrastructural organization of a basement membrane (lens capsule). *Proc R Soc Lond B Biol Sci* 1976; 193:335–358.
17. Tsukimoto K, Mathieu-Costello O, Prediletto R, et al. Ultrastructural appearances of pulmonary capillaries at high transmural pressures. *J Appl Physiol* 1991;71:573–582.
18. Costello ML, Mathieu-Costello O, West JB. Stress failure of alveolar epithelial cells studied by scanning electron microscopy. *Am Rev Respir Dis* 1992;145:1446–1455.
19. Fu Z, Costello ML, Tsukimoto K, et al. High lung volume increases stress failure in pulmonary capillaries. *J Appl Physiol* 1992;73:123–133.
20. Birks EK, Mathieu-Costello O, Fu Z, et al. Comparative aspects of the strength of pulmonary capillaries in rabbit, dog and horse. *Respir Physiol* 1994;97:235–246.
21. Mathieu-Costello O, Willford DC, Fu Z, et al. Pulmonary capillaries are more resistant to stress failure in dog than in rabbit. *J Appl Physiol* 1995; 79:908–917.
22. Birks EK, Mathieu-Costello O, Fu Z, et al. Very high pressures are required to cause stress failure of pulmonary capillaries in thoroughbred racehorses. *J Appl Physiol* 1997;82:1584–1592.

23. Neal CR, Michel CC. Openings in frog microvascular endothelium induced by high intravascular pressures. *J Physiol (Lond)* 1996;492:39–52.
24. Elliott AR, Fu Z, Tsukimoto K, et al. Short-term reversibility of ultrastructural changes in pulmonary capillaries caused by stress failure. *J Appl Physiol* 1992;73:1150–1158.
25. Dempsey JA, Hanson PG, Henderson KS. Exercise-induced alveolar hypoxemia in healthy human subjects at sea-level. *J Physiol (Lond)* 1984;355:161–175.
26. Wagner PD, Gillespie JR, Landgren GL, et al. Mechanism of exercise-induced hypoxemia in horses. *J Appl Physiol* 1989;66:1227–1233.
27. Whitwell KE, Greet TRC. Collection and evaluation of tracheobronchial washes in the horse. *Equine Vet J* 1984;16:499–508.
28. Jones JH, Smith BL, Birks EK, et al. Left atrial and pulmonary arterial pressures in exercising horses. (Abstract) *FASEB J* 1992;6:A2020.
29. Erickson BK, Erickson HH, Coffman JR. Pulmonary artery, aortic and oesophageal pressure changes during high intensity treadmill exercise in the horse: A possible relation to exercise-induced pulmonary haemorrhage. *Equine Vet J* 1990;9(suppl):47–52.
30. Manohar M. Pulmonary artery wedge pressure increases with high-intensity exercise in horses. *Am J Vet Res* 1993;54:142–146.
31. West JB, Mathieu-Costello O. Stress failure of pulmonary capillaries as a mechanism for exercise-induced pulmonary hemorrhage: A review. *Equine Vet J* 1994;26:441–447.
32. Hopkins SR, Schoene RB, Martin TR, et al. Intense exercise increases the permeability of the lung blood-gas barrier in elite athletes. *Am J Respir Crit Care Med* 1997;155:1090–1094.
33. Schoene RB, Hackett PH, Henderson WR, et al. High-altitude pulmonary edema. Characteristics of lung lavage fluid. *J Am Med Assoc* 1986;256:63–69.
34. Tsukimoto K, Yoshimura N, Ichioka M, et al. Protein, cell, and LTB_4 concentrations of lung edema fluid produced by high capillary pressures in rabbit. *J Appl Physiol* 1994;76:321–327.
35. Meyrick B, Reid L. The effect of continued hypoxia on rat pulmonary arterial circulation. An ultrastructural study. *Lab Invest* 1978;38:188–200.
36. Meyrick B, Reid L. Hypoxia-induced structural changes in the media and adventitia of the rat hilar pulmonary artery and their regression. *Am J Pathol* 1980;100:151–178.
37. Tozzi CA, Wilson FJ, Yu SY, et al. Vascular connective tissue is rapidly degraded during early regression of pulmonary hypertension. *Chest* 1991;99(suppl 3):41S–42S.
38. Tozzi CA, Poiani GJ, Harangozo AM, et al. Pressure-induced connective tissue synthesis in pulmonary artery segments is dependent on intact endothelium. *J Clin Invest* 1989;84:1005–1012.
39. West JB, Colice GL, Lee Y-J, et al. Pathogenesis of high-altitude pulmonary oedema: Direct evidence of stress failure of pulmonary capillaries. *Eur Respir J* 1995;8:523–529.
40. Haworth SG, Hall SM, Patel M. Peripheral pulmonary vascular and airway abnormalities in adolescents with rheumatic mitral stenosis. *Int J Cardiol* 1988;18:405–416.
41. Lee Y. Electron microscopic studies of the alveolar-capillary barrier in the patients of chronic pulmonary edema. *Jpn Circ J* 1979;43:945–954.
42. Berg JT, Fu Z, Breen EC, et al. High lung inflation increases mRNA levels of ECM components and growth factors in lung parenchyma. *J Appl Physiol* 1997;83:120–128.

Chapter 12

Effect of the Distribution of Vascular Pressures on Pulmonary Edema

J. Usha Raj, MD

In the pulmonary circulation there are three main longitudinal vascular segments: the arteries, the microvessels, and the veins. It is generally appreciated that most of baseline lung fluid filtration occurs across alveolar wall capillaries, ie, at least 50% and more of total fluid flux occurs at this site. However, considerable experimental evidence exists to show that fluid filtration also occurs across the thin-walled corner vessels, the extra-alveolar precapillary arterioles, and the postcapillary venules.[1,2] Because the pressure is higher in the upstream arterioles than in the venules, a greater amount of fluid may be filtered through these vessels. Therefore, the pre- and postcapillary corner vessels and the alveolar septal capillaries are the main sites of fluid filtration, and this middle portion of the pulmonary circulation can be referred to as the filtering segment. The forces responsible for fluid and protein fluxes between the pulmonary microcirculation and the interstitium are described in Starling's equation, $Jv=K[(^{P}mv-^{P}int)-\sigma(^{\pi}mv-^{\pi}int)]$.[3] The major force that alters fluid balance in the lung is capillary hydrostatic pressure. The magnitude of capillary pressure is directly influenced by the resistances in the precapillary arterial segment and the postcapillary venous segment as well as the pressures in the pulmonary artery and left atrium. Usually, a lumped value for the overall average capillary pressure is calculated using the equation of Gaar and Taylor,[4] which assumes that 60% of the resistance in the pul-

This work was supported by a grant from National Heart, Lung, and Blood Institute # 38438.

From: Weir EK, Reeves JT (eds). *Pulmonary Edema*. Armonk, NY: Futura Publishing Company, Inc.; ©1998.

monary circulation lies upstream from the midpoint of the alveolar wall capillaries, ie, the filtering segment of the lung vasculature, and 40% lies downstream. However, this pattern of distribution of resistances is not constant and may vary depending on a variety of factors.[5,6] Hence, a better knowledge of the distribution of resistances between the upstream and downstream vascular segments is useful in determining the actual forces that govern fluid filtration. When pressures are elevated in any particular vascular segment of the lung, an increase in fluid filtration is likely to occur. In general, a change in arterial resistance without any change in resistance or pressures elsewhere is unlikely to affect fluid filtration pressures significantly and hence, for the purposes of regulation of fluid filtration, changes in arterial tone are not that relevant. But any change in resistance and/or pressures in the downstream segment, viz, the veins and in the alveolar wall capillaries themselves, will certainly affect fluid and protein filtration. In any case, the actual amount of fluid filtered will depend on the balance between vascular pressures and the other forces that are operating at that site, such as the hydrostatic pressure in the interstitium surrounding the vessels and the absorptive pressure of the plasma protein in plasma and interstitium that surrounds the blood vessels. It is important to realize that potentially there can be two patients with identical pressures in the pulmonary artery and left atrium, and yet depending on a variety of variables that affect the pulmonary circulation, the pressures in the filtering segment may be quite different, such that one patient may be tending towards fulminant pulmonary edema and the other not. In such a situation, calculation of capillary hydrostatic pressure using the Gaar and Taylor equation would yield identical pressures in the two patients and be very misleading.

From experimental data it is known that the distribution of resistances in the longitudinal vascular segments of the lung depends on the age of the animal studied, the species, as well as on a variety of active and passive forces acting on the blood vessels. Age seems to affect the distribution of resistances in the lung such that veins contribute a larger proportion to total resistance in the younger animal than in the adult. Lungs that have a high fractional venous resistance under baseline conditions will have higher baseline fluid filtration rates. In general, the more immature lung appears to have a higher fractional resistance in veins,[5,7] as compared to the adult lung.[8-10] In neonatal lamb lungs that were isolated and perfused with blood, Raj and Chen[5] determined the profile of pressures in the lung by micropuncture and reported that ~40 of total vascular resistance was in veins. This relatively high fractional venous resistance may result in high microvascular pressures under resting conditions in the lamb and might explain the higher baseline lung lymph flow rates as compared to those in adult sheep.[11] A high baseline fractional venous resistance seems to be a characteristic of the developing lung. For example, in neonatal rabbit lungs, 30% of total vascular resistance is in veins[7] as compared to only 15% in adult rabbits (Figure 1).[8] There also appears to be a wide range in fractional venous resistance in lungs of different species (Figure 2),[12] ranging from 10% in some dog lung lobes to as high as 45% to 55% in neonatal lambs. In sheep, fractional venous resistance decreases with age. This finding is consistent in data obtained in isolated perfused lungs taken from lambs at different ages as well as in data obtained in awake, unanesthetized lambs and adult sheep in vivo (Figure 3). A high basal fractional venous resistance has considerable significance in the patho-

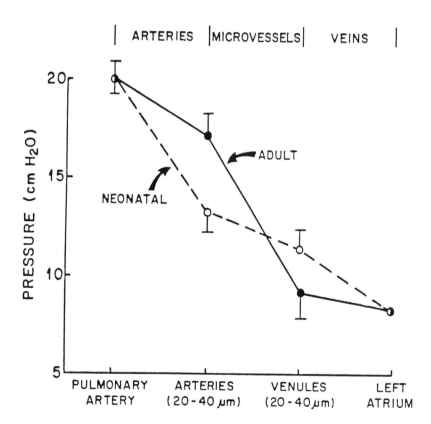

Figure 1. Vascular pressure profile in isolated perfused lungs of neonatal and adult rabbits. Lungs were perfused with blood, under zone 3 conditions (airway pressure = 5 cm H_2O, left atrial pressure = 7 cm H_2O), and flow rate was adjusted so that total pulmonary vascular pressure drop was similar in both groups of rabbit lungs (13 cm H_2O). In adult lungs, the main site of vascular pressure drop was the microvascular segment, whereas in neonatal lungs, arteries and veins contributed significantly to total vascular pressure drop.

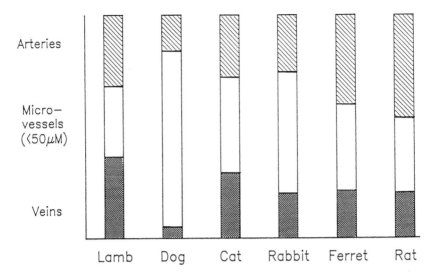

Figure 2. Comparison of fractional segmental vascular resistance in lungs of six species. Data for the dog are from Reference 9; data for the cat are from Reference 19; for the rabbit, from Reference 8; for the lamb, from Reference 5, and for the rat, from Reference 10. See text for details.

genesis of pulmonary edema, since any further venous constriction resulting from pathological situations such as hypoxemia, sepsis, etc, may further increase microvascular pressures for fluid filtration and may precipitate fulminant edema.

Vascular geometry and changes in active vasomotor tone primarily affect venous resistance, whereas passive factors primarily alter capillary resistance. There are contractile interstitial cells present adjacent to the capillaries that may, by changing their shape, alter capillary resistance in some instances.[13] Since changes in venous resistance primarily alter microvascular pressures, it is important to recognize and detect venous constriction in pathological conditions. Hypoxia can result in venous constriction and increased microvascular pressures for fluid filtration in some species at all ages, and in other species, only in the developing animal. The arteries, especially the small precapillary arterioles, have always been thought to be the primary site of constriction during hypoxia. In the ovine species, hypoxia results in an increase in lung fluid filtration and lung lymph flow in newborn lambs[14] but not in adult sheep.[15] One explanation for the increase in lymph flow may be that there is an increase in blood flow through a few vessels at the top of the lung, resulting in higher microvascular pressures in the overperfused vessels and greater fluid filtration,[16] and the other is that ac-

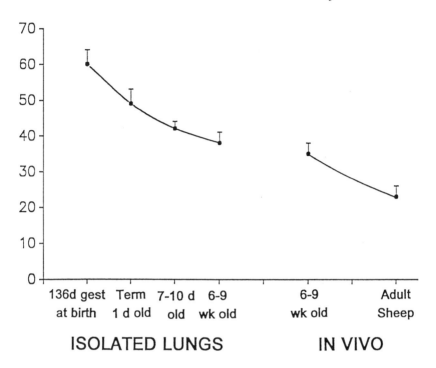

Figure 3. Influence of age on fractional venous resistance in ovine lungs. Sixty percent of total vascular resistance was contributed by veins in isolated per-fused preterm lamb lungs; this dropped to 40% by 6 weeks to 9 weeks of age. When venous resistance was partitioned in vivo using small catheters to obtain small venular pressures in awake, unanesthetized, chronically catheterized sheep, veins contributed 38% to total vascular resistance in 6- to 9-week-old sheep and only 23% in adult sheep.

tive venoconstriction may occur during hypoxia, resulting in higher microvascular pressures and increased fluid and protein filtration during hypoxia.[6] Venoconstriction during hypoxia is also seen in lungs of other species such as the ferret (Figure 4),[17] pig,[18] and cat,[19] but not in the rabbit.[20] Thus, hypoxic venoconstriction can greatly aggravate the tendency to edema formation. The pulmonary veins also constrict vigorously in response to a variety of vasoactive mediators such as platelet activating factor,[21] thromboxane,[22] and endothelin.[23] Therefore, in pathological conditions such as sepsis, where increased amounts of these mediators may be synthesized locally, active venoconstriction will increase microvascular pressures for fluid filtration and increase the tendency to pulmonary edema formation.

Passive factors may also alter the distribution of pressures such that the pressures in the filtering sites are closer to pulmonary artery pressure than under baseline conditions. An increase in blood flow rate

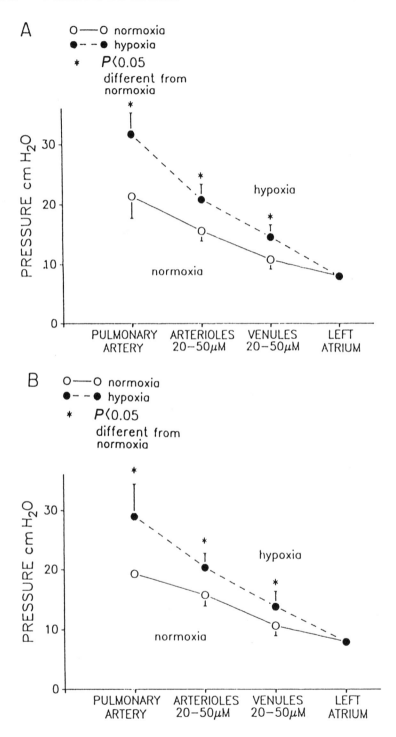

does not always affect pressures in the filtering segment. The effect of an increase in blood flow on microvascular pressures depends on the initial state of the pulmonary vascular bed, ie, the state of recruitment of the capillary bed. In adult sheep, Coates et al[24] found that when cardiac output was increased by infusion of isoproterenol without any change in ventilation, there was no increase in pulmonary artery or left atrial pressures and no suggestion of an increase in microvascular filtration pressures, indicating that when the lung vascular bed is only partially recruited, large increases in blood flow are accommodated with increases in the perfused surface area in the filtering segment and there may be little change in vascular pressures. Similarly, in neonatal lambs, when blood flow through the lungs was increased by the opening of an external shunt between the carotid artery and the jugular vein, lymph flow increased without a change in lymph protein concentration, indicating no change in microvascular pressures.[25] However, under conditions of maximal or submaximal recruitment, increases in blood flow can cause significant increases in microvascular and venous pressures, both in the neonatal[5,26] and adult[27,28] lung. Also, in situations where fractional venous resistance is high[5] or venous distensibility is low,[29] increases in blood flow rate will shift the filtration midpoint upstream toward the pulmonary artery,[30] resulting in microvascular filtration pressures that approach the pressure in the pulmonary artery (Figure 5). Very large increases in pulmonary blood flow and a shift of microvascular pressures toward the pulmonary artery pressure may account for the development of pulmonary edema in elite athletes and in racehorses.[31]

The resistance to flow in the circulation is determined by both vascular geometry and blood viscosity. Hematocrit is an important determinant of blood viscosity, and in the macrocirculation the effect of an increase in hematocrit is an increase in resistance to blood flow to many organs, including the lungs.[32–35] At the microcirculatory level, however, little is known about how the increase in hematocrit affects the distribution of pressures in the filtering segment of the lung. Considerable work has been done on the effects of hematocrit on the systemic microvessels, although these data cannot be used to explain the events in the pulmonary microcirculation. In fact, in the pulmonary capillary bed there may be large numbers of unrecruited capillaries for transit of

---

Figure 4. Effect of hypoxia on pulmonary vascular pressures in isolated perfused adult (n=5) and 3- to 5-week-old (n=5) ferret lungs. During perfusion, left atrial pressure was kept constant at 8 cm H_2O. In both groups of lungs, with hypoxia, pressure rose significantly in pulmonary arteries, arterioles, and venules.

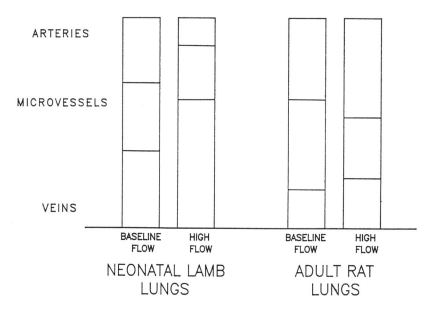

Figure 5. When fractional venous resistance is high under baseline conditions (lamb lungs), the effect of a threefold increase in blood flow rate is to push microvascular pressures closer to pulmonary artery pressure. In lungs with low fractional venous resistance as in the rat, this effect is not so prominent.

the trapped red blood cells. Also, the size and distensibility of pulmonary capillaries are probably larger than those of the systemic circulation. The effect of perfusate hematocrit and apparent viscosity on pulmonary microvascular pressures in isolated perfused rabbit lungs was studied by Raj et al.[36] They found that with an increase in perfusate hematocrit, there was an increase in total pulmonary vascular resistance, mainly due to an increase in resistance in small arteries and veins (Figure 6). Surprisingly, there was no effect of hematocrit in small capillaries and in large conduit arteries and veins. The effect of the large increase in small venous resistance is an increase in pressures in the upstream fluid filtration sites in capillaries and in small arterioles that results in increased fluid filtration. This nonhomogenous effect of an increase in perfusate hematocrit in the different longitudinal segments of the pulmonary circulation is important, since the very large increase in resistance in small veins greatly increases hydrostatic pressures at upstream filtration sites. The larger increase in resistance in small veins as compared to small arteries may be due to the fact that intraluminal pressures are lower in veins than in arteries, resulting in smaller transmural diameters in these vessels and a greater hindrance.

The lack of an effect of hematocrit in capillaries may have several

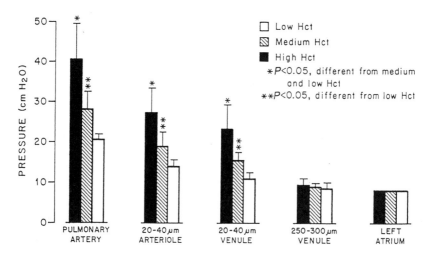

Figure 6. With an increase in perfusate hematocrit, total pulmonary vascular resistance increased significantly mainly because of an increase in resistance in arteries and small veins. Resistance in microvessels and that in large veins did not change appreciably with increases in hematocrit.

explanations: a significant Fahraeus and Lindqvist effect[37] in the pulmonary capillaries as in systemic capillaries, ie, a reduction in hematocrit in small vessels so that there is very little change in small vessel viscosity. Alternately, there may have been significant capillary distention and, thus, a compensation for the increase in perfusate hematocrit, such that actual resistance to flow is maintained the same in the capillaries. At any rate, in a lung where venous resistance is already high due to hypoxia and the presence of vasoconstrictor inflammatory mediators, the presence of a high hematocrit may tip the scales toward very high venous resistance, high microvascular pressures, increased fluid filtration, and pulmonary edema.

Other passive factors that alter the longitudinal distribution of vascular resistances include alveolar surface tension, which alters interstitial liquid pressure around capillaries[38] and thus, the distending pressures for capillaries and capillary resistance. Lung volume and alveolar gas pressure also affect the distribution of pressures,[39] and thus moment to moment changes in fluid filtration levels may be effected by changes in ventilatory patterns.

The distribution of pressures in pulmonary microcirculation not only affects fluid filtration and edema formation, but it also affects the entry of fluid back into the circulation. At the time of birth, the volume of fetal lung liquid in the potential airspaces is cleared from the lungs by 6 hours of age.[40] A brief increase in lung lymph flow accounts for only 10% of total volume of liquid cleared, so that most of the fluid seems to be cleared by the pulmonary circulation. The presence of increased microvascular filtration pressures and increased fluid filtration rates in the lung at the time of birth potentially slows the clearance of liquid and/or results in an increased contribution of lymphatics. To determine this, the effect of an increase in left atrial pressure and raised microvascular filtration pressures on the rate of liquid clearance was studied in neonatal lambs.[41] Presence of increased pulmonary microvascular pressures resulted in a delay in clearance of the lung liquid, especially during the first 2 hours, but by 6 hours most of the lung liquid was cleared. A small transient increase in lymph flow accounted for approximately 6% of the total volume of fluid cleared, indicating that lung lymphatics play a minor role in clearance of lung liquid, even under conditions of increased microvascular pressures.

References

1. Conhaim RL, Lai-Fook SJ, Staub NC. Sequence of perivascular liquid accumulation in liquid-inflated dog lung lobes. *J Appl Physiol* 1986;60: 513–520.
2. Mitzner W, Robatham JL. Distribution of interstitial compliance and filtration coefficient in canine lung. *Lymphology* 1979;12:140–148.
3. Starling EH. On the absorption of fluids from the connective tissue spaces. *J Physiol* 1896;19:312–326.
4. Gaar KA, Taylor AE, Owens LJ, Guyton AC. Pulmonary capillary pressure and filtration coefficient in the isolated perfused lung. *Am J Physiol* 1967;213:910–914.
5. Raj JU, Chen P. Microvascular pressures measured by micropuncture in isolated perfused lamb lungs. *J Appl Physiol* 1986;61:2194–2201.
6. Raj JU, Chen P. Micropuncture measurement of microvascular pressures in lamb lungs during hypoxia. *Circ Res* 1986;59:398–404.
7. Raj JU, Chen P, Navazo L. Micropuncture measurement of lung microvascular pressure profile in 3–4 week old rabbits. *Ped Res* 1986;20: 1107–1111.
8. Raj JU, Bland RD, Lai-Fook SJ. Microvascular pressures measured by micropipette in isolated edematous rabbit lungs. *J Appl Physiol* 1986;60: 539–545.
9. Bhattacharya J, Staub NC. Direct measurement of microvascular pressures in the isolated perfused dog lung. *Science* 1980;210:327–328.
10. Hillyard R, Anderson J, Raj JU. Segmental vascular resistance in isolated perfused rat lungs. Influence of vasomotor tone and cyclooxygenase and lipoxygenase inhibition. *Circ Res* 1991;68:1020–1026.
11. Bland RD, Hansen TN, Hazinski TA, Haberkern CM, Bressack MA. Studies of lung fluid balance in newborn lambs. *Ann N Y Acad Sci* 1982;384: 126–144.
12. Raj JU, Hillyard R, Kaapa P, Anderson J, Gropper M. Pulmonary vascular pressure profile in 2–3 week old, 5–6 week old, and adult ferrets. *Respir Physiol* 1990;82:307–317.

13. Kapanci Y, Assimacopoulos A, Irle C, Zwahlem A, Gabbiani G. Contractile interstitial cells in pulmonary alveolar septa. A possible regulator of ventilation/perfusion ratio. *J Cell Biol* 1974;60:375–392.
14. Bressack MA, Bland RD. Alveolar hypoxia increases lung fluid filtration in unanesthetized newborn lambs. *Circ Res* 1980;46:111–116.
15. Bland RD, Demling RH, Selinger SL, Staub NC. Effects of alveolar hypoxia on lung fluid and protein transport in unanesthetized sheep. *Circ Res* 1976;40:269–274.
16. Hansen TN, LeBlanc AL, Gest AL. Hypoxia and angiotensin II infusion redistribute lung blood flow in lambs. *J Appl Physiol* 1985;58:812–818.
17. Raj JU, Hillyard R, Kaapa P, Anderson J, Gropper M. Pulmonary arterial and venous constriction during hypoxia in 3–5 week old and adult ferrets. *J Appl Physiol* 1990;69:2183–2189.
18. Fike CD, Kaplowitz MR. Pulmonary venous pressure increases during alveolar hypoxia in isolated lungs of newborn pigs. *J Appl Physiol* 1992; 73:552–556.
19. Nagasaka Y, Bhattacharya J, Nanjo S, Gropper MA, Staub NC. Micropuncture measurement of lung microvascular pressure profile during hypoxia in cats. *Circ Res* 1984;54:90–95.
20. Fike CD, Lai-Fook SJ, Bland RD. Microvascular pressures during hypoxia in isolated lungs of newborn rabbits. *J Appl Physiol* 1988;65:283–287.
21. Toga H, Hitler S, Ibe BO, Raj JU. Vascular effects of platelet activating factor: Role of cyclo- and lipoxygenase. *J Appl Physiol* 1992;73:2559–2566.
22. Raj JU, Toga H, Ibe BO, Anderson J. Effects of endothelin, platelet activating factor and thromboxane A2 in ferret lungs. *Respir Physiol* 1992;88: 129–140.
23. Toga H, Ibe BO, Raj JU. In vitro responses of ovine intrapulmonary arteries and veins to endothelin-1: Effect of age. *Am J Physiol* 1992;263:15–21.
24. Coates G, O'Brodovich H, Jeffries AL, Wyatt DG. Effects of exercise on lung lymph flow in sheep and goats during normoxia and hypoxia. *J Clin Invest* 1984;74:133–141.
25. Feltes TF, Hansen TN. Effects of a large aorticopulmonary shunt on lung fluid balance in newborn lambs. *Pediatr Res* 1989;26:94–97.
26. Teague WG, Berner ME, Bland RD. Effect of pulmonary perfusion on lung fluid filtration in young lambs. *Am J Physiol* 1988;255:H1336–H1341.
27. Hyman AL. Effects of large increases in pulmonary blood flow on pulmonary venous pressure. *J Appl Physiol* 1969;27:179–185.
28. Landolt CC, Matthay MA. Overperfusion, hypoxia, and increased pressure cause only hydrostatic pulmonary edema in anesthetized sheep. *Circ Res* 1983;52:335–341.
29. Fike CD, Kaplowitz MR. Effect of blood flow rate and blood flow history on the newborn pulmonary circulation. *Am J Physiol* 1991;261:271–279.
30. Younes M, Bshouty Z, Ali J. Longitudinal distribution of pulmonary vascular resistance with very high pulmonary blood flow. *J Appl Physiol* 1987;62:344–358.
31. West JB, Mathieu-Costello O. Stress failure of pulmonary capillaries: Role in lung and heart disease. *Lancet* 1992;340:762–767.
32. Benis AM, Tavares P, Mortara F, Lockhart A. Effect of hematocrit on pressure flow relations for isolated perfused lobes of the canine lung. *Pflügers Arch* 1970;314:347–360.
33. Julien M, Hakim TS, Vahi R, Chang HK. Effect of hematocrit on vascular pressure profile in dog lungs. *J Appl Physiol* 1985;58:743–748.

34. Murray JF, Karp RB, Nadel JA. Viscosity effects on pressure flow relations and vascular resistance in dog lungs. *J Appl Physiol* 1969;27:336–341.
35. Nihill MR, McNamara DN, Vick RL. The effects of increased blood viscosity on pulmonary vascular resistance. *Am Heart J* 1976;92:65–72.
36. Raj JU, Ramanathan R, Chen P, Anderson J. Effect of hematocrit on microvascular pressures in 3-to 5-wk-old rabbit lungs. *Am J Physiol* 1989;256: H766–H771.
37. Fahraeus R, Lindqvist R. The viscosity of the blood in narrow capillary tubes. *Am J Physiol* 1931;96:562–568.
38. Raj JU. Alveolar liquid pressure measured by micropuncture in isolated lungs of mature and immature fetal rabbits. *J Clin Invest* 1987;79:1579–1588.
39. Raj JU, Chen P, Navazo L. Effect of inflation on microvascular pressures in lungs of young rabbits. *Am J Physiol* 1987;252:H80–H84.
40. Bland RD, Hansen TN, Haberkern CM, et al. Lung fluid balance in lambs before and after birth. *J Appl Physiol* 1982;53:992–1004.
41. Raj JU, Bland RD. Lung luminal liquid clearance in newborn lambs. Effect of pulmonary microvascular pressure elevation. *Am Rev Respir Dis* 1986; 134:305–310.

Chapter 13

Effects of Sustained Hydrostatic Pressure on the Expression of Endothelial Cell-Leukocyte Adhesion Molecules

Eric A. Schwartz, BS, Rena Bizios, PhD, and Mary E. Gerritsen, PhD

Introduction

In the mammalian cardiovascular system, endothelial cells are exposed to three types of mechanical forces: shear stresses, resulting from the flow of blood at the cell surface; tensile stresses, resulting from the pulsatile nature of blood flow and the compliance of the vessel wall; and hydrostatic pressure, resulting from containment of blood within the vasculature. These forces are detected by and transduced by the endothelial cells into various biological responses; for example, the morphology of endothelial cells in arteries is the result of exposure to shear stresses of specific direction and magnitude.[1-4] The responses of endothelial cells to fluid shear stresses and tensile stresses have been extensively studied in vitro.[5-8] In response to fluid shear, endothelial cells rearrange cytoskeletal stress fibers, elongate, and align their long axes in the direction of flow.[5-7] In contrast, endothelial cells respond to cyclic stretch by elongating perpendicularly to the direction of stretch.[8] Fluid shear and cyclic stretch elicit cellular and biochemical responses including cell proliferation,[5] changes in ion flux,[9-11] synthesis, and release of vasoactive compounds,[8,12-14] as well as altered expression of surface adhesion molecules.[15-17] Moreover, shear-sensitive transcription factors have been implicated in the upregulation of gene expression, and

From: Weir EK, Reeves JT (eds). *Pulmonary Edema*. Armonk, NY: Futura Publishing Company, Inc.; ©1998.

a putative, cis-acting shear stress response element in the promoter region of the gene for platelet-derived growth factor has recently been identified.[18-20]

The response of endothelial cells to hydrostatic pressure has only recently received attention.[21-23] Exposure of either subconfluent bovine pulmonary artery endothelial cells to 1.5 cm H_2O to 15 cm H_2O sustained hydrostatic pressure for time periods of up to 7 days[21]; subconfluent bovine aortic endothelial cells to 40 mm Hg to 80 mm Hg (54 cm H_2O to 109 cm H_2O) sustained hydrostatic pressure for time periods of 1 day to 9 days[22]; or confluent bovine aortic endothelial cells to flow (either oscillatory shear stress of time-averaged amplitude of 0.2 dynes/cm^2 and an oscillatory component of ± 15 dynes/cm^2 or steady shear stress of 0.2 dynes/cm^2) concurrent with hydrostatic pressure of 40 mm Hg (54 cm H_2O) for 12 hours to 48 hours[23] results in reorganization of the cytoskeleton, characterized by linear alignment of stress fibers, and reduction or loss of the characteristic peripheral actin band.[21-23] Furthermore, exposure of subconfluent bovine pulmonary artery endothelial cells[21] and bovine aortic endothelial cells[22] to sustained hydrostatic pressure results in cell elongation[21,22] and an increased proliferative rate, associated with formation of multiple layers.[21] This increased proliferation results, at least in part, from secretion of basic fibroblast growth factor (bFGF) from internal stores.[21]

The demonstration of morphological changes and growth factor secretion by endothelial cells exposed to sustained hydrostatic pressure suggests that there may be additional alterations in endothelial cell phenotype. This chapter investigates expression of several cell surface molecules, specifically intercellular adhesion molecule 1 (ICAM-1 or CD54), vascular cell adhesion molecule 1 (VCAM-1 or CD106), E-selectin (CD62E), platelet-endothelial cell adhesion molecule (PECAM or CD31), and the constitutive endothelial cell surface antigen, p96, by human umbilical vein endothelial cells (HUVEC) to sustained hydrostatic pressure.

Pressure Experiments: Cell Surface Molecules

HUVEC (Clonetics, San Diego, CA) were cultured in Medium 199 (Gibco, Gaithersburg, MD), supplemented with 10% fetal bovine serum (HyClone, Provo, UT), 90 U/mL heparin (Fisher, Springfield, NJ), and bovine brain extract (Clonetics) on gelatin- (1.5% w/w; Sigma, St. Louis, MO) coated tissue culture flasks (Becton-Dickinson, Franklin Lakes, NJ) under standard, sterile cell culture conditions in a 37°C, humidified, 5% CO_2/95% air environment.

The effect of sustained hydrostatic pressure on the expression of cell surface molecules (specifically, ICAM-1, VCAM-1, E-Selectin,

CD31, and p96) was examined by exposure of confluent HUVEC (passage 3–9) to hydrostatic heads of culture media, at a pressure of 4 cm H_2O, for 24 hours. Controls consisted of parallel cultures, seeded at similar cell densities and grown on identical substrates (to the HUVEC exposed to 4 cm H_2O pressure), but subsequently maintained in culture media under standard cell culture conditions (0.2 cm H_2O pressure; 37°C; humidified; 5% CO_2/95% air environment) for 24 hours. For studies aimed at examination of cell surface molecule response to sustained hydrostatic pressure in combination with endothelial activation, cells were either exposed simultaneously to pressure (4 cm H_2O) and to 100 ng/mL *E. coli* lipopolysaccharide (LPS; Sigma) or to each one of the two stimuli separately (controls).

Following the 24-hour incubation under these conditions, the culture media were removed and the cells washed with Versene (Gibco). Cells were trypsinized, washed, and incubated with either phycoerythrin-conjugated monoclonal antibodies to ICAM-1 (C78.5; Bayer, West Haven, CT), VCAM-1 (C313.4; Bayer), or E-Selectin (H18/7; kindly donated by Dr. M.A. Gimbrone, Jr., Brigham and Women's Hospital, Boston, MA), or with unlabeled primary mouse monoclonal antibodies to either CD31 (Dako, Carpinteria, CA), or p96 (also donated by Dr. M.A. Gimbrone, Jr.). After washing and incubating with fluorescein-conjugated rabbit antimouse antisera (in the case of unlabeled primary antibodies), expression of cell surface antigens was assessed by fluorescence activated cell sorting (FACS®) with use of a Becton-Dickinson FACScan.

In this study, the effects of sustained hydrostatic pressure on endothelial cells under basal (media alone) and activated (media containing 100 ng/mL LPS) conditions were evaluated. The effects of these conditions on two constitutive endothelial cell antigens, CD31 and p96 were examined. Neither pressure, LPS, nor the combination of the two stimuli altered the surface expression of CD31, a constitutively expressed endothelial cell antigen that has a role both in adhesion of leukocytes to the endothelium and, possibly, in angiogenesis, wound healing, and early cardiovascular development.[24] Previous studies have shown that CD31 is not upregulated by cytokines[25] or shear stress.[14] Another constitutive surface antigen expressed by endothelial cells, p96,[26] was also unaffected by either hydrostatic pressure or LPS, separately and in combination (Figure 1 and Table 1).

Results

The expression of the adhesion molecules ICAM-1, VCAM-1, and E-selectin (which mediate endothelium/leukocyte interactions) can be modulated by a number of external stimuli. ICAM-1, which demon-

Table 1

Effects of Sustained Hydrostatic Pressure and LPS on the Expression of Constitutive Surface Antigens by Endothelial Cells

	Mean Fluorescent Intensity			
Surface Antigen	Control	Pressure	LPS	LPS + Pressure
CD31	97.6	98.5	92.4	101.2
p96	54.5	55.1	65.1	62.8

HUVEC were either maintained under control (0.2 cm H_2O) pressure conditions (in the presence and absence of 100 ng/mL LPS) or exposed to 4 cm H_2O sustained hydrostatic pressure (in the presence and absence of 100 ng/mL LPS) for 24 hours. HUVEC were either immunofluorescently labeled with primary antibodies for CD31 and p96, or were left unlabeled; all samples were subsequently stained with fluorescent secondary antisera. Fluorescent intensities were read for 10,000 cells using a FACS® analyzer. LPS = lipopolysaccharide; HUVEC = human umbilical vein endothelial cells; FACS = fluorescence-activated cell sorting.

strates constitutive expression, is upregulated by cytokines[16,27–32] (interleukin-1, tumor necrosis factor, LPS), oxidants,[32] and fluid shear.[15,33] Little or no VCAM-1 and E-selectin are expressed under basal conditions,[16,33] but both can be markedly upregulated by inflammatory cytokines.[16,28] Physical forces, however, affect these molecules differently: VCAM-1 is either up-or downregulated, depending on the details of loading (ie, shear or stretch, cyclic or steady, laminar or turbulent, and high or low stress).[16,33–36] In contrast, E-selectin is unaffected by shear.[16,33]

Exposure of endothelial cells to sustained hydrostatic pressure had no effect on the basal expression of either E-selectin, VCAM-1, or ICAM-1 (Figure 1). In agreement with earlier studies, treatment of HUVEC with LPS resulted in increased expression of ICAM-1, VCAM-1, and E-selectin (Figure 1 and Table 2). Hydrostatic pressure had no effect on LPS-induced ICAM-1 and VCAM-1 expression. However, pressure did appear to have a modest effect on the magnitude of the E-selectin response to LPS (Figure 1 and Table 2). This result may be due to prolongation of surface E-selectin expression. Normally, cytokine-induced upregulation of E-selectin is maximal at 4 hours to 6 hours, and by 24 hours it is decreasing toward baseline levels.[29]

Many pathophysiological conditions of endothelial cells in vivo are linked to increased pressures; for example, hypertension leading to atherosclerosis,[37] glaucoma leading to retinal microangiopathy,[10,38]

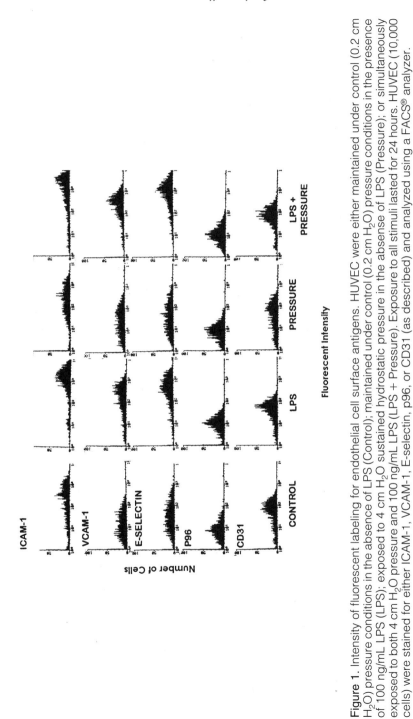

Figure 1. Intensity of fluorescent labeling for endothelial cell surface antigens. HUVEC were either maintained under control (0.2 cm H$_2$O) pressure conditions in the absence of LPS (Control); maintained under control (0.2 cm H$_2$O) pressure conditions in the presence of 100 ng/mL LPS (LPS); exposed to 4 cm H$_2$O sustained hydrostatic pressure in the absense of LPS (Pressure); or simultaneously exposed to both 4 cm H$_2$O pressure and 100 ng/mL LPS (LPS + Pressure). Exposure to all stimuli lasted for 24 hours. HUVEC (10,000 cells) were stained for either ICAM-1, VCAM-1, E-selectin, p96, or CD31 (as described) and analyzed using a FACS® analyzer.

Table 2

Effects of Sustained Hydrostatic Pressure and LPS on the Expression of Endothelial Cell-Leukocyte Adhesion Molecules

	Mean Fluorescent Intensity			
Surface Antigen	Control	Pressure	LPS	LPS + Pressure
ICAM-1	126.4	131.9	186.0	181.9
VCAM-1	78.2	83.1	131.5	140.4
E-Selectin	88.5	92.8	156.8	186.5
No primary antibody	63.16	59.2	61.4	64.1

HUVEC were either maintained under control (0.2 cm H_2O) pressure conditions (in the presence and absence of 100 ng/mL LPS) or exposed to 4 cm H_2O sustained hydrostatic pressure (in the presence and absence of 100 ng/mL LPS) for 24 hours. HUVEC were immunofluorescently labeled either with fluorescent primary antibodies for ICAM-1, VCAM-1, and E-selectin, or with fluorescent rabbit anit-mouse antisera. Fluorescent intensities were read for 10,000 cells using a FACS® analyzer.

LPS = lipopolysaccharide; HUVEC = human umbilical vein endothelial cells; ICAM = intercellular adhesion molecule; VCAM = vascular cell adhesion molecule; FACS = fluorescence-activated cell sorting.

and constrained tumor growth leading to angiogenesis and metastasis.[39] Accumulating data have documented the effects of fluid shear and of blood vessel wall stretch on a variety of endothelial properties (reviewed in Reference 14). However, the effects of hydrostatic pressure (the most pertinent force in pressure-related illnesses) on vascular cell function has been addressed only recently.[21-23]

The results of the present study confirm that endothelial cell responses to physical forces are specific and selective. As with shear,[14] surface expression of the constitutive endothelial cell surface molecule CD31 does not change in response to sustained hydrostatic pressure. In contrast to shear stress, sustained hydrostatic pressure does not increase the surface expression of the adhesion molecule ICAM-1, nor does pressure alter surface expression of VCAM-1. Furthermore, hydrostatic pressure does not contribute to the expression of ICAM-1 and VCAM-1, but it may have a modest effect on the E-selectin response to LPS.

Further studies comparing and contrasting the effects of physical forces on endothelial cells may provide important clues toward an improved understanding of how these clinically important environmental stimuli are integrated by the endothelial cell under normal and pathological states.

Acknowledgments   The authors acknowledge the Whitaker Foundation for a graduate fellowship to E.A. Schwartz.

References

1. Flaherty JT, Pierce JE, Ferrans VJ, et al. Endothelial nuclear patterns in the canine arterial tree with particular reference to hemodynamic events. *Circ Res* 1972;30:23–33.
2. Langille BL, Adamson SL. Relationship between blood flow direction and endothelial cell orientation at arterial branch sites in rabbits and mice. *Circ Res* 1981;48:481–488.
3. Nerem RM, Levesque MJ, Cornhill JF. Vascular endothelial morphology as an indicator of the pattern of blood flow. *J Biomech Eng* 1981;103: 172–177.
4. Levesque MJ, Liepsch D, Moravec S, et al. Correlation of endothelial cell shape and wall shear stress in a stenosed dog aorta. *Arteriosclerosis* 1986;6: 220–229.
5. Dewey CJ Jr, Bussolari SR, Gimbrone MA Jr, et al. The dynamic response of vascular endothelial cells to fluid shear stress. *J Biomech Eng* 1981;103: 177–185.
6. Eskin SG, Ives CL, McIntire LV, et al. Response of cultured endothelial cells to steady flow. *Microvasc Res* 1984;28:87–93.
7. Levesque MJ, Nerem RM. The elongation and orientation of cultured endothelial cells in response to shear stress. *J Biomech Eng* 1985;176:341–347.
8. Carosi JA, Eskin SG, McIntire LV. Cyclical strain effects on the production of vasoactive materials in cultured endothelial cells. *J Cell Physiol* 1992;151: 29–36.
9. Ando J, Komatsuda T, Kamiya A. Cytoplasmic calcium response to fluid shear stress in cultured vascular endothelial cells. *In Vitro Cell Dev Biol Anim* 1988;24:871–877.
10. Nakabayashi M, Kishida K, Okazaki H. Effect of experimental ocular hypertension on macrovacuolization in Schlemm's canal endothelial cells of monkey eyes. *Ophthalmic Res* 1991;23:177–186.
11. Schwarz G, Callewaert G, Droogmans G, et al. Shear stress-induced calcium transients in endothelial cells from human umbilical cord veins. *J Physiol (Lond)* 1992;458:527–538.
12. Diamond SL, Eskin SG, McIntire LV. Fluid flow stimulates tissue plasminogen activator secretion by cultured human endothelial cells. *Science* 1989;243:1483–1485.
13. Frangos JA, Eskin SG, McIntire LV, et al. Flow effects on prostacyclin production by cultured human endothelial cells. *Science* 1985;227:1477–1479.
14. Patrick CW Jr, McIntire LV. Shear stress and cyclic strain modulation of gene expression in vascular endothelial cells. *Blood Purif* 1995;13:112–124.
15. Nagel T, Resnick N, Atkinson WJ, et al. Shear stress selectively upregulates intercellular adhesion molecule-1 expression in cultured human vascular endothelial cells. *J Clin Invest* 1994;94:885–891.
16. Sampath R, Kukielka GL, Smith CW, et al. Shear stress-mediated changes in the expression of leukocyte adhesion receptors on human umbilical vein endothelial cells in vitro. *Ann Biomed Eng* 1995;23:247–256.
17. Jones DA, Smith CW, McIntire LV. Leucocyte adhesion under flow conditions: Principles important in tissue engineering. *Biomaterials* 1996;17: 337–347.
18. Resnick N, Gimbrone MA Jr. Hemodynamic forces are complex regulators of endothelial gene expression. *FASEB J* 1995;9:874–882.
19. Lan Q, Mercurius KO, Davies PF. Stimulation of transcription factors NF

kappa B and AP1 in endothelial cells subjected to shear stress. *Biochem Biophys Res Commun* 1994;201:950–956.

20. Resnick N, Collins T, Atkinson W, et al. Platelet-derived growth factor b chain promoter contains a cis-acting fluid shear-stress-responsive-element. *Proc Natl Acad Sci U S A* 1993;90:4591–4595.

21. Acevedo AD, Bowser SS, Gerritsen ME, et al. Morphological and proliferative responses of endothelial cells to hydrostatic pressure: Role of fibroblast growth factor. *J Cell Physiol* 1993;157:603–614.

22. Sumpio BE, Widmann MD, Ricotta J, et al. Increased ambient pressure stimulates proliferation and morphologic changes in cultured endothelial cells. *J Cell Physiol* 1994;158:133–138.

23. Thoumine O, Nerem RM, Girard PR. Oscillatory shear stress and hydrostatic pressure modulate cell-matrix attachment proteins in cultured endothelial cells. *In Vitro Cell Dev Biol Anim* 1995;31:45–54.

24. DeLisser MH, Newman PJ, Albeda SM. Platelet endothelial cell adhesion molecule (CD31). *Curr Top Microbiol Immunol* 1993;184:37–45.

25. Romer LH, McLean NV, Yan HC, et al. IFN-gamma and TNF-alpha induce redistribution of PECAM-1 (CD31) on human endothelial cells. *J Immunol* 1995;154:6582–6592.

26. Read MA, Neish AS, Luscinskas FW, et al. The proteasome pathway is required for cytokine-induced endothelial-leukocyte adhesion molecule expression. *Immunity* 1995;2:493–506.

27. Dustin ML, Rothlein R, Bhan AK, et al. Induction by IL-1 and interferon-gamma: Tissue distribution, biochemistry, and function of a natural adherence molecule (ICAM-1). *J Immunol* 1986;137:245–254.

28. Pober JS, Gimbrone MA Jr, Lapierre LA, et al. Overlapping patterns of activation of human endothelial cells by interleukin 1, tumor necrosis factor, and immune interferon. *J Immunol* 1986;137:1893–1896.

29. Bevilacqua MP, Stengelin S, Gimbrone MA Jr, et al. Endothelial leukocyte adhesion molecule-1: An inducible receptor for neutrophils related to complement regulatory proteins and lectins. *Science* 1989;243:1160–1165.

30. Rice GE, Munro JM, Bevilacqua MP. Inducible cell adhesion molecule 110 (INCAM-110) is an endothelial receptor for lymphocytes. A CD11/CD18 independent adhesion mechanism. *J Exp Med* 1990;171:1369–1374.

31. Sluiter W, Pietersma A, Lamers JM, et al. Leukocyte adhesion molecules on the vascular endothelium: Their role in the pathogenesis of cardiovascular disease and the mechanisms underlying their expression. *J Cardiovasc Pharmacol* 1993;22:S37–S44.

32. Roebuck KA, Rahman A, Lakshminarayanan V, et al. H_2O_2 and tumor necrosis factor-alpha activate intercellular adhesion molecule 1 (ICAM-1) gene transcription through distinct cis-regulatory elements within the ICAM-1 promoter. *J Biol Chem* 1995;270:18966–18974.

33. Morigi M, Zoja C, Figliuzzi M, et al. Fluid shear stress modulates surface expression of adhesion molecules by endothelial cells. *Blood* 1995;85:1696–1703.

34. Davies PF, Remuzzi A, Dewey CF, et al. Turbulent fluid shear stress induces vascular endothelial cell turnover in vitro. *Proc Natl Acad Sci U S A* 1986;83:2114–2118.

35. Ohtsuka A, Ando J, Korenaga A, et al. The effect of flow on the expression of vascular cell adhesion molecule-1 by cultured mouse endothelial cells. *Biochem Biophys Res Commun* 1993;193:303–310.

36. Walpola PL, Gotleib AI, Cybulsky MI, et al. Expression of ICAM-1 and

VCAM-1 and monocyte adherence in arteries exposed to altered shear stress. *Arterioscler Thromb* 1995;15:2–10.

37. Thubrikar MJ, Robicsek F. Pressure-induced arterial wall stress and atherosclerosis. *Ann Thorac Surg* 1995;683:1594–1603.

38. Aiello LP, Avery RL, Arrigg PG. Vascular endothelial growth factor in ocular fluid of patients with diabetic retinopathy and other retinal diseases. *N Engl J Med* 1994;331:1480–1487.

39. Nathanson SD, Nelson L. Interstitial fluid pressure in breast cancer, benign breast conditions, and breast parenchyma. *Ann Surg Oncol* 1994;1: 333–338.

Increased Permeability and Pulmonary Edema

Chapter 14

Mechanisms of Receptor-Initiated Changes in Endothelial Permeability

D. Michael Shasby, MD and Alan B. Moy, MD

Inflammatory edema is an important immunologic and physiological response that facilitates the transfer of immunologically competent elements of plasma to the extravascular space. It is characterized by the loss of focal adhesion of adjacent endothelial cells.[1] Several agonists that can cause inflammatory edema have been identified, including serotonin, histamine, substance P, and products of polymorphonuclear leukocytes. In their recent studies, the authors have focused on changes in endothelial cells caused by histamine receptor activation, in order to more precisely identify the signaling pathways that have evolved to cause the changes in endothelial function that result in edema, and at the same time to avoid the confounding irrelevant effects of pluripotent proteases and oxidants.

In vivo, histamine causes a rapidly reversible loss of focal apposition of adjacent endothelial cells. After application of histamine, small gaps develop between adjacent cells, and they reseal within 3 to 5 minutes.[2] Histamine also causes an increase in the permeability to albumin of monolayers of cultured human umbilical vein endothelial (HUVE) cells and, as discussed later in this chapter, the response of HUVE cells to histamine is also transitory with restoration of the barrier within 3 to 5 minutes.[3]

The authors examined the response of HUVE cells to histamine in order to build a model in which histamine alters the focal apposition of

The work reported in this chapter was completed during Dr. Moy's tenure as a Clinician Scientist of the American Heart Association. It was supported by NIH grant HL33540.

From: Weir EK, Reeves JT (eds). *Pulmonary Edema*. Armonk, NY: Futura Publishing Company, Inc.; ©1998.

Model of centrifugal and centripetal forces acting to determine endothelial cell shape.

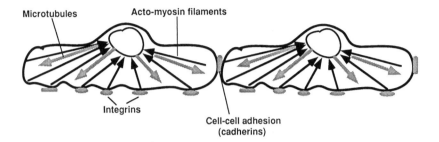

Figure 1. Model of forces acting to determine shape of endothelial cells.

adjacent cells by altering a balance of centripetal and centrifugal forces. In the model, the centripetal forces are determined largely by acto-myosin filaments. The centrifugal forces are determined principally by microtubules and by tethering of the cells at sites of focal adhesion between adjacent cells and between cells and substrate (Figure 1).

Role of Resting Centripetal Tension

Based on the model, histamine alters detectable endothelial focal adhesion by increasing centripetal tension, by decreasing centrifugal forces, or by altering both. Chelation of extracellular calcium causes a reversible loss of endothelial focal adhesion, detectable as an increase in endothelial permeability.[4,5] This effect is mediated, at least in part, by loss of tethering of cells to each other and to substrate because of the loss of calcium-dependent cadherin and integrin binding with chelation of extracellular calcium. The extent of myosin light chain (MLC) phosphorylation is a determinant of resting centripetal tension in HUVE cells.[6,7] The authors asked if the resting tension was necessary and sufficient to cause a detectable decrease in focal adhesion (measured as albumin flux across a monolayer) of adjacent HUVE cells. When MLC phosphorylation was reduced to very low levels (<0.1 mol phosphate per mol MLC), the decrease in focal adhesion detected as an increase in albumin flux across the monolayer was much less than it was in control cells.[8] This indicates that the resting tension was sufficient to cause a change in detectable focal adhesion of endothelial cells and that histamine could increase endothelial permeability by decreasing tethering without increasing centripetal tension.

Effect of Histamine on Tension

The next logical step was to measure centripetal tension in HUVE cells stimulated with histamine. Since MLC phosphorylation is an important determinant of centripetal tension, the authors also measured MLC phosphorylation in response to histamine. As a positive control, they also examined the effects of thrombin on MLC phosphorylation and centripetal tension. Histamine caused a small and very transitory increase in MLC phosphorylation, while thrombin increased phosphorylation by more than twice as much, and the duration of the increase was much longer (Figure 2).[6] The increase in MLC phosphorylation caused by thrombin can be prevented by pretreating the cells with ML-7, an inhibitor of myosin light chain kinase (MLCK) (Figure 3).[6] Thrombin increased the centripetal tension developed by HUVE cells, and this was prevented by pretreating the cells with ML-7. Hence, the thrombin-induced increase in tension was dependent on increased MLC phosphorylation.

In contrast to thrombin, histamine did not increase centripetal tension of HUVE cells (Figure 3).[6] Monolayers that did not show an increase in tension in response to histamine did increase tension when subsequently exposed to thrombin.[6] Hence, histamine causes a very small and transitory increase in MLC phosphorylation that does not increase centripetal tension of HUVE cells.

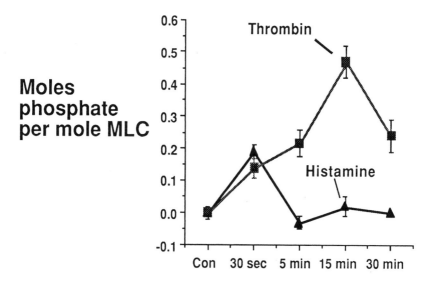

Figure 2. Phosphorylation of endothelial cell (HUVE cell) myosin light chain in response to histamine and thrombin.

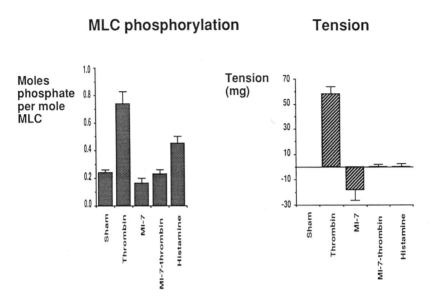

Figure 3. Phosphorylation of HUVE cell myosin light chain in response to thrombin (7 units/mL), an inhibitor of myosin light chain kinase-ML-7 (100 μmol/L), ML-7 (100 μmol/L) pretreatment followed by thrombin (7 units/mL), and histamine (1 × 10^{-5} mol/L).

Relationship of Increased Tension to Decrease in Endothelial Focal Adhesion

The authors were interested in determining how histamine altered focal adhesion. They concluded that since histamine did not increase tension, it must alter focal adhesion independent of an increase in centripetal tension. While the permeability assay was a reflection of changes in focal adhesion, it had poor resolution in time and magnitude. To improve the resolution of their measurements of focal adhesion, they adapted a method originated by Giaever and Keese.[9] Cells covering a small gold electrode increase the impedance of the electrode. The impedance is created by the resistances between cells, the resistance between cells and matrix, and the capacitance of the cell membrane. A model that incorporates these elements into a circuit closely predicts the responses of the cells to stimuli, which predictably affect one of the elements. This system measures focal adhesion in real time with microsecond resolution. As discussed below, it also allows us to resolve the impedance into its individual elements and determine which sites of focal adhesion are altered.

Histamine caused a prompt, but short-lived, 30% decrease in

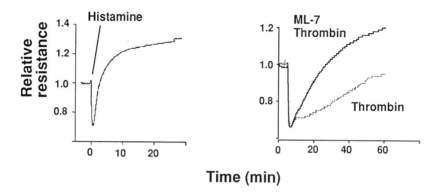

Time (min)

Figure 4. Change in resistance of monolayers of HUVE cells in response to histamine (1×10^{-5} mol/L), thrombin (7 units/mL), or pretreatment with the myosin light chain kinase inhibitor ML-7 (100 μmol/L) followed by thrombin (7 units/mL).

HUVE cell focal adhesion (Figure 4). The resistance was restored to basal levels within 3 to 5 minutes and consistently increased to 20% to 30% above basal levels within 20 to 30 minutes. In contrast to histamine, thrombin caused an approximately 40% decrease in resistance, and this persisted, remaining below basal levels for approximately 50 minutes. When MLC phosphorylation was inhibited with ML-7, thrombin caused a decrease in resistance that was the same as in cells not pretreated with ML-7, but after ML-7 pretreatment the decrease in resistance did not persist as long. In addition, after pretreatment with ML-7, the resistance increased to above basal levels as it did with histamine, a pattern that did not occur with thrombin alone (Figure 4).

Hence, histamine decreases endothelial focal adhesion independent of increases in centripetal tension. The changes in endothelial focal adhesion monitored as the impedance of a cell-covered electrode closely mimic the time course of the changes in endothelial focal adhesion documented in vivo. Thrombin also decreases cultured endothelial cell focal adhesion independent of an increase in centripetal tension. However, inhibition of MLC phosphorylation reduces the duration of the thrombin-initiated decrease in focal adhesion.

Sites at Which Histamine Decreases Focal Adhesion

Since histamine appears to directly decrease tethering independent of changes in centripetal tension, it was important to identify the sites of tethering that were affected by histamine. When the impedance of the endothelium was modeled as a capacitor and resistor in series, with the components of the circuit being the resistance between the cells, the resistance between the cell and matrix, and the capacitance of the cell membrane, it was possible to calculate a value for each of these entities.[9] The authors tested this model by making interventions that would have predictable effects on the different components of the model and then determining if the model responded appropriately. They first added antibody to cadherin-5 to the system. Cadherin-5 is thought to be the principal cadherin, mediating cell-to-cell adhesion in endothelium. The antibody caused a 30% decrease in total resistance. When this decrease was broken into its component parts, there was a 60% to 70% decrease in cell-to-cell resistance and a 10% decrease in cell-matrix resistance that lagged behind the overall decrease in resistance. This was interpreted as increased stress on cortical cell-matrix sites due to loss of cell-to-cell adhesion from the direct action of the antibody on cell-to-cell tethering because the small decrease in cell-matrix resistance lagged behind the drop in total resistance. These data support the ability of the model to reflect the behavior of the system.

The effects of chelation of extracellular calcium were also tested. This resulted in loss of both cell-to-cell and cell-matrix resistances, consistent with the calcium requirement of both cadherin and integrin binding.

When histamine was added to the cell-covered electrode, the changes in resistance were very similar to those caused by antibody to cadherin-5. There was a 30% decrease in total resistance with most of the change due to a 60% to 70% decrease in cell-to-cell resistance. Again there was a small, approximately 10%, decrease in cell-matrix resistance that was interpreted as representing stress on cortical cell matrix sites due to loss of cell-to-cell tethering. The restoration of the total resistance was led by restoration of the small decrease in cell-matrix resistance followed by restoration, and then an increase to above basal levels, of the cell-to-cell resistance. Hence, most of the effect of histamine was on the cell-to-cell resistance.

To further support the validity of the measurements, the authors examined the changes in impedance that occurred when nonconfluent cells were exposed to histamine. Since the cells were not confluent, there was no cell-to-cell component to the resistance. When these cells were exposed to histamine, there was no decrease in the resistance, but there was a 10% increase in resistance, indicating that histamine directly increased cell-matrix resistance. Again, the model interpreted the cells' behavior accurately.

Summary

Histamine is a well-recognized physiological mediator of increased vascular permeability. In the studies reported, the authors examined the ways that histamine alters endothelial cell function to permit the development of small breaches in the endothelial barrier. They found that histamine caused a small, but very short-lived, increase in MLC phosphorylation. Despite this increase in MLC phosphorylation, histamine did not increase centripetal tension of HUVE cells. The level of MLC phosphorylation (0.4 mol phosphate per mol MLC) and the lack of an increase in tension following histamine is in agreement with the observations of Pereschini and Hartshorne[10] that myosin ATPase activity does not increase until the light chain is phosphorylated to approximately 0.5 mol phosphate per mol light chain.

While histamine did not increase centripetal tension, it did decrease focal adhesion of HUVE cells in a reversible fashion that closely mimicked the kinetics of histamine's effect on the microvasculature in vivo.[2] Histamine predominantly decreased the adhesion between cells and had a very limited effect on the adhesion of cells to matrix. Histamine also had the interesting effect of markedly increasing the adhesion of cells to each other during the recovery phase. The authors believe that examination of this phase will be helpful in determining how the endothelial barrier is restored after the onset of an edematous response, and that it may lead to improved therapy.

While histamine did not increase centripetal tension in HUVE cells, thrombin did. The thrombin-induced increase in tension was dependent on MLC phosphorylation. However, the thrombin-induced decrease in cell focal adhesion was not dependent on the increase in tension. Hence, both histamine and thrombin initiate a decrease in cell-to-cell adhesion independent of an increase in centripetal tension. Thrombin decreased focal adhesion longer than histamine did, and the duration of this decrease in adhesion was shortened by inhibiting MLC phosphorylation. Whether this decrease in the duration of the fall in adhesion is due to increased centripetal tension or perhaps to increased stiffness of the cell when MLC is phosphorylated remains uncertain.

References

1. Majno G, Palade G. Studies on inflammation. 1. Effect of histamine and serotonin on vascular permeability: An electron microscopic study. *J Biophys Biochem Cytol* 1961;11:571–605.
2. Wu NZ, Baldwin AL. Transient venular permeability increase and endothelial gap formation induced by histamine. *Am J Physiol* 1992;262: H1238–H1247.
3. Carson M, Shasby S, Shasby DM. Histamine and inositol phosphate accumulation in endothelium: cAMP and G protein. *Am J Physiol* 1989;263: L664–L669.

4. Nicolaysen G. Intravascular concentration of calcium and magnesium ions and edema formation in isolated lungs. *Acta Physiol Scand* 1971;81: 325–339.
5. Shasby DM, Shasby S. Effects of calcium on transendothelial albumin transfer and electrical resistance. *J Appl Physiol* 1986;60:71–79.
6. Moy AB, Van Englehoven J, Bodmer J, et al. Histamine and thrombin modulate endothelial focal adhesion through centripetal and centrifugal forces. *J Clin Invest* 1996;97:1020–1027.
7. Goeckeler ZM, Wysolmerski RB. Myosin light chain kinase regulated endothelial cell contraction: The relationship between isometric tension, actin polymerization and myosin phosphorylation. *J Cell Biol* 1995;130: 613–627.
8. Sheldon R, Moy A, Lindsley K, Shasby S, Shasby DM. Role of myosin light-chain phosphorylation in endothelial cell retraction. *Am J Physiol* 1993;265:L606–L612.
9. Giaever I, Keese CR. Monitoring fibroblast behavior in tissue culture with an applied electrical field. *Proc Natl Acad Sci U S A* 1984;81:3761–3764.
10. Persechini A, Hartshorne D. Phosphorylation of smooth muscle myosin: Evidence for cooperativity between the myosin heads. *Science* 1981;213: 1383–1385.

Chapter 15

Regulation of Alveolar Capillary Barrier Function by Neutrophils

Claire M. Doerschuk, MD, Hiroshi Kubo, MD, Phd, Hideaki Motosugi, MD, PhD, Nicholas A. Doyle, MA, William M. Quinlan, BA, and Gregory J. Kutkoski, BS

Introduction

Acute lung injury resulting from endothelial injury and increased pulmonary vascular permeability often results in a series of clinical abnormalities referred to as the adult respiratory distress syndrome (ARDS) and multiple organ failure. Neutrophils usually contribute to both the pathogenesis and the evolution of this syndrome.[1-9] Neutrophils produce proteolytic enzymes and reactive oxygen intermediates that often initiate and perpetuate endothelial and epithelial cell damage. These same products are also the mechanisms of host defense against superimposed bacterial infection, and they are required for the resolution of the lung injury. Neutrophils are, therefore, both destructive and beneficial, and the effort of many investigators has been directed toward understanding the mechanisms of the neutrophil response.

The pathogenesis of ARDS has been extensively studied in vivo and in vitro using a variety of approaches. The effect of mediators on neutrophil-endothelial or neutrophil-epithelial cell interactions in vitro have been fruitful, as have studies investigating neutrophil and alveolar

Claire M. Doerschuk was a recipient of a Career Investigator Award from the American Lung Association. These studies were supported by HL48160, HL52466, and HL33009.

From: Weir EK, Reeves JT (eds). *Pulmonary Edema*. Armonk, NY: Futura Publishing Company, Inc.;©1998.

macrophage function. Intravascular injection of either complex stimuli, including endotoxin and live organisms, or individual mediators has been used to simulate the initial stages of ARDS in animals. These studies have made critical contributions to the understanding of the pathogenesis of this syndrome, but many important questions remain.

Studies have focused primarily on the initial events of neutrophil sequestration and adhesion to pulmonary microvascular endothelial cells in vivo. Intravascular complement fragments and other stimuli were used to initiate these processes. Intravascular infusion of complement fragments induces a rapid onset of neutropenia due to sequestration of neutrophils within the capillaries of many organs but primarily the lung, because the pulmonary circulation receives the entire cardiac output.[10] The circulating neutrophil counts remain low until the infusion of complement fragments is stopped. Following clearance of the fragments, a neutrophilia occurs and the circulating neutrophil counts subsequently return to initial values.

Brief infusions of complement fragments lasting 10 to 15 minutes do not result in pulmonary edema, as measured by isotopic or gravimetric methods.[11] However, even these short infusions initiate an injury to the alveolo-capillary membrane when measured with sensitive techniques that do not require the formation of frank edema. For example, infusion of complement fragments for 10 minutes induced an increase in the clearance of nebulized fluorescein isothiocyanate-(FITC) labeled dextran from the airspace into the blood.[11] This increase required neutrophils and was inhibited when rabbits were pretreated with indomethacin, suggesting that a cyclooxygenase-derived product was important in this injury.[11]

Recent studies have focused on understanding the mechanisms that mediate the initial sequestration of neutrophils, as well as understanding the process through which sequestered neutrophils remain within the lung and induce endothelial cell injury.[12–15] In particular, the roles of neutrophil-endothelial cell adhesion and changes in the biomechanical properties of neutrophils have been examined. The mechanisms involved in neutrophil-induced endothelial cell injury are also discussed in this chapter.

Neutrophil Adhesion to Pulmonary Capillary Endothelium

The adhesion molecules that mediate neutrophil-endothelial cell interactions include members of the selectin, integrin, and immunoglobulin-like families.[16] L-selectin is expressed on neutrophils, primarily at the tips of the microvillar processes, and is shed early in the response of neutrophils to inflammatory stimuli. P-selectin is expressed by endothelial cells and platelets. In endothelial cells, P-selectin is stored in Weibel-Palade bodies and can be upregulated to the plasma membrane without requiring protein synthesis. Immunohistochemical studies suggest that it is localized primarily in arterioles and venules but not pulmonary capillary endothelial cells. E-selectin is expressed only on endothelial cells and is not expressed constitutively. Since protein synthesis is required for expression, E-selectin is unlikely to mediate the rapid neutrophil sequestration that occurs when complement fragments are infused. The selectin family is thought to mediate rolling of neutrophils along postcapillary venular endothelium in the systemic circulation.[17-20] However, the site of neutrophil sequestration in the lungs is the capillary bed, where rolling does not occur due to the narrow diameter of these vessels.[21-22] The contribution of selectin-mediated adhesion in the pulmonary capillaries is not clear.

Integrins expressed on leukocytes include the CD11/CD18 complex. These molecules are expressed on the plasma membranes and within granules of neutrophils. The amount of CD11/CD18 expressed on the plasma membrane is sufficient, following a conformational change, to mediate adhesion, although upregulation of CD11/CD18 from the granules to the surface also occurs.[16] Intercellular adhesion molecule-1 (ICAM-1), a member of the immunoglobulin-like family of adhesion molecules, is expressed by endothelial cells. It is one important ligand for CD11/CD18 on endothelial cells, although other unidentified ligands exist. CD11/CD18-ICAM-1 interactions are thought to mediate firm adhesion between neutrophils and endothelial cells and follow loose interactions mediated through selectins in the systemic microvasculature.[16-20]

Initial questions focused on understanding the role of CD11/CD18 in neutrophil sequestration induced by infusion of complement fragments. These studies showed that neutrophil sequestration induced by infusion of complement fragments in rabbits pretreated with a blocking antibody against CD18 occurred as rapidly and to the same degree as that observed in rabbits treated with a control antibody.[13] Surprisingly, however, the neutropenia did not continue throughout the infusion of complement fragments in the anti-CD18 antibody-treated rabbits, but rather the circulating neutrophil counts began to increase by 7 minutes after infusion.[13] Neutrophil sequestration within the pulmonary capillaries at 15 minutes of infusion was almost completely inhibited by blockade of CD11/CD18 (Figure 1). These studies indicated that neutrophil sequestration and adhesion are complex events that occur in sequential steps. The initial se-

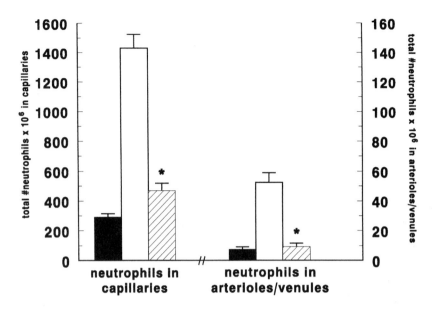

Figure 1. Neutrophil sequestration within the pulmonary capillaries. Infusion of complement fragments in rabbits for 15 minutes induced a fivefold increase in the number of neutrophils sequestered within the pulmonary capillaries. This increase was inhibited by 90% when the rabbits were pretreated with a blocking antibody against CD18.[13] Solid bars = rabbits pretreated with nonimmune IgG given infusion of saline; open bars = rabbits pretreated with nonimmune IgG given infusion of complement fragments; striped bars = rabbits pretreated with anti-CD18 antibodies given infusion of complement fragments.

questration does not require the CD11/CD18 adhesion complex. However, this complex was necessary to maintain the sequestered neutrophils within the pulmonary capillary bed for more than a few minutes.

The role of selectins in neutrophil sequestration was also investigated because studies of the response of neutrophils to inflammatory stimuli in the systemic postcapillary venules indicated that leukocyte rolling, the initial step, required selectins. Since the blocking anti-L-selectin antibodies activate neutrophils and alter the behavior, other routes of studying these molecules were pursued. Jutila and colleagues[23] showed that L-selectin is sensitive to chymotrypsin and is completely cleaved from the neutrophil membrane at low concentrations and short incubation times. When radiolabeled chymotrypsin-treated rabbit neutrophils were reinjected into the vasculature of rabbits, they sequestered similarly to control neutrophils in response to complement fragments.[24] Studies showed that the circulating neutrophil counts in L-selectin-deficient mice decreased to the same degree as those of wild-type mice in response to intravenous injection of complement fragments.[25] Finally, pretreatment of rabbits with fucoidin, an inhibitor of L- and P-selectin, or an anti-P-selectin antibody also did not inhibit complement fragment-induced neutropenia.[26] These studies suggest that neither L-selectin nor P-selectin mediates the initial sequestration. However, the number of sequestered neutrophils in the lungs of L-selectin mutant mice 5 minutes after injection was significantly less than in wild-type mice, and pretreatment with fucoidin inhibited neutrophil sequestration compared to that in control rabbits at 15 minutes of infusion.[25,26] In contrast, the anti-P-selectin antibody had no effect on either the initial neutropenia or the prolonged sequestration. These data suggest that adhesion mediated through L-selectin, but not through P-selectin, does occur following the initial sequestration.

Taken together, these data indicate that the initial process of neutrophil sequestration within the pulmonary capillary bed that results in neutropenia does not require either L-selectin, P-selectin, or CD11/CD18. Maintaining these sequestered neutrophils within the lungs for more than 5 to 7 minutes requires adhesive events that are mediated through L-selectin and CD11/CD18. Whether these adhesion molecules are used in tandem or sequentially remains to be determined.

Inflammatory Stimulus-Induced Changes in Biomechanical Properties of Neutrophils

Alternative mechanisms were considered because none of the known adhesion molecules appear to be important in the initial processes of neutrophil sequestration. Many inflammatory mediators, including C5a, platelet activating factor (PAF), leukotriene B$_4$ (LTB$_4$), IL-8, and formyl-methionyl-leucyl-phenylalanine (fMLP), induce a rapid stiffening of the cytoskeleton of neutrophils that results in a decreased ability of neutrophils to deform and enter narrow capillaries.[12,14,27–38] This stiffening is thought to be due to the events initiated when the inflammatory mediator binds to receptors on the plasma membrane of neutrophils and initiates the formation of actin microfilaments in the submembrane region of the cytoplasm. The stiffening can be prevented by pretreating neutrophils with cytochalasins, but not with colchicine; this suggests that changes in actin microfilaments but not microtubules are required.[14]

Neutrophils must elongate to pass through the capillary bed because many of the pulmonary capillary segments are smaller in diameter than spherical neutrophils.[22] A decrease in the deformability of neutrophils is likely to delay or prevent their passage through the pulmonary capillary pathways, resulting in neutrophil sequestration.[12,15] These observations suggested the hypothesis that circulating inflammatory mediators induce neutropenia by binding to their receptors on the neutrophil plasma membrane and causing decreased deformability of neutrophils and rapid sequestration within the capillary bed.

To test this hypothesis, the shape of neutrophils within the pulmonary capillary bed following a 1.5 minute infusion of complement fragments was compared to that in the lungs of saline-treated animals with use of confocal microscopy. These studies showed that the number of spherical or nearly spherical neutrophils was increased in the complement fragment-treated animals (Figure 2).[15] In fact, the number of spherical cells in the pulmonary capillaries was similar to the total

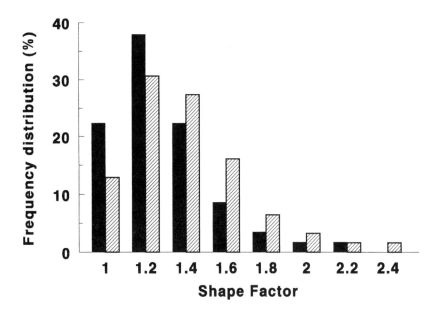

Figure 2. Frequency distribution describing the shape of neutrophils within the pulmonary capillaries. Confocal microscopy was used to evaluate the shape of neutrophils in the lungs of rabbits treated with complement fragments (solid bars) or saline (striped bars) for 1.5 minutes. Neutrophil shape was evaluated by measuring the longest axis of the neutrophil in a plane parallel to the capillary wall and the axis perpendicular to this longest axis at its midpoint. The shape factor was calculated as the longest axis/perpendicular axis. There was a significant increase in the number of neutrophils with a shape factor of 1.0 to 1.2 in rabbits that received a 1.5 minute infusion of complement fragments than in rabbits given an infusion of saline.[15]

number of circulating neutrophils that were available for sequestration. At later times when adhesion molecules were required, there was an increase in the number of flattened neutrophils.[15] These studies suggested that increased stiffening and decreased deformability may be the mechanism through which neutrophils sequester and that this stiffening is short-lived.

The mechanism through which this stiffening occurs has been attributed to the polymerization of soluble actin monomers (G-actin) to microfilaments (F-actin).[14,15,27–38] The signal-transduction pathways leading from occupancy of the receptors to polymerization of F-actin are complex and are thought to involve phosphatidylinositol-(4,5) diphosphate and the uncapping of F-actin barbed ends.[39–44] Studies have investigated the distribution of actin in neutrophils by use of ultrastructural immunohistochemistry and colloidal gold labeling with an antibody that recognized actin in both forms. Neutrophils within the pulmonary capillaries of normal rabbits contained 2.5 times as much actin in the submembrane rim beneath the plasma membrane as was present in the central regions of the cell.[15] In sequestered neutrophils of animals given infusion of complement fragments, this ratio increased to 5.1.[15] Surprisingly, more actin was present in the microvillar processes of neutrophils in complement fragment-treated lungs than in control lungs. These data suggested that actin monomers rapidly relocated from the central to the submembrane regions and the microvillar processes following activation. Because microvillar processes must flatten during the deformation process to accommodate the cytosolic volume, these studies also led to the novel hypothesis that increased stiffening might be due in part to a decreased ability of microvilli to flatten during deformation. These studies indicated that an increased concentration of actin was present in the submembrane region, supporting the hypothesis that increased concentration and F-actin formation results in stiffening.

When the studies that describe the roles of biomechanical properties of neutrophil and adhesive interactions between neutrophils and endothelial cells are considered together, the process of neutrophil sequestration is likely to involve a sequence of events as described in Figure 3. The mechanism underlying sequestration is likely to involve a stimulus-induced decrease in the ability of neutrophils to deform and pass through the narrow pulmonary capillary bed. In contrast to the venules of the systemic microvasculature, neutrophil sequestration within the capillary bed appears to be a mechanical event without a requirement for rolling. This decrease in deformability results in delayed transit and sequestration of neutrophils, but adhesion molecules are required to maintain the sequestered neutrophils within the capillary bed. Both L-selectin and CD11/CD18 appear to play a role in adhesion.

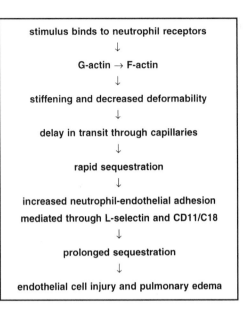

stimulus binds to neutrophil receptors
↓
G-actin → F-actin
↓
stiffening and decreased deformability
↓
delay in transit through capillaries
↓
rapid sequestration
↓
increased neutrophil-endothelial adhesion
mediated through L-selectin and CD11/C18
↓
prolonged sequestration
↓
endothelial cell injury and pulmonary edema

Figure 3. Postulated mechanism through which neutrophil sequestration occurs.

The Role of Adhesion Molecules in Neutrophil-Mediated Lung Injury

The role of adhesion molecules in lung injury induced by intravenous injection of cobra venom factor has been studied by Ward and colleagues.[45–56] Cobra venom factor induces neutrophil sequestration, neutrophil-mediated endothelial cell injury, and the formation of edema without emigration of neutrophils. The injury requires complement, neutrophils, platelets, and reactive oxygen intermediates.[45–49] In addition, adhesion molecules are required, particularly L-selectin, P-selectin, CD11/CD18, and ICAM-1, as evaluated with use of blocking antibodies, soluble adhesion molecule-IgG chimeras, and oligosaccharides.[50–56]

Recent studies have extended these observations by evaluating the role of adhesion molecules in cobra venom factor-induced lung injury with use of mice that are deficient in one or more adhesion molecules. When wild-type mice were given either anti-P-selectin antibody or anti-ICAM-1 antibody, neutrophil sequestration and edema formation were largely inhibited.[55] However, ICAM-1-deficient and P-selectin-deficient mice showed no decrease in lung injury compared to wild-type mice. When the mutant mice were pretreated with an antibody against the molecule they were missing, lung injury was not prevented. These data indicate that the antibodies were not inhibiting nonspecifically, and suggest that residual expression could not account for the discrepancy between the role of adhesion molecules when studied using antibodies compared to mutant mice. In fact, when P-selectin/ ICAM-1 double mutant mice received cobra venom factor, there was also no inhibition of lung injury, indicating that these molecules are not substituting for each other.[55]

Current studies are focused on understanding this discrepancy in the observed function of an adhesion molecule, depending on the method through which its function is inhibited. Although it is possible that antibodies have a greater effect than solely inhibition of their respective antigens, it appears more likely that mutant mice use alternative pathways to mediate neutrophil adhesion and lung injury. First, this discrepancy was observed when the role of ICAM-1 was evaluated in *E. coli* endotoxin-induced pneumonia, as neutrophil emigration was inhibited by 65% to 75% when mice were pretreated with either of two anti-ICAM-1 antibodies while ICAM-1 mutant showed no defect in neutrophil emigration.[57] Pretreatment with antisense oligonucleotides targeted to ICAM-1 to prevent ICAM-1 expression inhibited neutrophil emigration to a similar degree as did pretreatment with anti-ICAM-1 antibodies.[57] These observations suggest that genetic deletion resulted in use of alternative pathways that were not available when adhesion molecules were inhibited acutely. Second, several recent studies have suggested that the pathways mediating neutrophil emigration in chronic inflammatory responses are different than those mediating acute neutrophil emigration. For example, Winn and Harlan[58] showed that neutrophil emigration in response to endotoxin in rabbits was inhibited by an anti-CD18 antibody at 4 hours but not at 24 hours after instillation. Studies have shown that neutrophil emigration during acute *Pseudomonas aeruginosa*-induced pneumonia occurred through CD11/ CD18-dependent pathways, while neutrophil emigration in recurrent infection by this organism occurred through pathways that are at least particularly CD18-independent.[59] These alternative pathways may be similar to those used by mutant mice. Current studies are focused on understanding the mechanisms involved in the selection of an adhesion pathway and the molecules that mediate CD11/CD18-independent adhesion.

The Role of Oxidants in Lung Injury

Reactive oxygen intermediates result in cell injury through a variety of mechanisms including oxidation of membrane lipids,[60] injury to the interstitial matrix and basement membranes of the lung, and destruction of anti-inflammatory molecules including α_1-proteinase inhibitor and α_2-macroglobulin (reviewed in References 5 through 8). In addition to injuring the parenchymal cells of the lung, they induce the production of chemotactic factors and other mediators. Lipid peroxidation products have been identified in the lavage fluid in experimental studies of ARDS; the levels of reduced glutathione in the bronchoalveolar lavage fluid of patients is decreased.[61–63] Many studies that examine the role of oxidants in vivo have been performed in animals. For example, studies by Bernard and colleagues[64] have shown that pretreatment of sheep with the antioxidant, N-acetylcysteine, ameliorated edema formation in endotoxin-induced lung injury in sheep. Cobra venom factor-induced lung injury was inhibited when rats were pretreated with catalase, desferroxamine, or superoxide dismutase.[45–47] These studies suggest that reactive oxygen intermediates participate in the lung injury.

Recent studies have examined the role of nicotinamide-adenine dinucleotide phosphate (reduced form) (NADPH) oxidase-derived radicals in cobra venom factor-induced lung injury.[49] This enzyme catalyzes the formation of superoxide. Superoxide dismutase subsequently catalyzed the formation of hydrogen peroxide. In the presence of iron (Fe^{2+}), hydrogen peroxide forms hydroxyl radical. Any of these reactive oxygen intermediates are capable of inducing cell injury.

NADPH oxidase-deficient mice were generated by a mutation in the X-linked gene for the 91 kd subunit of NADPH oxidase.[65] This deficiency resulted in mice with chronic granulomatous disease similar to that observed in patients, including an increased susceptibility to *Staphylococcus aureus* and *Aspergillus fumigatus*.[66] Surprisingly, the NADPH oxidase-deficient mice showed no inhibition of lung injury induced by cobra venom factor when compared to wild-type mice.[49] When mice were depleted of neutrophils by use of cyclophosphamide, cobra venom factor-induced lung injury was inhibited in both NADPH oxidase-deficient and wild-type mice. Allopurinol inhibited injury in both types of mice. However, the particular reactive oxygen species that were important in the lung injury appeared to change in the NADPH oxidase-deficient mice. In particular, catalase, a scavenger of hydrogen peroxide, completely inhibited the lung injury in wild-type mice but had no effect in the NADPH oxidase-deficient mice. In contrast, N_G-methyl-L-arginine (L-NMA), an inhibitor of nitric oxide production, inhibited lung injury in the NADPH oxidase-deficient but not wild-type mice.[49] These studies suggest that the NADPH oxidase-deficient mice were using alternative pathways to generate reactive oxygen intermediates. Neutrophils from NADPH oxidase-deficient mice may produce nitric oxide, which combines with superoxide generated through xanthine oxidase in endothelial cells to form peroxynitrite and nitrogen dioxide, two potent inducers of cell injury.[9,67,68]

Importantly, as in the case of the adhesion molecule mutations, these studies indicate that mice, deficient in an important molecule, may not provide clear information about the role of that molecule due to the use of alternative pathways. However, these mice do provide valuable information about the regulation of oxidant-producing pathways. These studies also suggest that nitric oxide synthase-derived oxidants are capable of inducing endothelial cell injury and pulmonary edema.

The conflicting roles of nitric oxide as a vasodilator and as a source of oxidants have been difficult to resolve. The beneficial effects of nitric oxide in at least some patients with ARDS,[69] as well as studies by the authors demonstrating that L-NMA did not inhibit cobra venom factor-induced lung injury in wild-type mice, suggest that when all oxidant-generating enzyme systems are present and functioning, the balance of the effects of nitric oxide are to benefit the patient. Future studies will further evaluate the use of nitric oxide as a therapeutic modality.

The Role of Elastase in Lung Injury

The granules of neutrophils contain several proteinases including neutrophil elastase. The role of elastase in chronic obstructive lung disease, particularly emphysema, cystic fibrosis, and other destructive lung diseases, has been described.[70] Elastase also appears to contribute to lung injury during ARDS.[70–72] For example, studies by Sakamaki and colleagues[73] using the inhibitor, ONO-5046, prevented both the formation of edema and neutrophil emigration. These studies suggest that elastase may play a role in the development of ARDS, either by facilitating neutrophil migration between cells and through connective tissue or by contributing to lung parenchymal injury.

New Opportunities for Therapeutic Intervention

The observation that neutrophil accumulation within the capillary bed occurs through a process that involves at least two steps, each with a unique mechanism, leads to many opportunities for therapeutic intervention. An understanding of the mechanisms through which neutrophils become stiff will allow for therapies to be targeted at inhibiting a critical step. For example, $PI(4,5)P_2$ appears important in the uncapping of actin microfilaments.[40,41,44] Molecules that inhibit the activity of the phosphatidylinositol-4 phosphate-5 kinase or molecules that recognize and bind newly generated phosphatidylinositides may inhibit neutrophil sequestration within the lungs and the subsequent lung injury.

Therapy focused on inhibiting adhesion molecules may also prove beneficial because engagement of adhesion molecules is likely to be required before neutrophil-endothelial cell injury can occur. The role of adhesion molecules has been investigated in several lung injuries with varying effects (reviewed in References 3,4,62,63,78,79). These studies suggest that the benefit of a particular anti-adhesion molecule therapy may depend upon the particular pathogenetic mechanism underlying the lung injury. The molecule to be targeted appears critical.

Several different and exciting approaches to therapeutic intervention are currently being considered. As mentioned above, a novel approach that has not yet been examined is focused on inhibiting the changes in biomechanical properties of neutrophils to prevent sequestration. Other signal-transduction pathways may also be eligible sites for inhibition.[74-78] Inhibitors of cytokines including tumor necrosis factor-α (TNF-α) and interleukin-1 (IL-1) are being evaluated and to date have shown mixed results.[79,80] Inhibitors of chemokines, molecules that form chemotactic/haptotactic gradients for neutrophil emigration and that are important activators of neutrophils, are also the focus of considerable interest.[81] Developmental efforts are also currently focusing on blocking the function of adhesion molecules by either inhibiting expression using antisense oligonucleotides, post-translational events using leumedins, or recognition of ligand using competitive antagonists. Inhibitors of neutrophil effector molecules, including elastase and other proteases and oxidants, are another locus for intervention. The pharmaceutical approaches that are presently under investigation include antisense oligonucleotides targeted to endothelial adhesion molecules or to cytokines that prevent expression of protein; humanized antibodies that recognize and block the function of adhesion molecules, chemokines, or cytokines; naturally occurring or synthetic peptides or proteins that block integrin function, complement activation, or cytokine function; and oligosaccharides that inhibit the interactions between selectins and their ligands.

The risks of inhibiting host defense and preventing the normal response of neutrophils to infection are difficult to evaluate. Patients with genetic deficiencies in the expression of CD11/CD18 (leukocyte adhesion deficiency type I) have severe defects in the inflammatory response, which usually result in death at a young age.[82] Patients with a defect in the function of selectins (leukocyte adhesion deficiency type II) appear to have fewer infections.[83] In addition, redundancies in some adhesion pathways may lead to a smaller risk of infection compared to others, when these pathways are inhibited, but the effect on ameliorating injury may be less. The duration of treatment, the molecule(s) to be inhibited, and the efficacy of a particular therapeutic agent are likely to be critical in balancing the risk of infection with the inhibition of injury.

Summary

The processes through which neutrophils sequester in the lungs, adhere to endothelium, and either initiate, perpetuate, or resolve lung injury are becoming clear. Each process offers a potential approach for therapeutic intervention. Much of our understanding, however, is based on acute injuries in previously healthy animals. Chronic inflammation or acute inflammation superimposed on chronic inflammatory processes may occur through different pathways. Mice that are deficient in single or combinations of molecules may help to elucidate these alternative pathways and mechanisms.

Acknowledgment   The authors wish to thank Patrice Ayers for her help in preparation of the manuscript.

References

1. Harlan JM. Leukocyte-endothelial interactions. *Blood* 1985;65:513–525.
2. Tate RM, Repine JE. Neutrophils and the adult respiratory distress syndrome. *Am Rev Respir Dis* 1983;128:552–559.
3. Wortel CH, Doerschuk CM. Neutrophils and neutrophil-endothelial cell adhesion in ARDS. *New Horiz* 1993;1:631–637.
4. Strieter RM, Kunkel SL. Acute lung injury: The role of cytokines in the elicitation of neutrophils. *J Invest Med* 1994;42:640–651.
5. Simpson R, Hechtman HB. Pulmonary injury following sepsis. *Prog Clin Biol Res* 1994;388:265–275.
6. Reid PT, Donnelly SC, Haslett C. Inflammatory predictors for the development of the adult respiratory distress syndrome. *Thorax* 1995;50:1023–1026.
7. Fujishima S, Aikawa N. Neutrophil-mediated tissue injury and its modulation. *Int Care Med* 1995;21:277–285.
8. Demling RH. The modern version of adult respiratory distress syndrome. *Ann Rev Med* 1995;46:193–202.
9. Fulkerson WJ, MacIntyre N, Stamler J, Crapo JD. Pathogenesis and treatment of the adult respiratory distress syndrome. *Arch Intern Med* 1996; 156:29–38.
10. Doerschuk CM, Allard MF, Hogg JC. Neutrophil kinetics in rabbits during infusion of zymosan-activated plasma. *J Appl Physiol* 1989;67:88–95.
11. Gie RP, Doerschuk CM, English D, Coxson HO, Hogg JC. Neutrophil-associated lung injury following the infusion of activated plasma. *J Appl Physiol* 1991;70:1271–1278.
12. Worthen GS, Schwab B, Elson EL, Downey GP. Mechanics of stimulated neutrophils: Cell stiffening induces retention in capillaries. *Science* 1989; 245:183–185.
13. Doerschuk CM. The role of CD18-mediated adhesion in neutrophil sequestration induced by infusion of activated plasma in rabbits. *Am J Respir Cell Mol Biol* 1992;7:140–148.
14. Inano H, English D, Doerschuk CM. Effect of zymosan-activated plasma on the deformability of rabbit polymorphonuclear leukocytes and the role of the cytoskeleton. *J Appl Physiol* 1992;73:1370–1376.

15. Motosugi H, Graham L, Noblitt TW, et al. Changes in neutrophil actin and shape during sequestration induced by complement fragments in rabbits. *Am J Pathol* 1996;149:963–973.
16. Carlos TM, Harlan JM. Leukocyte-endothelial adhesion molecules. *Blood* 1994;84:2068–2101.
17. Von Andrian UH, Chambers JD, McEvoy LM, Bargatze RF, Arfors KE, Butcher EC. Two-step model of leukocyte-endothelial cell interaction in inflammation: Distinct roles for LECAM-1 and the leukocyte beta 2 integrins in vivo. *Proc Natl Acad Sci U S A* 1991;88:7538–7542.
18. Abbassi O, Lane CL, Krater SS, et al. Canine neutrophil margination mediated by lectin adhesion molecule-1 in vitro. *J Immunol* 1991;147: 2107–2115.
19. Butcher EC. Leukocyte-endothelial cell adhesion as an active, multi-step process: A combinatorial mechanism for specificity and diversity in leukocyte targeting. In: Gupta S, Waldmann TA (eds): *Mechanisms of Lymphocyte Activation and Immune Regulation IV: Cellular Communications.* New York: Plenum Press; 1992;181–194.
20. Butcher EC. Leukocyte-endothelial cell recognition: Three (or more) steps to specificity and diversity. *Cell* 1991;67:1033–1036.
21. Gebb SA, Graham JA, Hanger CC, et al. Sites of leukocyte sequestration in the pulmonary microcirculation. *J Appl Physiol* 1995;79:493–497.
22. Doerschuk CM, Beyers N, Coxson HO, Wiggs B, Hogg JC. Comparison of neutrophil and capillary diameters and their relation to neutrophil sequestration in the lung. *J Appl Physiol* 1993;74:3040–3045.
23. Jutila MA, Kishimoto TK, Finken M. Low-dose chymotrypsin treatment inhibits neutrophil migration into sites of inflammation in vivo: Effects of Mac-1 and MEL-14 adhesion protein expression and function. *Cell Immunol* 1991;132:201–214.
24. Doyle NA, Quinlan WM, Graham L, Doerschuk CM. The role of LECAM-1 in neutrophil sequestration induced by infusion of complement fragments. (Abstract) *Am Rev Respir Dis* 1992;145:A187.
25. Doyle NA, Tedder TF, Doerschuk CM. The role of L-selectin in neutrophil sequestration and emigration in murine lungs. (Abstract) *Am J Respir Crit Care Med* 1995;153:A.
26. Kubo H, Doyle NA, Doerschuk CM. The role of P-selectin in complement fragment-induced neutrophil sequestration. (Abstract) *Am J Respir Crit Care Med* 1995;151:A455.
27. Downey GP, Worthen GS. Neutrophil retention in model capillaries: Deformability, geometry, and hydrodynamic forces. *J Appl Physiol* 1988;65: 1861–1871.
28. Buttrum SM, Drost EM, MacNee W, et al. Rheological response of neutrophils to different types of stimulation. *J Appl Physiol* 1994;77:1801–1810.
29. Chien S. Blood cell deformability and interactions: From molecules to micromechanics and microcirculation. *Microvasc Res* 1992;44:243–254.
30. Zhelev DV, Hochmuth RM. Mechanically stimulated cytoskeleton rearrangement and cortical contraction in human neutrophils. *Biophys J* 1995;68:2004–2014.
31. Kawaoka EJ, Miller ME, Cheung ATW. Chemotactic factor-induced effects upon deformability of human polymorphonuclear leukocytes. *J Clin Immunol* 1981;1:41–44.
32. Watts RG, Crispens MA, Howard TH. A quantitative study of the role of F-actin in producing neutrophil shape. *Cell Motil Cytoskeleton* 1991;19: 159–168.

33. Packman CH, Lichtman MA. Activation of neutrophils: Measurement of actin conformational changes by flow cytometry. *Blood Cells* 1990;16: 193–207.
34. Wallace PJ, Weston RP, Packman CH, Lichtman MA. Chemotactic peptide-induced changes in neutrophil actin conformation. *J Cell Biol* 1984; 99:1060–1065.
35. Howard TH, Oresajo CO. The kinetics of chemotactic peptide-induced change in F-actin content, F-actin distribution, and the shape of neutrophils. *J Cell Biol* 1985;101:1078–1085.
36. Bochsler PN, Neilsen NR, Dean DF, Slauson DO. Stimulus-dependent actin polymerization in bovine neutrophils. *Inflammation* 1992;16:383–392.
37. Pecsvarady Z, Fisher TC, Fabok A, Coates TD, Meiselman HJ. Kinetics of granulocyte deformability following exposure to chemotactic stimuli. *Blood Cells* 1992;18:333–352.
38. Frank RS. Time-dependent alterations in the deformability of human neutrophils in response to chemotactic activation. *Blood* 1990;76:2606–2612.
39. Stossel TP. On the crawling of animal cells. *Science* 1993;260:1086–1094.
40. Barkalow K, Hartwig JH. The role of actin filament barbed-end exposure in cytoskeletal dynamics and cell motility. *Biochem Soc Trans* 1995;23:451–456.
41. Janmey PA. Phosphoinositides and calcium as regulators of cellular actin assembly and disassembly. *Ann Rev Physiol* 1994;56:169–191.
42. Janmey PA, Chaponnier C. Medical aspects of the actin cytoskeleton. *Curr Opin Cell Biol* 1995;7:111–117.
43. DiNubile MJ, Cassimeris L, Joyce M, Zigmond SH. Actin filament barbed-end capping activity in neutrophil lysates: The role of capping protein-beta2. *Mol Biol Cell* 1995;6:1659–1671.
44. Hartwig JH, Bokoch GM, Carpenter CL, et al. Thrombin receptor ligation and activated rac uncap actin filament barbed ends through phosphoinositide synthesis in permeabilized human platelets. *Cell* 1995;82: 643–653.
45. Till GO, Johnson KJ, Kunkel RG, Ward PA. Intravascular activation of complement and acute lung injury. Dependency on neutrophils and toxic oxygen metabolites. *J Clin Invest* 1982;69:1126–1135.
46. Ward PA, Till GO, Kunkel R, Beauchamp C. Evidence for role of hydroxyl radical in complement and neutrophil-dependent tissue injury. *J Clin Invest* 1983;72:789–801.
47. Tvedten HW, Till GO, Ward PA. Mediators of lung injury in mice following systemic activation of complement. *Am J Pathol* 1985;119:92–100.
48. Mulligan MS, Yeh CG, Rudolph AR, Ward PA. Protective effects of soluble CR1 in complement- and neutrophil-mediated tissue injury. *J Immunol* 1992;148:1479–1485.
49. Kubo H, Morgenstern D, Quinlan WM, Ward PA, Dinauer MC, Doerschuk CM. Preservation of complement-induced lung injury in mice with deficiency of NADPH oxidase. *J Clin Invest* 1996;97:2680–2684.
50. Mulligan MS, Varani J, Warren JS, et al. Roles of β_2 integrins of rat neutrophils in complement- and oxygen radical-mediated acute inflammatory injury. *J Immunol* 1992;148:1847–1857.
51. Mulligan MS, Smith CW, Anderson DC, et al. Role of leukocyte adhesion molecules in complement-induced lung injury. *J Immunol* 1993;150: 2401–2406.
52. Mulligan MS, Polley MJ, Bayer RJ, Nunn MF, Paulson JC, Ward PA. Neutrophil-dependent acute lung injury: Requirement for P-selectin (GMP-140). *J Clin Invest* 1992;90:1600–1607.

53. Mulligan MS, Watson SR, Fennie C, Ward PA. Protective effects of selectin chimeras in neutrophil-mediated lung injury. *J Immunol* 1993;151: 6410–6417.
54. Mulligan MS, Paulson JC, De Frees S, Zheng Z-L, Lowe JB, Ward PA. Protective effects of oligosaccharides in P-selectin-dependent lung injury. *Nature* 1993;364:149–151.
55. Doerschuk CM, Quinlan WM, Doyle NA, et al. The roles of P-selectin and ICAM-1 in acute lung injury as determined using blocking antibodies and mutant mice. *J Immunol* 1996;157:4609–4614.
56. Albelda SM, Smith CW, Ward PA. Adhesion molecules and inflammatory injury. *FASEB J* 1994;8:504–512.
57. Kumasaka T, Quinlan WM, Doyle NA, et al. The role of ICAM-1 in endotoxin-induced pneumonia evaluated using ICAM-1 antisense, anti-ICAM-1 antibodies, and ICAM-1 mutant mice. *J Clin Invest* 1996;97: 2362–2369.
58. Winn RK, Harlan JM. CD18-independent neutrophil and mononuclear leukocyte emigration into the peritoneum of rabbits. *J Clin Invest* 1993;92: 1168–1173.
59. Kumasaka T, Doyle NA, Quinlan WM, Graham L, Doerschuk CM. The role of CD11/CD18 in neutrophil emigration during acute and recurrent *Pseudomonas aeruginosa*-induced pneumonia in rabbits. *Am J Pathol* 1996; 148:1297–1305.
60. Freeman BA, Crapo JD. Biology of disease: Free radicals and tissue injury. *Lab Invest* 1982;47:412–426.
61. Pacht E, Timerman A, Lykens M, Merola AJ. Deficiency of alveolar fluid glutathione in patients with sepsis and the adult respiratory distress syndrome. *Chest* 1991;100:1397–1403.
62. Cochrane CG, Spragg RG, Revak DS, Cohen AB, Weinbaum G. The presence of neutrophil elastase and evidence of oxidation activity in bronchoalveolar lavage fluid of patients with adult respiratory distress syndrome. *Am Rev Respir Dis* 1983;127:S25–S27.
63. Ishizaka A, Stephens KE, Tazelaar HD, Hall EW, O'Hanley P, Raffin TA. Pulmonary edema after *Escherichia coli* peritonitis correlated with thiobarbituric acid reactive materials in bronchoalveolar lavage fluid. *Am Rev Respir Dis* 1988;137:783–789.
64. Bernard G, Lucht W, Niedermeyer M, Snapper JR, Ogletree ML, Brigham KL. Effect of N-acetylcysteine on the pulmonary response to endotoxin in the awake sheep and upon in vitro granulocyte function. *J Clin Invest* 1984;73:1772–1784.
65. Pollock, JD, Williams DA, Gifford MAC, et al. Mouse model of X-linked chronic granulomatous disease, an inherited defect in phagocyte superoxide production. *Nat Genet* 1995;9:202–209.
66. Dinauer MC, Orkin SH. Chronic granulomatous disease. *Annu Rev Med* 1992;43:117–124.
67. Moncada S, Higgs A. The L-arginine-nitric oxide pathway. *N Engl J Med* 1993;329:2002–2012.
68. Gaston B, Drazen JM, Loscalzo J, Stamler JS. The biology of nitrogen oxides in the airways. *Am J Respir Crit Care Med* 1994;149:538–551.
69. Chollet-Martin S, Gatecel C, Kermarrec N, Gougerot-Pocidalo M-A, Payen DM. Alveolar neutrophil functions and cytokine levels in patients with the adult respiratory distress syndrome during nitric oxide inhalation. *Am J Respir Crit Care Med* 1996;153:985–990.

70. Janoff A. Elastase in tissue injury. *Annu Rev Med* 1985;36:207–216.
71. Lee CT, Fein AM, Lippmann M, Holtzman H, Kimbel P, Weinbaum G. Elastolytic activity in pulmonary lavage fluid from patients with adult respiratory distress syndrome. *N Engl J Med* 1981;304:192–196.
72. Idell S, Kucich U, Fein A, et al. Neutrophil elastase-releasing factors in bronchoalveolar lavage from patients with adult respiratory distress syndrome. *Am Rev Respir Dis* 1985;132:1098–1105.
73. Sakamaki F, Ishizaka A, Urano T, et al. Effect of a specific neutrophil elastase inhibitor, ONO-5046, on endotoxin-induced acute lung injury. *Am J Respir Crit Care Med* 1996;153:391–397.
74. Talbott GA, Sharar SR, Harlan JM, Winn RK. Leukocyte-endothelial interactions and organ injury: The role of adhesion molecules. *New Horiz* 1994;2:545–554.
75. Albert RK. Mechanisms of the adult respiratory distress syndrome. *Thorax* 1995;50:S49–S52.
76. Worthen GS, Avdi N, Buhl AM, Suzuki N, Johnson GL. FMLP activates Ras and Raf in human neutrophils. *J Clin Invest* 1994;94:815–823.
77. Nick JA, Avdi NJ, Gerwins P, Johnson FL, Worthen GS. Activation of a p38 mitogen-activated kinase in human neutrophils by lipopolysaccharide. *J Immunol* 1996;156:4867–4875.
78. Knall C, Young S, Nick JA, Buhl AM, Worthen GS, Johnson GL. Interleukin-8 regulation of the ras/raf/mitogen-activated protein kinase pathway in human neutrophils. *J Biol Chem* 1996;271:2832–2838.
79. Bazzoni F, Beutler B. The tumor necrosis factor ligand and receptor families. *N Engl J Med* 1996;334:1717–1725.
80. Fisher CJ, Agosti JM, Opal SM, et al. Treatment of septic shock with the tumor necrosis factor: Fc fusion protein. *N Engl J Med* 1996;334:1697–1702.
81. Gura T. Chemokines take center stage in inflammatory ills. *Science* 1996; 272:954–956.
82. Arnaout MA. Leukocyte adhesion molecule deficiency: Its structural basis, pathophysiology, and implications for modulating the inflammatory response. *Immunol Rev* 1990;114:145–180.
83. Etzioni AM, Frydman S, Pollack S, et al. Recurrent severe infections caused by a novel leukocyte adhesion deficiency. *N Engl J Med* 1992; 327:1789–1792.

Chapter 16

Mechanisms of Ischemia-Reperfusion Injury in the Lung

Timothy M. Moore, PhD, Pavel L. Khimenko, MD, PhD, and Aubrey E. Taylor, PhD

Introduction

Microvascular injury, manifested as an increase in microvascular permeability to fluid and protein, occurs in tissues that are subjected to periods of ischemia followed by reperfusion (I/R). In 1981, Granger et al[1] proposed the first working hypothesis that described how reperfusion of ischemic tissues produced microvascular damage and tissue edema. These investigators showed that reintroduction of molecular O_2 during reperfusion of an ischemic ileal preparation resulted in superoxide (O_2^-), hydrogen peroxide (H_2O_2), and other radical species production, which mediated the microvascular injury. The oxygen radicals were proposed to be generated by increased xanthine oxidase activity and by activated granulocytes that were sequestered in the ischemic-reperfused (I/R) tissue.

It is now known that oxygen radicals mediate I/R-induced microvascular damage in all tissues. The lung is no exception. In addition to oxygen radicals, many other mediators of lung I/R injury have been identified by use of various experimental lung models. Lung I/R injury models have been designed to represent clinical situations where pulmonary blood flow is interrupted but lung ventilation continues, or when both pulmonary blood flow and ventilation cease and O_2 is not available to the lung during the ischemia. Results from studies that use these models have provided important information regarding the eti-

Support provided by NIH HL22549.

From: Weir EK, Reeves JT (eds). *Pulmonary Edema*. Armonk, NY: Futura Publishing Company, Inc.; ©1998.

ologies of lung injury following formation and clearance of pulmonary emboli and lung injury associated with transplantation.

This chapter presents the current knowledge of lung I/R injury based primarily on a model in which both pulmonary flow and ventilation are interrupted for a period of time and then flow and ventilation are restored. The following questions are addressed: (1) How does I/R damage the microvascular endothelial barrier and what are the major factors that control endothelial permeability? (2) Are endogenous factors that limit the severity of I/R-induced lung injury and edema formation released or activated? (3) What are potentially useful therapeutic strategies for correcting I/R-induced microvascular damage? The discussion begins with a brief description of the isolated rat lung model from Dr. Aubrey Taylor's laboratory,[6,7] and then the findings from use of this model are presented and compared to work by other investigators.

The Isolated Rat Lung Model

Investigators at Taylor's laboratory[6,7] have extensively studied I/R injury using an isolated, buffer-perfused rat lung model in which the physiological conditions of this ex vivo lung preparation can be carefully controlled. It is important to note that each experimental lung serves as its own control, ie, measurements of microvascular permeability (assessed by measuring the capillary filtration coefficient, $K_{f,c}$) and pulmonary vascular resistances are obtained both prior to and following a 45-minute period of ischemia and a 30-minute or 90-minute period of reperfusion in the same lung. This I/R model eliminates several problems that arise in the interpretation of data from in vivo lung models, since changes in microvascular permeability and vascular resistances can only be due to the direct I/R insult and are not influenced by systemic events. Furthermore, the hydrostatic effects of increased microvascular pressure on lung edema formation do not complicate the measurement of $K_{f,c}$, since pulmonary capillary pressure (P_c) is also measured (see Reference 2 for a review on microvascular fluid exchange).

Factors That Promote Increased Microvascular Permeability and Pulmonary Edema

Figure 1 summarizes the factors that promote increased microvascular permeability in the isolated, buffer-perfused rat lung subjected to I/R as discussed below.

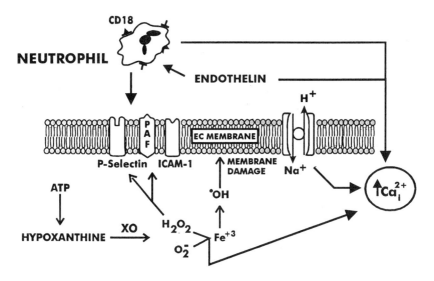

Figure 1. Factors that promote the microvascular permeability increase associated with lung ischemia and reperfusion. CD18 = neutrophil β_2 integrin common subunit; PAF = platelet activating factor; EC membrane = endothelial cell membrane; XO = xanthine oxidase; ICAM-1 = intercellular adhesion molecule-1.

Tissue Inflammation

Oxygen radical generation in the I/R lung is the major factor contributing to microvascular injury. Radicals such as O_2^- and H_2O_2 are released in response to both endothelial cell xanthine oxidase and granulocyte activation. In the presence of iron (Fe^{3+}), O_2^- and H_2O_2 react to produce the hydroxyl radical ($\cdot OH$), which in turn produces endothelial membrane damage. It is now well known that allopurinol (a xanthine oxidase inhibitor), superoxide dismutase (SOD) and catalase (O_2^- and H_2O_2 scavengers), and various $\cdot OH$ scavengers significantly reduce microvascular damage associated with lung I/R.[3-6]

In addition to producing endothelial membrane damage, oxygen radicals can stimulate the release of pro-inflammatory mediators such as platelet activating factor (PAF) and cyclooxygenase or lipoxygenase products. These inflammatory mediators can promote granulocyte adhesion to the microvascular endothelium and/or directly activate endothelial cell receptors, causing a modification of the endothelial barrier, which results in an increased microvascular permeability. The granulocyte-endothelial cell interactions that occur during I/R are mediated by adhesion molecules. Granulocytes first roll along the microvascular endothelium by an interaction of L-selectin (constituitively

expressed on granulocytes) with some endothelial-derived counter lig-
and. Additionally, endothelial-derived oxygen radicals mobilize preformed P-selectin, another rolling factor, to the endothelial cell surface.
Selectin-mediated interactions facilitate initial granulocyte tethering to
the endothelium and are important for initiating the inflammatory response. Immunoneutralization of P-selectin with a specific monoclonal
antibody (PB1.3) completely prevents I/R-induced microvascular
damage whereas immunoneutralization of L-selectin (HRL3) does not
provide protection.[6] These findings suggest that the I/R endothelium
initiates binding and subsequent activation of granulocytes during
lung I/R.

Endothelial-derived oxygen radicals can also promote endothelial
PAF production, which causes the P-selectin-tethered granulocytes to
become firmly adhered to endothelial cells. PAF promotes this firm adherence by facilitating leukocyte integrin (β_2 integrin family) binding to
endothelial cell-expressed integrin ligands. The granulocyte integrins
that mediate firm adherence are CD11a/CD18 and CD11b/CD18,
which are also known as LFA-1 and MAC-1, respectively. The endothe-
lial-expressed adherence factors belong to the immunoglobulin super-
family of proteins and are called intercellular adhesion molecules
(ICAMs). Firm adhesion of granulocytes to the endothelium causes the
release of more oxygen radicals and proteases from the granulocyte,
which in turn initiates a process that results in endothelial membrane
damage. Firm adherence and subsequent migration of granulocytes
across the endothelial barrier stimulates a Ca^{2+}-dependent active contraction of the endothelial cells. As a result of these effects, the microvascular barrier becomes overtly "leaky" to even large plasma proteins. Interstitial edema and then alveolar edema develop as a result of
this increased microvascular permeability. Immunoneutralization of
CD18 (common to both LFA-1 and MAC-1) with monoclonal antibody
CL26,[6] immunoneutralization of ICAM-1 with monoclonal antibody
1A29,[6] and antagonism of PAF receptors with WEB 2086 or BN52021[7]
significantly attenuate I/R-induced microvascular damage and lung
neutrophil sequestration. These findings are common findings in many
studies that evaluate the inflammatory response in lung I/R injury as
well as in other tissues studied under different conditions (see Reference
8 for a review on leukocyte adhesion and the inflammatory process).

Endothelin

It has been shown that endothelin, an endothelial cell-derived
vasoconstrictor, is released in the isolated guinea pig lung during is-
chemia/hypoxia and reperfusion, and that phosphoramidon, an en-

dothelin converting enzyme inhibitor, prevents this release when given prior to the induction of I/R.[9] Endothelin released from the I/R lung has a significant role in producing microvascular damage.[10,11] Endothelin exerts its biological effects by acting on at least two different receptor subtypes, ET_A and ET_B. Both an endothelin ET_A and a nonspecific receptor antagonist, when given prior to an ischemic period, prevent I/R-induced microvascular injury and reduce lung neutrophil sequestration,[10,11] although endothelin ET_B receptor antagonism does not prevent I/R damage from occurring.[10] The exact mechanism associated with endothelin participation in the injury process is presently unclear since endothelin infusion into normal lungs produces intense vasoconstriction and hydrostatic alveolar edema, but no apparent alteration in microvascular permeability.[10] Endothelin may act to promote granulocyte migration across the microvascular barrier[12] and/or directly increase endothelial cell intracellular Ca^{2+} levels in parallel with other permeability promoting factors.[13]

Na$^+$/H$^+$ Exchange Activation

It is well known that acidosis occurs in ischemic tissues. The changes in intracellular and extracellular pH that occur during both ischemia and reperfusion can have profound effects on the integrity of the microvascular barrier. Hayashi et al[14] have shown that lung intracellular pH decreases by approximately 0.19 pH units during a 30-minute period of anoxic ischemia, indicating that lung acid/base imbalance is present in lungs devoid of O_2. Investigators at Taylor's laboratory have now shown that the significant increase in microvascular permeability ($K_{f,c}$) that occurs after 45 minutes of ischemia followed by 30 minutes of reperfusion can be completely prevented by reperfusing the lung with slightly acidic perfusates (pH = 7.0 to 7.1).[15] This protective maneuver is due to the acidic perfusates inhibiting cellular Na$^+$/H$^+$ exchange activity, which is mimicked by direct inhibition of the Na$^+$/H$^+$ antiport protein with dimethyl amiloride (DMA).[15] Similar observations have been reported in studies of myocardial ischemia and reperfusion injury.[16] The authors hypothesize that lung acidosis occurring with ischemia establishes tissue conditions that favor the activation of endothelial cell Na$^+$/H$^+$ exchange when physiological pH is restored during reperfusion. The movement of Na$^+$ into the cell in exchange for H$^+$ extrusion leads to an activation of the Na$^+$/Ca^{2-} exchanger in a manner that promotes an increase in endothelial Ca^{2+} levels. The end result is endothelial contraction and microvascular permeability increase. An alternative hypothesis is that Na^+/H exchange is activated in marginated granulocytes and this is necessary for the I/R-induced inflammatory response to occur.[17] They have yet to test these hypotheses completely, but regardless of the outcome, their studies clearly show that activation of the Na^+/H^+ antiporter is necessary for microvascular injury to occur with lung I/R.

Ca^{2+}-Calmodulin and Myosin Light Chain Kinase

The I/R-induced microvascular injury requires activation of the Ca^{2+}-binding protein, calmodulin. Activated calmodulin stimulates myosin light chain kinase (MLCK), causing endothelial cells to contract. Contraction of endothelial cells increases intercellular gap size producing an increase in microvascular permeability. Both a calmodulin antagonist (trifluoperazine) and an MLCK inhibitor (ML-7) significantly reduce the increased permeability that occurs after reperfusion of ischemic lungs.[18] These findings agree with studies that use cultured endothelial monolayers to show endothelial cell shape to be regulated in part by MLCK activity.[19] The stimulus for the Ca^{2+}-calmodulin-mediated MLCK activation is not presently clear, but all of the previous permeability-promoting factors discussed above increase intracellular Ca^{2+} levels in endothelium. Therefore, the final common pathway leading to I/R-induced microvascular permeability increase is elevated endothelial cell Ca^{2+} levels.

Factors That Limit Pulmonary Edema After Ischemia and Reperfusion

Alveolar Epithelial Transport Mechanisms

Figure 2 shows that interfering with Na^+-dependent fluid removal from the alveolar spaces during I/R causes an exacerbation of lung edema formation.[20] Edema fluid is transported from the alveolar spaces into the interstitial spaces and vascular spaces by amiloride-sensitive Na^+ transport driven by the activity of the Na^+/K^+ ATPase. The edema resolution during I/R is not dependent on an $Na^+/glucose$ transport system. These data simply indicate that the lung possesses an active edema safety factor that is important during I/R for limiting the amount of alveolar edema, but is not sufficient to prevent alveolar edema from occurring. Future studies should be directed at finding ways to enhance alveolar epithelial fluid transport systems in order to oppose I/R-induced pulmonary edema.

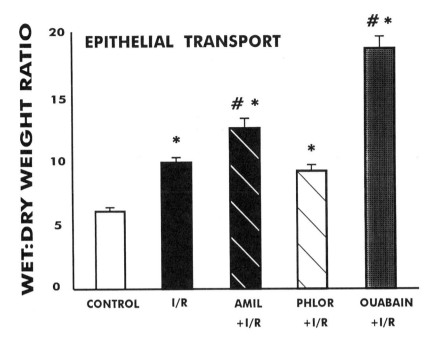

Figure 2. Wet-to-dry weight ratios of lungs not subjected to ischemia and reperfusion (I/R) (CONTROL), lungs subjected to I/R, lungs pretreated with amiloride and subjected to I/R (AMIL + I/R), lungs pretreated with phloridzin and subjected to I/R (PHLOR + I/R), and lungs pretreated with ouabain and subjected to I/R (OUABAIN + I/R). *Significant difference as compared to CONTROL; #significant difference as compared to I/R ($P<0.05$).

Factors That Prevent or Reverse Increased Permeability and Pulmonary Edema

Figure 3 summarizes the factors that can either prevent or reverse increased microvascular permeability in the isolated, buffer-perfused rat lung subjected to I/R as discussed below. Also, shown on the left-hand side of Figure 3 is a summary of the factors that promote increased microvascular permeability.

Cyclic Adenosine Monophosphate Elevation

The effects of adenosine-3',5'-cyclic monophosphate (cAMP) on I/R-induced lung injury have been extensively studied. Not only can this intracellular second messenger protect against lung injury, but it can actually reverse preexisting damage. Adkins et al[21] first observed

DAMAGING FACTORS   PROTECTIVE INTERVENTIONS

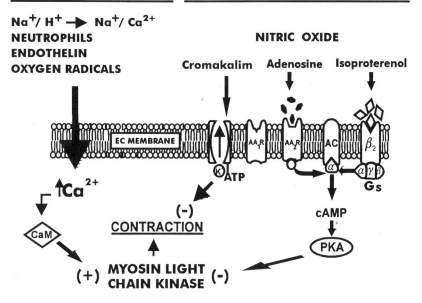

Figure 3. The proposed mechanism by which lung ischemia and reperfusion induces microvascular injury and the protective interventions into the injury process. Na^+/H^+ = Na^+/H^+ exchange activation; Na^+/Ca^{2+} = Na^+/Ca^{2+} exchange activation; EC membrane = endothelial cell membrane; CaM = calmodulin; K^+ATP = ATP-sensitive K^+ channel; AA_1R = adenosine A_1 receptor subtype; AA_2R = adenosine A_2 receptor subtype; AC = adenylyl cyclase; G_s = G-stimulatory protein with its subunits; β_2 = beta-adrenergic receptor subtype 2; PKA = protein kinase A.

that cAMP-elevating compounds such as isoproterenol (a β_2-adrenergic receptor agonist), forskolin (a direct activator of adenylyl cyclase), and dibutyryl-cAMP (a nonhydrolyzable cAMP analog) prevent increases in microvascular permeability associated with lung I/R. Seibert et al[22] later showed that isoproterenol, forskolin, or dibutyryl-cAMP can reverse the preexisting microvascular injury caused by I/R. Barnard et al[23] further showed that inhibitors of cAMP phosphodiesterase (PDE), which prevent degradation of cAMP, also reverse I/R-induced microvascular injury. In fact, histologic examination of lungs subjected to I/R indicate that endothelial cell shape is affected by the PDE treatment, such that endothelial cells appear more rounded after I/R and become more flattened in appearance after cAMP elevation. This study by Barnard et al[23] demonstrated a very important positive correlation between the functional protective effects of cAMP on the microvascular barrier and the observed microscopic changes in endothelial cell shape. The protective effects of cAMP on lung I/R injury can also be achieved by activation of the adenosine A_2 receptor subtype. Hsu et al[24] have shown that ATP-MgCl$_2$ protects isolated rat lungs from I/R injury by stimulating adenosine A_2 receptors. Khimenko et al[25] also showed that elevation of cAMP by adenosine acting on A_2 receptors reverses I/R-induced microvascular injury. This reversal effect was also shown to be protein kinase A (PKA)-dependent.[25]

Other than the PKA requirement, the exact mechanism by which cAMP reverses I/R-induced lung microvascular injury is unknown. The prevailing hypothesis, based upon several observations, is that cAMP and PKA mediate their permeability reversal effects by causing endothelial cell relaxation by interfering with the Ca^{++}-calmodulin-MLCK contractile system. Furthermore, it is possible that cAMP could affect the microfilament component of the endothelial cell cytoskeleton, which plays an important role in maintaining normal microvascular permeability.[26] Actin filaments in endothelial cell monolayers can be disrupted during an energy-depleted state, ie, ischemia, and they appear as F-actin fragments in the endothelial cell cytosol.[27] This fragmentation causes monolayers to become permeable to protein, but increasing cAMP levels can stimulate F-actin stabilization and restore normal monolayer permeability.[28]

Activation of ATP-Sensitive K⁺ Channels

Studies by Khimenko et al[29] have shown that activation of K^+_{ATP} channels prevents I/R-induced increases in microvascular permeability. Furthermore, addition of cromakalim (a K^+_{ATP} channel agonist) to lungs already injured by 45 minutes of ischemia and 30 minutes' reperfusion reverses the I/R-induced injury. This effect of cromakalim on microvascular permeability is identical to the effect of cAMP elevation (ie, inhibition of endothelial contraction), but activation of K^+_{ATP} channels does not result from PKA activation by cAMP. This conclusion is based on the observation that isoproterenol produces a reversal of preexisting microvascular damage even in the presence of a K^+_{ATP} channel antagonist (glybenclimide).[29] Additional work is required to determine how K^+_{ATP} channel activation causes protection and reversal of I/R-induced microvascular injury.

Nitric Oxide

The effects of nitric oxide (NO) in lung I/R injury are difficult to summarize, since several conflicting reports have been published. There are basically three different hypotheses that describe the relationship between NO and lung I/R injury: (1) endogenous NO production in the postischemic lung mediates tissue injury after I/R, (2) endogenous NO production in the postischemic lung limits the severity of I/R-induced microvascular injury, and (3) endogenous NO production in the postischemic lung neither limits nor mediates microvascular injury after I/R, but exogenous NO administration prevents microvascular injury through some as yet unidentified mechanism. Recent studies tend to agree with the latter of these hypotheses, but a role for endogenous NO production in regulating postreperfusion pulmonary vascular resistance has been described.

Is Endogenous NO Injurious?

The reaction between NO and O_2^- represents an alternative mechanism by which ·OH can be produced in ischemic-reperfused tissues[30]

$$\text{L-arginine} + O_2 \text{ —NOS} \rightarrow \text{L-citrulline} + \cdot\text{NO} \tag{1}$$

$$O_2^- + \cdot\text{NO} \rightarrow \text{ONOO}^- \tag{2}$$

$$\text{ONOO}^- + \text{H}^+ \leftrightarrow \text{ONOOH} \tag{3}$$

$$\text{ONOOH} \rightarrow \cdot\textbf{OH} + \text{NO}_2 \qquad \dots(4)$$

The conversion of L-arginine to L-citrulline in the presence of O_2 generates NO, and this conversion is mediated by nitric oxide synthase (NOS). NO can then combine with O_2^- to form peroxynitrite (ONOO$^-$) which, once protonated, decomposes to produce hydroxyl radicals. Ischiropoulos et al[31] addressed the involvement of peroxynitrite in mediation of I/R-induced lung tissue oxidation. In this study, isolated and buffer-perfused rat lungs were subjected to 60 minutes of ischemia (but ventilated with 95% O_2 + 5% CO_2) and 60 minutes of reperfusion. Thirty minutes prior to ischemia, an NOS inhibitor (N^G-Nitro-L-Arginine methyl ester [L-NAME]) was injected into the trachea, and lung thiobarbituric acid reactive substances (TBARS), conjugated diene levels, dinitrophenol- (DNP) reactive protein carbonyl levels, and nitrotyrosine levels were measured to assess lung tissue oxidation. The NOS inhibitor decreased the production of all measures of oxidant production, causing these investigators to conclude that peroxynitrite contributed to oxidative injury associated with I/R in rat lungs.

Is Endogenous Nitric Oxide Protective?

Pinsky et al,[32] with use of a rat lung transplant model, showed that reperfusion of the transplanted lung tissue diminished NO production as measured at the lung's surface. Detectable NO could be restored when SOD was superfused over the lung's surface, indicating that superoxide was responsible for reducing the endogenous NO levels at reperfusion and implying that peroxynitrite was formed. A nonhydrolyzable cGMP analog was added to the ischemic lung's preservation solution and lung function was significantly improved. This study suggested that endogenous NO production and subsequent cyclic guanine monophosphate (cGMP) generation act to limit lung injury. Superoxide production facilitates removal of NO from the microcirculation, promoting lung injury, but peroxynitrite is merely an inconsequential product of the NO-O_2^- reaction.

Is Exogenous Nitric Oxide Protective?

In a study by Naka et al,[33] it was shown that addition of an NO donor, nitroglycerin, to hypothermic preserved (6 hours) and reperfused rat lungs provided a more functional lung. Furthermore, nitroglycerin addition to the lung preservation solution was also able to decrease sequestration of neutrophils. However, Matsuzaki et al,[34] who studied I/R injury in an in situ rabbit lung model, failed to show a protective effect of sodium nitroprusside on I/R-induced lung edema formation when lung wet-to-dry weight ratios were used to assess lung damage. Sodium nitroprusside also failed to reduce neutrophil sequestration in the lung tissue. The differences in the findings of these two studies are difficult to explain since different measurements were used to assess lung injury.

In studies conducted in Taylor's lab, it has been shown that NO donors, but not NO synthase inhibitors, prevent the microvascular permeability increase associated with I/R.[35] Three different L-arginine analogs, given at concentrations sufficient to inhibit NO synthase, failed to prevent the I/R-induced increase in $K_{f,c}$. Furthermore, none of the NOS inhibitors produced an exacerbation of the I/R-induced permeability increase, but postreperfusion vascular resistances were significantly elevated. Interestingly, very high concentrations of L-NAME or N^G-monomethyl-L-arginine (L-NMA) protected lungs against I/R injury, but by a mechanism not specific for NO synthase inhibition because both D-NAME and D-NMA at the same molar concentrations produced equal levels of protection. Furthermore, both L- and D-NAME (5 mmol/L concentrations), used as a hydrochloric acid (HCl) salt, produced significant decreases in lung perfusate pH. The decreased perfusate pH was responsible for providing protection against the I/R-induced microvascular damage, as discussed previously. In contrast to the results from the NOS inhibitor studies, NO-donating compounds, ($\pm$)-S-Nitroso-N-acetylpenicillamine (SNAP) and spermine-NO, prevented I/R-induced microvascular injury from occurring when they were given to lungs at the onset of reperfusion. Barbotin-Larrieu et al[36] have also shown that ventilation of postischemic neonatal pig lungs with NO prevents I/R-induced microvascular injury and lung sequestration of neutrophils. Based upon these findings, the authors therefore hypothesize the following: (1) endogenous NO and subsequent peroxynitrite production in postischemic lung tissue does not contribute to I/R-induced increases in microvascular permeability, (2) endogenous NO production in the postischemic lung limits I/R-induced resistance increase, but not I/R-induced microvascular damage, and (3) exogenous NO, whether given in the vascular system or administered via the airways, is highly protective against I/R-induced microvascular damage. The exact mechanism by which exogenously administered NO prevents reperfusion-induced microvascular damage is still not known. Future studies should be designed to further evaluate how NO mediates protection, since the results from these studies could have important clinical implications.

Summary

This chapter presents the factors that promote, limit, and prevent I/R-induced lung microvascular injury. The scope of this chapter is somewhat space limited and the authors acknowledge the fact that there exist other important studies that are relevant to the mechanisms of lung I/R injury besides those specifically mentioned here (see Reference 37 for a more comprehensive review of the lung I/R injury literature). Knowledge of how lung I/R injury affects the microvascular barrier has been considerably extended over just the past 5 years. Several important discoveries, such as the reversal effects of cAMP and the protective effects of NO, may eventually influence the clinical therapies for lung I/R injury. Of course, there is still much to be learned about this phenomenon and hopefully, research devoted to understanding the physiology and pathophysiology of the lung's microcirculation will continue to expand.

References

1. Granger DN, Rutili G, McCord JM. Superoxide radicals in feline intestinal ischemia. *Gastroenterology* 1981;79:474–480.
2. Taylor AE, Adkins WK, Wilson PS, et al. Regulation of capillary exchange of fluid and protein. In: Ayres SM, Grenvik A, Holbrook P, et al (eds): *Textbook of Critical Medicine*. Philadelphia: W.B. Saunders; 1995;659–673.
3. Adkins WK, Taylor AE. Role of xanthine oxidase and neutrophils in is-

chemia-reperfusion injury in the rabbit lung. *J Appl Physiol* 1990;69: 2012–2018.

4. Allison RC, Kyle J, Adkins WK, et al. Effect of ischemia reperfusion or hypoxia reoxygenation on lung vascular permeability and resistance. *J Appl Physiol* 1990;69:597–603.

5. Fisher PW, Huang Y-CT, Kennedy TP, et al. PO_2-dependent hydroxyl radical production during ischemia-reperfusion lung injury. *Am J Physiol* 1993;265:L279–L285.

6. Moore TM, Khimenko PL, Adkins WK, et al. Adhesion molecules contribute to ischemia and reperfusion-induced injury in the isolated rat lung. *J Appl Physiol* 1995;78:2245–2252.

7. Moore TM, Khimenko PL, Wilson PS, et al. PAF antagonists attenuate I-R-induced microvascular injury in the isolated rat lung. *FASEB J* 1996;10: A–109.

8. Granger DN, Schmid-Schonbein GW. *Physiology and Pathophysiology of Leukocyte Adhesion.* New York, Oxford: Oxford University Press; 1995;1–498.

9. Vemulapalli S, Rivelli M, Chiu PJ, et al. Phosphoramidon abolishes the increases in endothelin-1 release induced by ischemia-hypoxia in isolated perfused guinea pig lungs. *J Pharmacol Exp Ther* 1992;262:1062–1069.

10. Khimenko PL, Moore TM, Taylor AE. Blocking ET_A receptors prevents ischemia and reperfusion injury in rat lungs. *J Appl Physiol* 1996;80:203–207.

11. Okada M, Yamashita C, Okada M, et al. Contribution of endothelin-1 to warm ischemia/reperfusion injury of the rat lung. *Am J Respir Crit Care Med* 1995;152:2105–2110.

12. Elferink JGR, de Koster BM. Endothelin-induced activation of neutrophil migration. *Biochem Pharmacol* 1994;48:865–871.

13. Yanagisawa M, Kurihara H, Kimura Y, et al. A novel potent vasoconstrictor peptide produced by vascular endothelial cells. *Nature* 1988;322: 411–436.

14. Hayashi Y, Inubushi T, Nioka S, et al. ^{31}P-NMR spectroscopy of isolated perfused rat lung. *J Appl Physiol* 1993;74:1549–1554.

15. Moore TM, Khimenko PL, Taylor AE. Restoration of normal pH triggers ischemia-reperfusion injury in lung by Na^+/H^+ exchange activation. *Am J Physiol* 1995;269:H1501–H1505.

16. Bond JM, Harper IS, Chacon E, et al. The pH paradox in the pathophysiology of reperfusion injury to rat neonatal cardiac myocytes. *Ann N Y Acad Sci* 1994;723:25–37.

17. Molski TFP, Naccache PH, Borgeat P, et al. Similarities in the mechanisms by which formyl-methionyl-leucyl-phenylalanine, arachidonic acid, and leukotriene B_4 increase calcium and sodium influxes in rabbit neutrophils. *Biochem Biophys Res Commun* 1981;103:227–232.

18. Khimenko PL, Moore TM, Wilson PS, et al. Role of calmodulin and myosin light-chain kinase in lung ischemia/reperfusion injury. *Am J Physiol* 1996;271:L121–L125.

19. Sheldon R, Moy A, Lindsley K, et al. Role of myosin light-chain phosphorylation in endothelial cell retraction. *Am J Physiol* 1993;265:L606–L612.

20. Khimenko PL, Barnard JW, Moore TM, et al. Vascular permeability and epithelial transport effects on lung edema formation in ischemia and reperfusion. *J Appl Physiol* 1994;77:1116–1121.

21. Adkins WK, Barnard JW, May S, et al. Compounds that increase cAMP prevent ischemia-reperfusion pulmonary capillary injury. *J Appl Physiol* 1992;72:492–497.

22. Seibert AF, Thompson WJ, Taylor AE, et al. Reversal of increased microvascular permeability associated with ischemia-reperfusion: Role of cAMP. *J Appl Physiol* 1992;72:389–395.
23. Barnard JW, Seibert AF, Prasad VR, et al. Reversal of pulmonary capillary ischemia-reperfusion injury by rolipram, a cAMP phosphodiesterase inhibitor. *J Appl Physiol* 1994;77:774–781.
24. Hsu K, Wang D, Wu S-Y, et al. Ischemia-reperfusion lung injury attenuated by ATP-MgCl$_2$ in rats. *J Appl Physiol* 1994;76:545–552.
25. Khimenko PL, Moore TM, Hill LW, et al. Adenosine A$_2$-receptors reverse ischemia-reperfusion lung injury independent of β-receptors. *J Appl Physiol* 1995;78:990–996.
26. Shasby DM, Shasby SS, Sullivan JM, et al. Role of endothelial cytoskeleton in control of endothelial permeability. *Circ Res* 1982;51:657–661.
27. Kuhne W, Besselman M, Noll T, et al. Disintegration of cytoskeletal structure of actin filaments in energy-depleted endothelial cells. *Am J Physiol* 1993;264:H1599–H1608.
28. Minnear FL, DeMichelle MAA, Moon DG, et al. Isoproterenol reduces thrombin-induced pulmonary endothelial permeability in vitro. *Am J Physiol* 1989;257:H1613–H1623.
29. Khimenko PL, Moore TM, Taylor AE. ATP-sensitive K$^+$ channels are not involved in ischemia-reperfusion lung endothelial injury. *J Appl Physiol* 1995;79:554–559.
30. Beckman JS, Beckman TW, Chen J, et al. Apparent hydroxyl radical production by peroxynitrite: Implications for endothelial injury from nitric oxide and superoxide. *Proc Natl Acad Sci U S A* 1990;87:1620–1624.
31. Ischiropoulos H, Al-Mehdi A, Fisher AB. Reactive species in ischemic rat lung injury: Contribution of peroxynitrite. *Am J Physiol* 1995;269:L158–L164.
32. Pinsky DJ, Naka Y, Chowdhury NP, et al. The nitric oxide/cyclic GMP pathway in organ transplantation: Critical role in successful lung preservation. *Proc Natl Acad Sci U S A* 1994;91:12086–12090.
33. Naka Y, Chowdhury NC, Liao H, et al. Enhanced preservation of orthotopically transplanted rat lungs by nitroglycerin but not hydralazine. *Circ Res* 1995;76:900–906.
34. Matsuzaki Y, Waddell TK, Puskas JD, et al. Amelioration of post-ischemia lung reperfusion injury by prostaglandin E$_1$. *Am Rev Respir Dis* 1993;148:882–889.
35. Moore TM, Khimenko PL, Wilson PS, Taylor AE. The role of nitric oxide in lung ischemia and reperfusion injury. *Am J Physiol* 1996;271:H1970–H1977.
36. Barbotin-Larrieu F, Mazmanian M, Baudet B, et al. Prevention of ischemia-reperfusion lung injury by inhaled nitric oxide in neonatal piglets. *J Appl Physiol* 1996;80:782–788.
37. Moore TM, Khimenko PL, Taylor AE. Endothelial damage caused by ischemia and reperfusion and different ventilatory strategies in the lung. *Chin J Physiol* 1996;39:65–81.

Chapter 17

Endothelial Cell Activation and Barrier Dysfunction

Hazel Lum, PhD

Introduction

The endothelium orchestrates the homeostatic balance of blood vessels through the production of factors that regulate vessel tone, coagulation state, cell growth, cell death, leukocyte trafficking, and barrier function. Quiescent or nonactivated endothelial cells are metabolically active with low cell turnover rate, and are activated by a host of external stimuli, including receptor-binding mediators (eg, thrombin, cytokines),[1,2] oxidants,[3] as well as mechanical factors such as shear stress.[4] The activated endothelial cell presents characteristic features of inflammation including impaired barrier function, increased adhesiveness for leukocytes, elevated proliferative and angiogenic capacities, and increased secretory function.

The morphological manifestations of impaired endothelial barrier function are cell shape changes associated with intercellular gap formation, indicating disruption of cellular junctions.[1-3,5,6] Thus, the mechanism by which mediators cause increased endothelial permeability appears to be predominantly increased transport of proteins and liquid via the paracellular pathway. Central in the regulation of this increase in endothelial permeability is activation of the protein kinase C (PKC) cascade. This chapter discusses the current understanding of the paracellular transport pathways as potential targets for regulation by the PKC-signaling cascade in activated endothelium.

This work was supported by NIH grant HL45638 and a grant from the American Heart Association of Metropolitan Chicago.

From: Weir EK, Reeves JT (eds). *Pulmonary Edema*. Armonk, NY: Futura Publishing Company, Inc.; ©1998.

Structure of the Endothelial Barrier

Endothelial cells form junctional complexes consisting of tight junctions, adherens junctions, and gap junctions that serve as diffusive pathways for transport of solutes. Based on tracer studies in animal models as well as in cultured endothelial cells, it is proposed that molecules are transported through hypothesized "pores" in a size-selective manner.[7,8] The tight junctions provide the primary barrier to diffusion of solutes across epithelium and endothelium. Tight junctions of endothelium contain a 225 kd protein (ZO-1) located on the cytoplasmic side of the junction[9] and a 65 kd integral membrane protein (occludin),[10] both of which may be important in regulating the endothelial barrier. The recent identification of occludin has been proposed to represent the intramembranous strands observed with freeze-fracture replicas of tight junctions which seal the outer membrane leaflets and effectively impart the barrier property to the endothelium and epithelium. Endothelial junctions are in general less restrictive than epithelial junctional complexes, which may likely be attributed to the fact that endothelium has a less complex organization of these intramembranous strands than epithelium.[11]

The adherens junctions of endothelium are composed of cadherins, a supergene family of cell-to-cell adhesion molecules, several intermediate proteins (particularly, α-, β-, and γ-catenins), and prominent bundles of actin microfilaments.[12] Cadherins are responsible for Ca^{2+}-dependent homophilic cell adhesion (ie, cadherin of one cell binds to another cadherin of the adjacent cell), and this cell recognition function is believed to be important for formation of not only adherens junctions, but also gap junctions and tight junctions.[13,14] Based on crystal structure analysis, the extracellular NH_2 terminus of cadherin has five tandem repeat sequences of $\approx$110 amino acids each, with the first repeat containing the recognition site (Figure 1, panel a).[15] This recognition sequence has been identified as the tripeptide, His-Ala-Val, a relatively conserved sequence for most cadherins.[16] However, in the endothelial-specific VE-cadherin (cadherin 5), recognition function is not dependent on this tripeptide.[17] Ca^{2++} binding sites are also identified in the NH_2 terminus, and the binding of Ca^{2+} is proposed to rigidify the adhesive interactions.[15]

Interruption of cadherin-to-cadherin adhesion impairs barrier function. Monoclonal antibodies directed against an extracellular domain of cadherin has inhibited the formation of tight junctions in Madin Darby Canine Kidney epithelial cells, resulting in decreased transepithelial electrical resistance.[13] Similarly, in endothelial cells, incubation with antibodies directed against the extracellular domain of

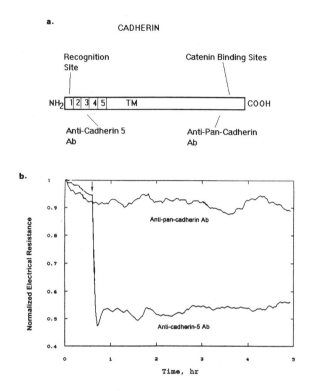

Figure 1. (a) Diagram of the general primary structure of cadherin. Numbers 1 to 5 indicate the five extracellular repeats of the NH_2 terminus; TM = transmembrane domain. Anti-cadherin 5 Ab was directed against residues 26–194; anti-pan-cadherin Abs against the cytoplasmic domain. (b) Effects of anti-cadherin 5 and anti-pan-cadherin Abs on the transendothelial electrical resistance across human microvascular endothelial cells. Arrow indicates time of addition of the Abs.

cadherin 5 decreased the transendothelial electrical resistance, whereas the control antibody, directed against the cytoplasmic domain, was ineffective in decreasing the resistance (Figure 1, panels a and b). The anti-cadherin 5 antibody as well as antibody directed against the extracellular domain of N-cadherin, another endothelial cadherin, also increased endothelial permeability of tracer proteins across endothelial monolayers.[18,19] These observations indicate that cadherins are crucial for tethering one endothelial cell to another.

The cell-to-cell adhesion function of cadherins is also dependent on formation of complexes of cadherins with the cytoplasmic proteins α-catenins, β-catenins, and γ-catenins and with actin microfilaments. The highly conserved cytoplasmic domain of cadherins binds at least two of the catenins: γ-catenins and β-catenins. When the cadherin cytoplasmic domain is deleted, these truncated cadherins are unable to bind to catenins and cause impaired cell-to-cell adhesion and barrier function.[20,21] Since α-catenin contains actin-binding activity, this protein may be particularly important for linkage of cadherin to the actin cytoskeleton. The function of γ-catenin may provide the intermediate linkage between cadherin and α-catenin, since it has binding sites for α-catenin. Therefore, disruption of these protein-to-protein interactions may lead to barrier dysfunction.

Activated Endothelium and Increased Permeability

The vascular endothelium is responsive to a host of extracellular stimuli and its subsequent activation engages sophisticated transduction processes by which cellular signals are amplified, integrated, and targeted to regulate cellular activities. Different endothelial activation factors (ie, oxidants, cytokines, growth factors, vasoactive factors, shear stress) engage different strategies to transduce the external stimulus into chemical messengers, which signal the regulation of post-translational activities in the cytoplasm and/or of transcriptional processes in the nucleus. One of these messengers is PKC, a key regulatory enzyme in signal transduction, involved in diverse processes such as cell growth and differentiation, synaptic transmission, smooth muscle contraction and relaxation, endocrine and exocrine secretion, tumor promotion, and aging. Activation of PKC is also a critical factor in promoting leakiness of the endothelial barrier.

Protein Kinase C Activation in Endothelial Barrier Function

There is a substantial amount of evidence to support the thesis that activation of the PKC cascade is a crucial signaling pathway for mediator-induced increases in endothelial permeability. In cultured monolayers of bovine pulmonary artery endothelial cells, thrombin caused a dose-dependent increase of endothelial permeability in association with activation of PKC.[22] Stimulation of endothelial cells with H_2O_2 also increases endothelial permeability with concomitant translocation of PKC to the membrane.[3] The importance of PKC has also been demonstrated with studies using inhibitors of PKC. Guinea pig lungs pretreated with H-7 (a PKC inhibitor that acts on the catalytic site of the enzyme)[23] produced a reduction in the H_2O_2-induced increase in pulmonary capillary filtration coefficient.[5] The bradykinin-induced increase in vascular permeability of fluorescein-labeled dextran in the hamster cheek pouch was also inhibited in the presence of PKC inhibitors sphingosine or H-7.[24] In bovine pulmonary microvascular endothelial monolayers, H-7 or calphostin C (which prevents PKC activation by binding the regulatory site of the enzyme) inhibited the increase in endothelial albumin permeability in response H_2O_2[3] and thrombin.[22,25]

Endothelial Protein Kinase C Isoforms

PKC is a multigene family consisting of at the least 11 isoforms known to date in mammalian cells. It catalyzes the phosphorylation of substrates at serine and threonine residues. Although 110 substrates of PKC have been reported,[26] the critical target substrates responsible for regulation of the endothelial barrier function are unknown.

Endothelial cells have Ca^{2+}-dependent PKCα and PKCβ isoforms and the Ca^{2+}-independent isoforms ε, ζ, and λ. Of these, PKCα and PKCβ isoforms may play predominant roles in modulating endothelial permeability. Stimulation of human umbilical vein endothelial cells with platelet activating factor (PAF) causes increase in permeability and the translocation of both of these isoforms, but not of PKCε.[27] Similarly, H_2O_2 treatment of bovine pulmonary microvascular endothelial cells causes increase in permeability and the translocation of PKCβ.[3] When PKCβ1 is overexpressed in human dermal microvascular endothelial cells by stable transfection of PKCβ1 cDNA, the threshold of the PMA-induced increase in albumin permeability is significantly lowered compared to nontransfected control cells (Figure 2, panel a). However, when the endothelial cells are transfected with antisense PKCβ1 cDNA to decrease PKCβ1 expression, the PMA-induced increase in permeability is decreased (Figure 2, panel b). These observations indicate that Ca^{2+}-dependent PKC isoforms may be the more important class of isoforms for endothelial barrier regulation.

Intracellular Activators of Protein Kinase C

The Ca^{2+}-dependent PKC isoforms constitute the conventional class of isoforms (cPKC)(α, βI, βII, and γ) that are activated by Ca^{2+}, phosphatidylserine (PS), and diacylglycerol (DAG); the new isoforms (nPKC) (α, δ, Θ, μ, and η) are Ca^{2+}-independent and are activated by PS and DAG; and the atypical isoforms (aPKC) (ζ and λ) are activated by PS but do not require DAG or Ca^{2+}.[26] Cis-unsaturated free fatty

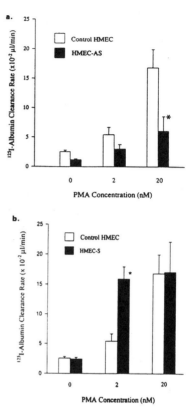

Figure 2. Effects of 2 nM and 20 nM PMA on the transendothelial ^{125}I-albumin clearance rate (index of endothelial permeability) in human microvascular endothelial cells transfected with the (a) antisense PKCβ1 (HMEC-AS) or (b) sense PKCβ1 (HMEC-S). Nontransfected HMEC served as control. Each group consisted of six monolayers; mean ±SE; nM = nmol/L.

acids (eg, arachidonic, linoleic) generated by phospholipase A_2- mediated hydrolysis of phospholipids also can activate isoforms in the cPKC, nPKC, and aPKC classes in the presence or absence of Ca^{2+}.[26,28] These fatty acids also potentiate PKC activity of isoforms that rely on DAG-dependent activation.[26,28] PKC can also be activated by intermediates of the phosphatidylinositol phosphate metabolic pathway.[26] Interestingly, the activation of phosphatidylinositol-3 kinase (PI-3 kinase), which associates with growth factor receptors via its SH2 domain, catalyzes the generation of phosphatidylinositol 3,4 bisphosphate and phosphatidylinositol 3,4,5 trisphosphate (which are specific activators of nPKCs),[26] providing a mechanism by which growth factor receptors (eg, Vascular Endothelial Growth Factor/Vascular Permeability Factor) can signal through the PKC cascade and regulate barrier function.

The importance of DAG-mediated activation of PKC in barrier function is demonstrated by the observation that direct treatment of endothelial cells with 1-oleoyl 2-acetyl glycerol (a 1,2-diacylglycerol analog) or phospholipase C (PLC) results in increased endothelial permeability to albumin in a dose-dependent manner.[22] DAG is transiently produced by the hydrolysis of phosphatidylinositol 4,5 bisphosphate (PIP_2) catalyzed by phosphatidylinositide-specific PLC (PI-PLC), and this is accompanied by an equimolar release of inositol-1,4,5-trisphosphate ($Ins(1,4,5)P_3$). The dominant substrates of PI-PLC are three common phosphoinositides (PIP_2, PIP [phosphatidylinositol 4-phosphate], and PI).[29] The hydrolysis of PIP and PI generates DAG, but not $Ins(1,4,5)P_3$. Only PI-PLC-mediated hydrolysis of PIP_2 generates the Ca^{2+}-mobilizing $Ins(1,4,5)P_3$ and DAG. The $Ins(1,4,5)P_3$ binds to receptors located on intracellular Ca^{2+} storage organelles and causes release of Ca^{2+}. In a study of bovine pulmonary artery endothelial cells,[1] thrombin increased $Ins(1,4,5)P_3$ levels within 10 seconds, and the value decreased to a baseline by 20 seconds,[1] which is typical for agonist-mediated generation of $Ins(1,4,5)P_3$. Increased endothelial permeability is a Ca^{2+}-dependent process, and the $Ins(1,4,5)P_3$-mobilized intracellular Ca^{2+}, together with Ca^{2+} influx, may contribute to regulation of barrier function.[31,32]

DAG can also be generated from sources other than PIP_2 hydrolysis. Phospholipase D (PLD) mediates the hydrolysis of phosphatidylcholine to yield phosphatidic acid, which can be converted to DAG by phosphatidic acid hydrolase.[33] Furthermore, PKC may activate PLD, producing a positive feedback pathway to generate additional DAG.[34] The PLD-mediated generation of DAG provides a greater amount of DAG than does the PLC-mediated hydrolysis of PIP_2, and the duration is prolonged, which can provide a sustained source of DAG for activating PKC.

Reversing the Increased Permeability

The increased permeability of activated endothelium is a reversible process. In time-course studies, the agonist-induced increase in endothelial permeability decreased to near basal levels 15 to 60 minutes after removal of the agonist from the incubating medium.[1,6,35] In the intact lung, continuous perfusion of thrombin caused increased capillary filtration coefficient that peaked at 10 minutes of stimulation; but by 40 minutes, the increase was returned to near baseline.[36] Morphologically, the number of intercellular gaps in vascular endothelium was observed to increase in response to histamine[32,35] and bradykinin,[37] which decreased to control numbers within 15 to 30 minutes after the stimulation. Similarly, in cultured endothelial cell monolayers, the thrombin-induced endothelial retraction and the increase in number of intercellular gaps were returned to control levels by 30 minutes.[6]

The mechanism of this "off-switch" may be regulated at multiple levels along the activated signaling cascade (eg, receptor desensitization, uncoupling of receptor-effector interaction). In thrombin-mediated activation responses, one potential negative regulatory pathway involves PKCβ functioning to limit activation of the PI-PLC cascade[38] and Ca^{2+} entry.[39] The basis of the negative regulation is likely caused by an uncoupling of the G protein with PI-PLC. This idea is supported by the observation that the isoform PLC-β was phosphorylated at serine 887 by PKC activation without a concomitant effect on the PLC-β activity, suggesting that the phosphorylation interfered with G protein-PLCβ interaction and not the catalytic activity.[40] This negative feedback regulation was also observed to modulate the effects of thrombin on the endothelial barrier function. In endothelial cells transfected with antisense PKCβ1 cDNA, the increases in $[Ca^{2+}]_i$ and albumin permeability in response to thrombin stimulation were greater than in nontransfected control cells.[40a]

Another mechanism for the reversal of the activated endothelium and the permeability increase is the activation of protein phosphatases and/or inhibition of protein kinases, both of which can reduce phosphorylation of substrate proteins responsible for increasing endothelial permeability. The activation of constitutive serine/threonine protein phosphatases (ser/thr PP) in endothelial cells may function to reverse the action of protein kinases. There are four main classes of ser/thr PP (ie, PP1, PP2A, PP2B, and PP2C), based on substrate (phosphorylase kinase) selectivity, sensitivity to specific inhibitors, and cation requirements.[41] Endothelial cells stimulated with thrombin show a decrease in the transendothelial electrical resistance within 1 to 3 minutes, and by 10 to 15 minutes, the resistance returns to near baseline (Figure 3, panel a). Calyculin A, inhibitor of PP1 and PP2A with equal potency, or FK506, inhibitor of PP2B, can impair this recovery (Figure 3, panel b), suggesting that dephosphorylation constitutes an important mechanism to return endothelial barrier function to normal. The substrate(s) regulated by PP1, PP2A, and PP2B in the endothelial barrier response remains to be determined. It has been proposed that endothelial cell contraction, controlled by the actin-myosin motor, provides the basis for cell shape change and impaired barrier function. Thus, the phosphorylation of myosin light chain (MLC) may be a key substrate regulated by these phosphatases, since calyculin A promoted MLC phosphorylation and PP1 has been found to be associated with myosin in endothelial cells.[42]

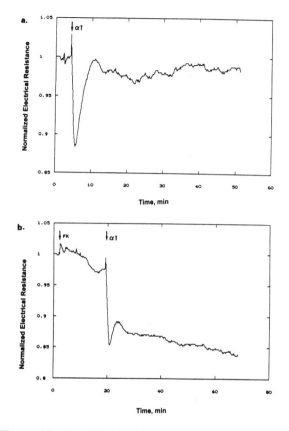

Figure 3. Effects of FK506 (PP2B inhibitor) on the thrombin-induced decrease in transendothelial electrical resistance. Arrows indicate time of addition of reagents. FK = 100 ng/mL FK506; αT = 100 nmol/L human α-thrombin. (a) α-thrombin alone; (b) FK506 followed by α-thrombin.

Cadherin Function in Activated Endothelium

The increase in permeability of activated endothelium occurs with striking changes in the organization of the actin cytoskeleton (ie, the peripheral F-actin band becomes less prominent and stress fibers spanning the cell increase in density).[1,3,6] Pretreatment of endothelial cells with 7-nitrobenz-2-oxa-1,3-diazole (NBD)-phallicidin (an actin-stabilizing agent) prevents the thrombin-induced loss of peripheral F-actin band, intercellular gap formation, and cell shape change as well as the increase in endothelial permeability to albumin.[43] These results indicate that this shift in actin microfilament distribution in the permeability response is a major factor in intercellular gap formation, cell shape change, and impairment of the endothelial barrier.

One important role of the actin microfilament system in promoting barrier function is related to the requirement of cadherin to be anchored to the microfilaments in order to maintain cadherin-to-cadherin interaction and tight cell-to-cell adhesion.[20,21] Therefore, a loss of actin microfilaments such as that with thrombin stimulation would impair cadherin-to-cadherin adhesion and promote increased permeability. Such actin redistribution is also associated with altered interactions with catenins. In endothelial cells, thrombin stimulation causes a time-dependent decrease in the amount of α-, β-, and γ-catenins associated with cadherin.[30] Catenins are essential intermediate proteins that link cadherin with actin microfilaments.[12] The decreased amount of catenins in association with cadherin suggests impairment of anchorage of cadherin to the actin cytoskeleton, resulting in decreased cell-to-cell adhesion and increased permeability. Indeed, the cadherin amount in the TritonX-100 insoluble cell fraction was observed to be lowered after endothelial cells were challenged with thrombin (H.L., unpublished data, 1996).

Evidence from studies of epithelial cells indicates that activation of tyrosine kinases may phosphorylate cadherin-associated proteins, leading to decreased cell-to-cell adhesive strength.[44,45] Although much

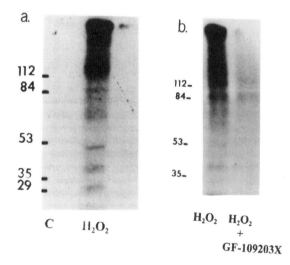

Figure 4. Autoradiogram of ^{32}P-labeled proteins immunoprecipitated with anti-pan-cadherin Ab from human microvascular endothelial cells treated for 10 minutes with (a) 100 μmol/L H_2O_2 or with (b) 100 μmol/L H_2O_2+5 μmol/L PKC inhibitor, GF109203X.

less is known regarding the role of phosphorylation in the function of cadherin/catenins in endothelial cells, there is evidence supporting PKC-mediated phosphorylation in the regulation of these junctional proteins. The PKC inhibitor, calphostin C, was shown to prevent the thrombin-induced dissociation of catenins from cadherins in endothelial cells,[30] suggesting that PKC-mediated phosphorylation regulates the cadherin/catenin system. When endothelial cells were activated by the oxidant, H_2O_2, with a concentration shown to increase permeability,[3] the cadherin immunocomplex of proteins was phosphorylated (Figure 4, panel a). With pretreatment with an inhibitor of Ca^{2+}-dependent PKC isoforms, GX 109203X, the H_2O_2-induced phosphorylation of the proteins was inhibited (Figure 4, panel b). These observations suggest that PKC-mediated phosphorylation of the cadherin and its associated proteins may be a mechanism by which increased permeability is regulated. Although the phosphorylated proteins have yet to be identified, the cadherin molecule is a potential PKC substrate since serine and threonine residues of its cytoplasmic tail can be phosphorylated.[46]

Conclusions

A wide range of external stimuli including thrombin, oxidants, shear stress, growth factors, and cytokines activate vascular endothelium, resulting in impaired barrier function. Morphologically, this increase in permeability is accompanied by reversible cell shape change and intercellular gap formation, suggesting that the increased transport is governed predominantly by diffusive pathways through cellular junctions. Current evidence indicates that interfering with the function of cadherins, the integral adhesion molecules of adherens junctions in endothelium, results in increased permeability. Thus, one mechanism that contributes to the increased permeability in response to activating stimuli may be altered cadherin function.

Activation of the PKC cascade is critical for the increased permeability, and the Ca^{2+}-dependent PKCα and β isoforms appear to be the more important isoforms in this permeability response. The precise role of PKC activation in regulation of the endothelial barrier is not known. An intriguing possibility is a direct modulation of the phosphorylation of the endothelial cadherin/catenin system by PKC. Future research is needed for the identification of key protein substrates of PKC activation, the function of their phosphorylation, and the role of individual PKC isoforms in regulation of the endothelial barrier function. Furthermore, since increases in permeability are reversible, it is important to determine these cellular "off-switch" mechanisms (eg, receptor desensitization, PKC-mediated negative feedback pathways, activation of protein phosphatases).

References

1. Lum H, Aschner JL, Phillips PG, et al. Time-course of thrombin-induced increase in endothelial permeability: Relationship to Ca^{2+}_i and inositol polyphosphates. *Am J Physiol* 1992;263:L219–L225.
2. Partridge CA, Horvath CJ, Delvecchio PJ, et al. Influence of extracellular matrix in tumor necrosis factor-induced increase in endothelial permeability. *Am J Physiol* 1992;263:L627–L633.
3. Siflinger-Birnboim A, Goligorsky MS, Delvecchio PJ, et al. Activation of protein kinase C pathway contributes to hydrogen peroxide-induced increase in endothelial permeability. *Lab Invest* 1992;67:24–30.
4. Jo H, Dull RO, Hollis TM, et al. Endothelial albumin permeability is shear dependent, time dependent, and reversible. *Am J Physiol* 1991;260:H1992–H1996.
5. Johnson A, Phillips P, Hocking D, et al. Protein kinase C inhibitor prevents pulmonary edema in response to H_2O_2. *Am J Physiol* 1989;256:H1012–H1022.
6. Garcia JGN, Siflinger-Birnboim A, Bizios R, et al. Thrombin-induced increase in albumin permeability across the endothelium. *J Cell Physiol* 1986;128:96–104.
7. Taylor AE, Granger DN. Exchange of macromolecules across the microcirculation. In: Renkin EM, Michel CC (eds): *Handbook of Physiology. The Cardiovascular System. Microcirculation.* Bethesda, MD: American Physiological Society; 1984;467–520.
8. Siflinger-Birnboim A, Delvecchio PJ, Cooper JA, et al. Molecular sieving characteristics of the cultured endothelial monolayer. *J Cell Physiol* 1987;132:111–117.
9. Li C, Poznansky MJ. Characterization of the ZO-1 protein in endothelial and other cell lines. *J Cell Sci* 1990;97:231–237.
10. Furuse M, Hirase T, Itoh M, et al. Occludin: A novel integral membrane protein localizing at tight junctions. *J Cell Biol* 1993;123:1777–1788.
11. Schneeberger EE, Lynch RD. Structure, function, and regulation of cellular tight junctions. *Am J Physiol* 1992;262:L647–L661.
12. Takeichi M. Cadherins: A molecular family important in selective cell-cell adhesion. *Annu Rev Biochem* 1990;59:237–252.
13. Gumbiner BM, Simons K. A functional assay for proteins involved in establishing an epithelial occluding barrier: Identification of a uvomorulin-like polypeptide. *J Cell Biol* 1986;102:457–468.
14. Jongen WMF, Fitzgerald DJ, Asamoto M, et al. Regulation of connexin 43-mediated gap junctional intercellular communication by Ca^{2+} in mouse epidermal cells is controlled by E-cadherin. *J Cell Biol* 1991;114:545–555.
15. Shapiro L, Fannon AM, Kwong PD, et al. Structural basis of cell-cell adhesion by cadherins. *Nature* 1995;374:327–337.
16. Lutz KL, Jois SDS, Siahaan TJ. Secondary structure of the HAV peptide which regulates cadherin-cadherin interaction. *J Biomol Struct Dyn* 1995;13:447–455.
17. Huber P, Dalmon J, Engiles J, et al. Genomic structure and chromosomal mapping of the mouse VE-cadherin gene (Cdh5). *Genomics* 1996;32:21–28.

18. Alexander JS, Blaschuk OW, Haselton FR. An N-cadherin-like protein contributes to solute barrier maintenance in cultured endothelium. *J Cell Physiol* 1993;156:610–618.

19. Lampugnani MG, Resnati M, Raiteri M, et al. A novel endothelial-specific membrane protein is a marker of cell-cell contacts. *J Cell Biol* 1992;118:1511–1522.

20. Fujimori T, Takeichi M. Disruption of epithelial cell-cell adhesion by exogenous expression of a mutated nonfunctional N-cadherin. *Mol Biol Cell* 1993;4:37–47.

21. Navarro P, Caveda L, Breviario F, et al. Catenin-dependent and -independent functions of vascular endothelial cadherin. *J Biol Chem* 1995;270:30965–30972.

22. Lynch JJ, Ferro TJ, Blumenstock FA, et al. Increased endothelial albumin permeability mediated by protein kinase C activation. *J Clin Invest* 1990;85:1991–1998.

23. Gescher A. Towards selective pharmacological modulation of protein kinase C: Opportunities for the development of novel antineoplastic agents. *Br J Cancer* 1992;66:10–19.

24. Murray MA, Heistad DD, Mayhan WG. Role of protein kinase C in bradykinin-induced increases in microvascular permeability. *Circ Res* 1991;68:1340–1348.

25. Tiruppathi C, Malik AB, Delvecchio PJ, et al. Electrical method for detection of endothelial cell shape change in real time: Assessment of endothelial barrier function. *Proc Natl Acad Sci U S A* 1992;89:7919–7923.

26. Liu JP. Protein kinase C and its substrates. *Mol Cell Endocrinol* 1996;116:1–29.

27. Bussolino F, Silvagno F, Garbarino G, et al. Human endothelial cells are targets for platelet-activating factor (PAF). Activation of α and β protein kinase C isozymes in endothelial cells stimulated by PAF. *J Biol Chem* 1994;269:2877–2886.

28. Nishizuka Y. Intracellular signaling by hydrolysis of phospholipids and activation of protein kinase C. *Science* 1992;258:607–614.

29. Fain JN. Regulation of phosphoinositide-specific phospholipase C. *Biochim Biophys Acta* 1990;1053:81–88.

30. Rabiet M-J, Plantier J-L, Rival Y, et al. Thrombin-induced increase in endothelial permeability is associated with changes in cell-to-cell junction organization. *Arterioscler Thromb Vasc Biol* 1996;16:488–496.

31. Lum H, Delvecchio PJ, Schneider AS, et al. Calcium dependence of the thrombin-induced increases in endothelial albumin permeability. *J Appl Physiol* 1989;66:1471–1476.

32. Mayhan WG, Joyner WL. The effect of altering the external calcium concentration and a calcium channel blocker, verapamil, on microvascular leaky sites and dextran clearance in the hamster cheek pouch. *Microvasc Res* 1984;28:159–179.

33. Billah MM, Anthes JC. The regulation and cellular functions of phosphatidylcholine hydrolysis. *Biochem J* 1990;269:281–291.

34. Conricode KM, Brewer KA, Exton JH. Activation of phospholipase D by protein kinase C. Evidence for a phosphorylation-independent mechanism. *J Biol Chem* 1992;267:7199–7202.

35. Wu NZ, Baldwin AL. Transient venular permeability increase and endothelial gap formation induced by histamine. *Am J Physiol* 1992;262:H1238–H1247.

36. Horgan MJ, Lum H, Malik AB. Pulmonary edema after pulmonary artery occlusion and reperfusion. *Am Rev Respir Dis* 1989;140:1421–1428.
37. Yong T, Gao XP, Koizumi S, et al. Role of peptidases in bradykinin-induced increase in vascular permeability in vivo. *Circ Res* 1992;70:952–959.
38. Pachter JA, Pai J-K, Mayer-Ezell R, et al. Differential regulation of phosphoinositide and phosphatidylcholine hydrolysis by protein kinase C-β1 overexpression. Effects on stimulation by α-thrombin, 5'-o-(thiotriphosphate), and calcium. *J Biol Chem* 1992;267:9826–9830.
39. Xu Y, Ware JA. Selective inhibition of thrombin receptor-mediated Ca^{2+} entry by protein kinase C β. *J Biol Chem* 1995;270:23887–23890.
40. Ryu SH, Kim U-H, Wah MI, et al. Feedback regulation of phospholipase C-β by protein kinase C. *J Biol Chem* 1990;265:17941–17945.
40a. Vuong PT, Malik AB, Nagpala PG, Lum H. Protein kinase Cβ modulates thrombin-induced Ca^{2+} signalling and endothelial permeability increase. *J Cell Physoil* 1997. In Press.
41. Sim ATR. The regulation and function of protein phosphatases in the brain. *Mol Neurobiol* 1992;5:229–246.
42. Verin AD, Patterson CE, Day MA, et al. Regulation of endothelial cell gap formation and barrier function by myosin-associated phosphatase activities. *Am J Physiol* 1995;269:L99–L108.
43. Phillips PG, Lum H, Malik AB, Tsan M-F. Phallacidin prevents thrombin-induced increases in endothelial permeability to albumin. *Am J Physiol* 1989;257:C562–C567.
44. Volberg T, Zick Y, Dror R, et al. The effect of tyrosine-specific protein phosphorylation on the assembly of adherens-type junctions. *EMBO J* 1992;11:1733–1742.
45. Takeda H, Nagafuchi A, Yonemura S, et al. V-src kinase shifts the cadherin-based cell adhesion from the strong to the weak state and beta catenin is not required for the shift. *J Cell Biol* 1995;131:1839–1847.
46. Cunningham BA, Leutzinger Y, Gallin WJ, et al. Linear organization of the liver cell adhesion molecule L-CAM. *Proc Natl Acad Sci U S A* 1984;81: 5787–5791.

Chapter 18

Regulation of Myosin Phosphorylation and Barrier Function in Endothelium

Joe G.N. Garcia, MD and
Lydia I. Gilbert-McClain, MD

Thrombin Model of Endothelial Cell Permeability

The vascular endothelium provides a nonthrombogenic surface and a semiselective cellular barrier between circulating proteins/cells and the interstitial tissues. A number of diverse inflammatory stimuli can produce profound alterations in endothelial cell integrity, resulting in intercellular gap formation, barrier dysfunction, tissue edema, and potentially life-threatening organ malfunction or failure. In prior studies the authors have described an in vitro model of endothelial cell activation evoked by the bioregulatory coagulant serine protease, thrombin, resulting in significant cellular shape changes, cellular contraction, and endothelial cell monolayer permeability.[1,2] Thrombin-induced endothelial cell activation and intercellular gap formation (Figure 1) required active proteolytic activity with cellular activation occurring through a novel mechanism involving receptor proteolysis linked to Gq-coupled, phospholipase C-mediated increases in diacylglycerol and inositol trisphosphate.[3,4] Synthetic thrombin receptor-activating peptides, whose sequences correspond to the newly exposed N-terminus of the cleaved receptor, were potent inducers of endothelial cell

This work was supported by grants from the National Heart, Lung, and Blood Institute, (HL57362, HL50533, HL57402, HL58064), the American Heart Association, the American Heart Association -Indiana Affiliate, the Veteran's Administration Medical Research Service, and awards from the American Lung Association.

From: Weir EK, Reeves JT (eds). *Pulmonary Edema*. Armonk, NY: Futura Publishing Company, Inc.; ©1998.

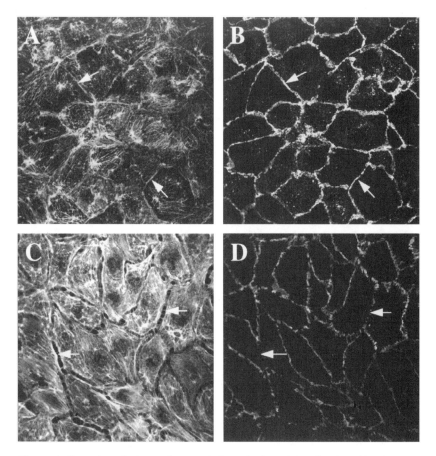

Figure 1. Alterations in the actin cytoskeleton in thrombin-stimulated bovine endothelium detected by confocal microscopy. Shown is the immunofluorescence of thrombin-stimulated bovine endothelial cells that have been stained with rhodamine phalloidin to detect F-actin and FITC-labeled α-catenin antibodies for colocalization. Actin staining in control cells reveals the presence of a dense peripheral band (Panel A) with α-catenin colocalization at cellular borders (Panel B). Thrombin exposure (10 min) induces interendothelial cell gap formation (arrows) (Panel C) , loss of the dense peripheral band, loss of α-catenin colocalization (Panel D), and prominent stress fiber assembly in the cytoplasm (Panel C).

barrier dysfunction consistent with receptor proteolysis and tethered ligand-induced signaling events involved in barrier dysfunction.[5]

Endothelial Cell Contraction:
Role of Myosin Phosphorylation

There are fairly persuasive arguments that the primary permeability pathway across the microvascular segment occurs via a paracellular pathway that is closely linked to intercellular gap formation between activated Endothelial cells. Over the past several years the concept has emerged that endothelial cell shape and intercellular gap formation govern endothelial cell barrier function via a dynamic equilibrium of competing adhesive and contractile forces that generate centripetal tension and are driven by an actomyosin molecular motor.[6] Constitutive tension exists, enabling the cell to be poised ready to respond to its biological environment. The cell-to-cell and cell-matrix processes, which constitute endothelial cell tethering forces, and the cellular contractile processes share linkage to the endothelial cell actin cytoskeleton. Actin and myosin comprise ~16% of endothelial cell proteins, and recent studies support the hypothesis that actin-myosin interactions control the paracellular pathway of vascular permeability.[1,7-9] Immunofluorescence studies have demonstrated prominent redistribution of actin microfilaments after thrombin stimulation (Figure 1) and biochemical studies have shown actin and myosin to be actively redistributed from a Triton detergent-soluble to a Triton-insoluble cellular fraction indicative of microfilament formation, a process generally understood to reflect phosphorylation.[2,8] The results of the authors' published studies[10] support the hypothesis that the actin-myosin cytoskeleton plays a critical role in maintaining the structural and mechanical integrity of the endothelial cell monolayer, and that activation of the contractile apparatus is a key event in thrombin-induced endothelial cell barrier dysfunction.

Although the exact regulatory and signaling events involved in endothelial cell contractile responses are unknown, substantial data now suggest that endothelial cells are similar to smooth muscle cells (SMCs) where phosphorylation of the regulatory light chain of SMC myosin catalyzed by Ca^{2+}/calmodulin (CaM)- dependent myosin light chain kinase (MLCK) is an obligatory event in SMC contraction. Endothelial cell gap formation was observed upon activation of endothelial cell MLCK (EC MLCK) in "skinned" or permeabilized endothelial cell monolayers, which was dependent on the availability of adenosine triphosphate (ATP), Ca^{2+}, and CaM.[11] A basal level of bovine or human endothelial cell centripetal tension is present at all times and is primarily driven by a low but consistent level of myosin light chain phosphorylation (0.3 to 0.4 mol phosphate per mol of myosin light chain), predominantly present as a monophosphorylated form.[10,19] Thrombin induces productive actomyosin interactions via rapid and substantial increases in mono- and diphosphorylated myosin light chains in human and bovine endothelium (Figure 2). Significant increases in phosphorylated myosin light chain species have been detected in endothelium as soon as 15 seconds after thrombin and myosin light chain phosphorylation was maximal at 1 minute to 2 minutes with 60% to 80% of myosin light chain species phosphorylated (0.9 to 1.1 mol/mol), predominantly as diphosphorylated myosin light chains.[10] Although human umbilical vein endothelial cells (HUVEC) and bovine pulmonary artery endothelial cells (BPAEC) appeared to respond similarly to agonists, five myosin light chain bands were reproducibly detected by the SMC myosin light chain antibody in HUVEC monolayers whereas only three BPAEC bands were identified, likely reflecting the presence of both smooth muscle and nonmuscle myosin light chain isoforms in the human venous cells.[10]

Figure 2 depicts the temporal relationship between thrombin-induced biochemical events and physiological responses. Panel A shows that the rapid thrombin-mediated increase in $Ca^{2+}{}_i$ precedes maximal myosin light chain phosphorylation as well as protein kinase C (PKC) activation. These biochemical events occur prior to endothelial cell gap formation, isometric force development, decreases in electrical resistance, and subsequent monolayer permeability (Figure 2, panel B). Attenuation of the agonist-stimulated rise in intracellular Ca^{2+}, antagonism of Ca^{2+}/CaM-dependent signal transduction pathways, and pharmacological inhibition of MLCK (with ML-7 or KT5926) all produced marked abrogation of agonist-stimulated myosin light chain phosphorylation and attenuation of the permeability response.[10] Thus, similar to SMC, phosphorylation of endothelial cell myosin catalyzed by the Ca^{2+}/CaM-dependent MLCK provides the molecular machinery for endothelial cell force generation and contraction and subsequent intercellular gap formation.

Increase in cyclic adenosine monophosphate (cAMP), accomplished either through stimulation of adenylate cyclase activity (such as with forskolin or cholera toxin) or by cell-permeable cAMP analogues, is well recognized as a barrier-promoting event under basal conditions, as well as a marked inhibition of agonist-induced gap formation and endothelial cell permeability.[13–15] Furthermore, these agents that increase cAMP attenuate both constitutive and agonist-induced myosin light chain phosphorylation in a manner that is tightly linked to profound barrier protection.[10] These results suggest that one mechanism by which cAMP accomplishes these protective effects on

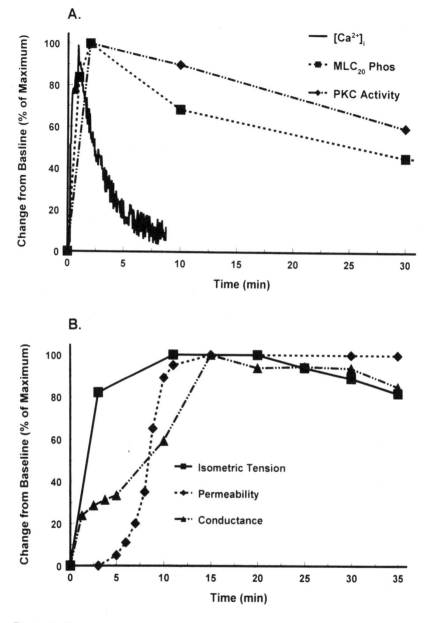

Figure 2. Temporal relationship of thrombin-stimulated biochemical events, signaling pathways, and physiological responses. Shown in panel A are the kinetics of Ca^{2+} mobilization, myosin light chain phosphorylation, and protein kinase C (PKC) activity following 100 nmol/L thrombin stimulation in bovine pulmonary artery endothelium. Panel B depicts the effect of thrombin on electrical resistance (cells grown on a gold electrode) shown as conductance (the reciprocal of resistance), isometric force development, and endothelial cell permeability to albumin.

endothelial cell permeability may be via partial attenuation of agonist-induced myosin light chain phosphorylation.

Cloning and Regulation of Endothelial Cell Myosin Light Chain Kinase

Despite the clear evidence that myosin light chain phosphorylation is a key event in endothelial cell paracellular gap formation and that this reaction is undoubtedly catalyzed by MLCK,[10] several lines of evidence suggested that EC MLCK activity may be unique. The first was the observation that, unlike other Ca^{2+}/CaM-dependent enzymes and SMC MLCK, EC MLCK appeared to be less sensitive to increases in cytosolic Ca^{2+}.[10,16] Increases in cytosolic Ca^{2+} via Ca^{2+} ionophores A23187[10] or ionomycin[16] not only failed to *increase* the level of phosphorylated myosin light chains (Figure 3, panel A) but they produced significant MLC *dephosphorylation*.[16] Second, as depicted in panel B, MLCK inhibition with KT5926 failed to provide significant protection against ionomycin-induced permeability in BPAEC monolayers. The third line of evidence for a unique endothelial MLCK isoform was the observation that the molecular weight of EC MLCK was significantly greater than any previously characterized SMC MLCK isoform. Gallagher et al[17] recently reported a high-molecular-weight MLCK isoform (208 kd) present in embryonic SMC tissues by immunoreactive detection. Smooth muscle MLCK derived from various tissues ranges in molecular weight from 130 kd to 160 kd depending upon the species and tissue source.[17] Using antisera to residues #102–293 of rabbit uterine smooth muscle MLCK, Garcia et al[17,18] demonstrated by Western blotting that bovine and human endothelium contain an immunoreactive MLCK protein whose molecular size is 214 kd. These data suggest

---

→

Figure 3. Effect of thrombin and ionomycin on bovine endothelial cell myosin light chain phosphorylation and permeability. Panel A depicts the effects of thrombin (100 nmol/L) and ionomycin (5 μmol/L) on myosin light chain (MLC) phosphorylation at 2 min and 10 min, respectively, determined by urea gel electrophoresis. Thrombin produced a sharp stoichiometric rise in MLC phosphorylation from 0.3 mol/mol to 0.9 mol/mol. Ionomycin reduced MLC phosphorylation to 0.1 mol/mol. Panel B depicts the albumin clearance of bovine pulmonary artery endothelial cells that have been pretreated with 10 μmol/L KT5926 and then challenged with thrombin or ionomycin at the concentrations noted above. Mysoin light chain kinase (MLCK) inhibition with KT5926 abolished thrombin-induced permeability but did not significantly reduce ionomycin-mediated endothelial cell barrier dysfunction.

A.
MLC Phosphorylation

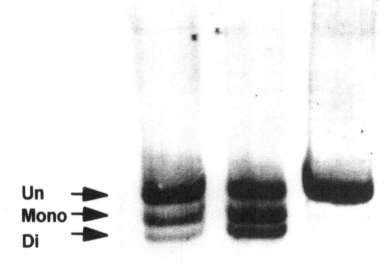

Un ➤
Mono ➤
Di ➤

C   Thr   Iono

B.

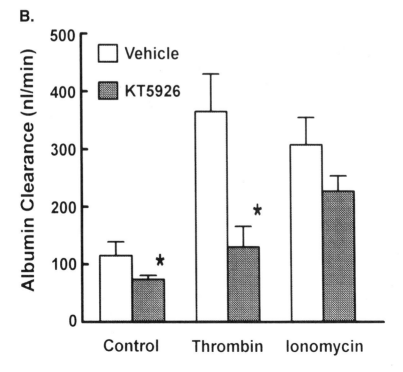

the distinct possibility that either a novel MLCK isotype is present in endothelium that is less sensitive to [Ca^{2+}] than MLCK from either smooth muscle or other nonmuscle cells or that EC MLCK activity requires specific regulatory elements in addition to Ca^{2+}/CaM availability. By use of both standard HUVEC cDNA library screening (deoxythymidine- [dT] primed and randomly primed libraries), as well as polymerase chain reaction (PCR) amplification techniques, Garcia et al[18] generated five overlapping fragments which span the entire coding region of EC MLCK (EMBL data base accession number V48959). The complete sequence of the 1914 amino acid protein computed to a predicted mass of 211 kd, indicating that this nonmuscle MLCK expressed in cultured bovine and human Endothelial cells is the longest CaM-dependent kinase reported.

Sequence analysis revealed that residues #923–1913 correspond directly to the smooth muscle MLCK (smMLCK) with high identity with bovine smMLCK (97%), rabbit smMLCK (90%), and nonmuscle chicken embryo fibroblast MLCK (65%).[18] As depicted in Figure 4, the regional motifs for EC MLCK are conserved throughout this portion of the molecule. To confirm that the derived open-reading frame represents an expressed protein, antisera was generated against a synthetic peptide antigen (V368) corresponding to the unique region (residues #368–374) of the amino acid sequence. In bovine and human endothelium, V368 antisera detects a single protein with an apparent molecular weight of 214 kd, which corresponds well to the 211 kd-computed

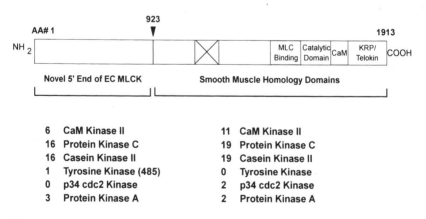

Figure 4. Schematic representation of the high molecular weight endothelial cell myosin light chain kinase isoform. The 1914 amino acid kinase has been depicted in regional motifs based on comparison with smooth muscle myosin light chain kinase (MLCK) from amino acid #922–1914. The number of sites for phosphorylation by specific kinases are shown for the novel 922 amino acid portion as well as for the region homologous to smooth muscle MLCK.

mass of the nonmuscle MLCK. To establish that the 214 kd protein is a member of the MLCK family, Verin et al performed CaM-binding studies with biotinylated CaM and confirmed the immunoreactive 214 kd protein as a CaM-binding protein.[21] They next immunoprecipitated BPAEC MLCK under denaturing conditions, using either V368 or an anti-MLCK antibody (D119) raised against the repeat region of the smMLCK isoform. Both V368 and D119 immunoprecipitates yielded a single 214 kd band visualized by Western immunoblotting with anti-kinase-related protein (KRP) antibodies (generated against the conserved C terminus), whereas no band was detected when nonimmune serum was used for immunoprecipitation.

Finally, to confirm that the 214 kd MLCK protein exhibits kinase activity, they preincubated D119 or V368 immunocomplexes with specific MLCK inhibitors, KT 5926 (10 μmol/L) or ML-7 (3 μmol/L) and measured myosin light chain phosphorylation. These studies revealed the presence of substantial MLCK activity, which was significantly decreased (~50%) by both MLCK-specific inhibitors. Together, these data indicate that a novel, high-molecular-weight MLCK isoform is present in human and bovine endothelium. Structure-function analysis of this important kinase may reveal potentially novel mechanisms of endothelial cell contraction.

Regulation of Myosin Dephosphorylation in Endothelium: Involvement of Type 1 and Type 2B Phosphatases

The rapidly increased levels of phosphorylated myosin light chains elicited by thrombin (maximal at 1 to 2 minutes) are diminished substantially by 30 minutes, and begin to approach baseline values by 60 minutes (Figure 2), indicating either MLCK inactivation, a significant induction of myosin-specific phosphatase activity, or both. This is particularly significant, as endothelial cell contraction, gap formation, and permeability responses remain constant for 90 minutes after thrombin, despite declining levels of phosphorylated myosin light chain. These results are in accordance with the report by Kolodney and Wysolmerski,[12] which demonstrates that thrombin increases endothelial cell centripetal tension from 0.65 to 1.3×10^5 dyne/cm^2, with peak tension developing after 5 minutes and persisting for longer than 40 minutes. This divergence between the level of myosin light chain phosphorylated and centripetal tension is strikingly similar to the "latch-bridge" state described in SMC, where maintenance of force/tension/contraction occurs despite myosin light chain dephosphorylation.

Given this background, myosin light chain dephosphorylation by a myosin-specific phosphatase would logically be a key element in the regulation of endothelial cell gap formation and barrier function. The authors have extensively studied myosin dephosphorylation in human and bovine endothelium with use of inhibitor data and partial purification of the endothelial cell myosin-associated phosphatase in their laboratory.[19] Their data indicate that of the four serine/threonine phosphatases (PPases) present in mammalian cells (PPases 1, 2A, 2B, 2C), a type 1 serine/threonine phosphatase appears to be at least partially responsible for myosin dephosphorylation similar to that described in SMC. For example, calyculin, an inhibitor equally selective for PPases type 1 and 2A, produced >95% dose-dependent inhibition of total bovine endothelial cell PPase activity using either ^{32}P-phosphorylase A or ^{32}P-rabbit skeletal muscle myosin light chain as PPase substrates.[19] In contrast, when okadaic acid, a PPase inhibitor with greater potency against type 2A than PPase 1, was added to endothelial cell homogenates, only 30% inhibition of total ^{32}P-phosphorylase A PPase activity was observed at concentrations specific for PPase 2A (<10 nmol/L) and only a marginal effect on ^{32}P-myosin was noted.[19] The contention that the PPase responsible for myosin dephosphorylation is likely a type 1 PPase and not type 2A is further supported by the additional observations that, unlike PPase 1, immunoreactive type 2A PPase, is virtually absent from a myosin-enriched pellet fraction, whereas both PPases have been readily observed (by Western blotting) in the myosin-depleted supernatant fraction.[19] PPase activity in the myosin-enriched pellet was insensitive to 2 nmol/L okadaic acid (0% inhibition) but sensitive to 5 nmol/L calyculin (>95% inhibition). As calyculin A (0.1 nmol/L to 10 nmol/L), but not okadaic acid (1nmol/L to 100 nmol/L), produced significant dose-dependent enhancement of both myosin light chain phosphorylation (three- to fourfold) and endothelial cell permeability (eightfold), the authors conclude that a type 1 myosin-associated PPase is involved in regulation of endothelial cell contractility and barrier function.[19]

Although available studies are limited, an induction of type 1 PPase activity in thrombin-stimulated endothelial cell homogenates has not been observed when compared to controls.[20] This suggests that the rapid dephosphorylation of myosin light chain that occurs after thrombin may either reflect MLCK deactivation combined with high endogenous type 1 PPase activity or the involvement of other PPases, such as the Ca^{2+}-dependent PPase 2B, may be susceptible to thrombin activation. Verin et al[20] have recently verified an induction of PPase 2B activity in bovine endothelium beginning 5 minutes after thrombin with peak activity noted at 15 minutes. This activity, which is susceptible to inhibition by PPase 2B inhibitors deltamethrin or cyclosporin, appears to be present in endothelial cell cytoskeletal fractions tightly associated with actin. Both deltamethrin and cyclosporin blunt MLC dephosphorylation after maximal thrombin stimulation and exacerbate thrombin-induced barrier dysfunction.[20]

Summary

As depicted in Figure 5, myosin light chain phosphorylation is regulated by constitutive and inducible activities of a novel EC MLCK and myosin-associated phosphatases which appear to include type 1 and type 2B serine/threonine phosphatases. As the phosphorylation status of myosin is a key determinant of cellular isometric centripetal tension, further studies that examine structure-function relationships of both the newly described MLCK as well as the catalytic and regulatory subunits of the endothelial cell myosin-specific phosphatases should greatly accelerate our understanding of endothelial cell contractile responses, gap formation, and barrier dysfunction.

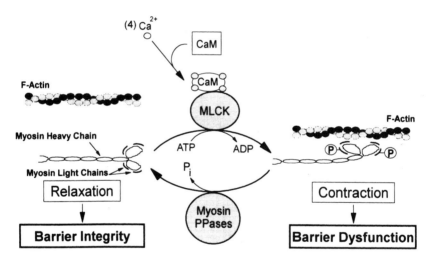

Figure 5. Proposed model of the regulation of endothelial cell contraction/relaxation via myosin light chain phosphorylation and dephosphorylation. A rise in endothelial cell Ca^{2+}_i results in Ca^{2+}-calmodulin (CaM) binding, a conformational change in CaM, and subsequent activation of the Ca^{2+}/CaM-dependent MLCK. The increase in myosin light chain (MLC) phosphorylation catalyzed by the high molecular weight 214 kd MLCK produces endothelial cell contraction and barrier dysfunction through paracellular gaps. These events are followed by subsequent MLC dephosphorylation accomplished via a cascade of serine/threonine protein phosphatases (PPase), which include a type 1 myosin-associated phosphatase and a type 2B PPase.[20,21] Together these kinase and phosphatase activities regulate the degree of productive actomyosin interaction and endothelial cell permeability.

Acknowledgements   The authors gratefully acknowledge Rebecca Snyder for expert secretarial assistance.

References

1. Garcia JGN, Siflinger-Birnboim A, Bizios R, Del Vecchio PJ, Fenton JW, Malik AB. Thrombin-induced increases in albumin permeability across cultured endothelial monolayers. *J Cell Physiol* 1986;128:96–104.
2. Garcia JGN, Pavalko F, Patterson CE. Vascular endothelial cell activation and permeability responses to thrombin. *Blood Coagul Fibrinolysis* 1995;6: 609–626.
3. Garcia JGN, Fenton JW, Natarajan V. Thrombin stimulation of human endothelial cell phospholipase D activity. Regulation by phospholipase C, protein kinase C, and cyclic adenosine 3′,5′-monophosphate. *Blood* 1992; 79:2056–2067.
4. Garcia JGN, Dominguez J, English D. Sodium fluoride induces phosphoinositide hydrolysis, Ca^{2+} mobilization, and prostacyclin synthesis in cultured human endothelium: Further evidence for regulation by a pertussis toxin-insensitive guanine nucleotide-binding protein. *Am J Respir Cell Mol Biol* 1991;5:113–124.
5. Garcia JGN, Patterson CE, Bahler C, Aschner J, Hart CM, English D. Thrombin receptor activating peptides induce Ca^{2+}_i mobilization, barrier dysfunction, prostaglandin synthesis, and platelet-derived growth factor mRNA expression in cultured endothelium. *J Cell Physiol* 1993;156: 541–549.
6. Moy AB, Engelenhoven JV, Bodmer J, et al. Histamine and thrombin modulate endothelial focal adhesion through centripetal and centrifugal forces. *J Clin Invest* 1996;97:1020–1027.
7. Schnittler HJ, Wilke A, Gress T, Suttorp N, Drenckhahn D. Role of actin and myosin in the control of paracellular permeability in pig, rat, and human vascular endothelium. *J Physiol* 1990;431:379–401.
8. Stasek JE, Patterson CE, Garcia JGN. Protein kinase C phosphorylates caldesmon$_{77}$ and vimentin and enhances albumin permeability across cultured bovine pulmonary artery endothelial cell monolayers. *J Cell Physiol* 1992;153:62–75.
9. Shasby DM, Shasby SS, Sullivan JM, Peach MJ. Role of endothelial cell cytoskeleton in control of endothelial permeability. *Circ Res* 1982;51: 657–661.
10. Garcia JGN, Davis HW, Patterson CE. Regulation of endothelial cell gap formation and barrier dysfunction: Role of myosin light chain phosphorylation. *J Cell Physiol* 1995;163:510–522.
11. Wysolmerski RB, Lagunoff D. Regulation of permeabilized endothelial cell retraction by myosin phosphorylation. *Am J Physiol* 1991;261: C32–C40.
12. Kolodney M, Wysolmerski R. Isometric contraction by fibroblasts and endothelial cells in tissue culture: A quantitative study. *J Cell Biol* 1992; 117:73–82.
13. Minnear FL, DeMichele MA, Moon DG, Rieder CL, Fenton JW. Isoproterenol reduces thrombin-induced pulmonary endothelial permeability in vitro. *Am J Physiol* 1990;257:H1613–H1623.
14. Moy AB, Shasby SS, Scott BD, Shasby DM. The effect of histamine and

cyclic adenosine monophosphate on myosin light chain phosphorylation in human umbilical vein endothelial cells. *J Clin Invest* 1993;92:1198–1206.

15. Patterson CE, Davis H, Schaphorst K, Garcia JGN. Mechanisms of cholera toxin prevention of thrombin- and PMA-induced endothelial cell barrier dysfunction. *Microvasc Res* 1994;48:212–235.

16. Garcia JGN, Schaphorst KL, Hart CM, et al. Mechanisms of ionomycin-induced endothelial cell barrier dysfunction. *Am J Physiol: Lung* 1997;273: L172–L184.

17. Gallagher PJ, Garcia JGN, Herring BP. Expression of a novel myosin light chain kinase in embryonic tissues and cultured cells. *J Biol Chem* 1995; 270:29090–29095.

18. Garcia JGN, Lazar V, Gilbert-McClain L, Gallagher PJ, Verin A. Myosin light chain kinase in endothelium: Molecular cloning and regulation. *Am J Respir Cell Mol Biol* 1997;16:489–494.

19. Verin AD, Patterson CE, Day ME, Garcia JGN. Regulation of endothelial cell gap formation and barrier function by myosin-associated phosphatase activities. *Am J Physiol* 1995;269:L99–L108.

20. Verin AD, Herenyiova M, Robles-Rivera L, Garcia JGN. Role of Ca^{2+}/ calmodulin-dependent phosphatase 2B in thrombin-induced endothelial cell contractile responses. *Am J Physiol: Lung* 1997; in press.

21. Verin AD, Gilbert-McClain LI, Patterson CE, Garcia JGN. Biochemical regulation of the non-muscle myosin light chain kinase isoform in bovine endothelium. *Am J Respir Cell Mol Biol* 1998. In Press.

Chapter 19

The Counteradhesive Proteins, SPARC and Thrombospondin-1, Regulate Endothelial Barrier Function Through Protein Tyrosine Phosphorylation

Simeon E. Goldblum, MD

Introduction to the Counteradhesive Proteins

The counteradhesive proteins are a small but growing group of structurally dissimilar multidomain proteins that have been grouped together solely on a functional basis.[1-3] Each of these proteins contains multiple domains, some of which can recognize and bind to multiple receptors on a given host cell. These receptor-ligand interactions can induce overlapping, or at times, conflicting biological responses. By definition each of these so-called counteradhesive proteins, at least under certain conditions, can inhibit cell-substrate interactions. This so-called anti-adhesive effect can include inhibition of cell adhesion to and spreading on extracellular matrix (ECM) proteins as well as focal adhesion (FA) disassembly. As a result, the affected cell assumes a

This work was supported in part by the office of Research and Development, Department of Veterans Affairs, the US Army Medical Research and Development Command (Grant DAMD 17–94-J-4117) and Grant DK48373 from the National Institutes of Health. The SPARC data was generated in collaboration with Dr. E. Helene Sage, University of Washington, Seattle, WA (grants GM-40711 and HL18645 from the NIH) and the thrombospondin work was performed in collaboration with Dr. Joann E. Murphy-Ullrich, University of Alabama at Birmingham, Birmingham, AL (grants HL44575 and HL50061 from the NIH).

From: Weir EK, Reeves JT (eds). *Pulmonary Edema*. Armonk, NY: Futura Publishing Company, Inc.; ©1998.

rounded cell phenotype. This emphasis on single-cell morphology and on the cell-matrix interface that requires specialized techniques such as interference reflection microscopy, has encouraged studies of cells under subconfluent conditions. Only recently has it been appreciated that the counteradhesive proteins may also influence cell-cell interactions.[4-10] Three principal members of the counteradhesive protein group that exert biological effects on the endothelial cell (EC) are SPARC (Secreted Protein Acidic and Rich in Cysteine), also known as osteonectin, thrombospondin (TSP), and tenascin. Only that information most relevant to endothelial barrier function is emphasized in this chapter because extensive reviews of these three proteins are available in the literature.[11-21] Within this context, data are available for SPARC, and less so for TSP-1. Accordingly, the discussion is restricted to these two proteins.

SPARC Regulates Pulmonary Vascular Endothelial Barrier Function Through Protein Tyrosine Phosphorylation

Background

SPARC, the only purely counteradhesive protein that has been described, was first demonstrated in bone in 1981.[11] This apparently multifunctional protein, expressed in a wide range of host tissues under diverse conditions, has been referred to by several names including osteonectin, 43K, BM-40, and "culture shock" protein.[11] SPARC is a 43 kd, highly acidic (pI$\approx$4.3) glycoprotein composed of four novel domains, including two Ca^{2+}-binding sites.[22] It is highly conserved across species lines. For example, bovine and murine SPARC share a 92% amino acid sequence identity.[11] SPARC contains at least one region that is homologous to a membrane-associated, albumin-binding protein, gp60, that is present on all continuous capillary endothelia.[23] In several studies, SPARC has been immunolocalized to cytoplasmic granules in a perinuclear distribution.[24,25] As the name SPARC suggests, it is a highly secreted protein.[11,24] Under basal conditions, SPARC accounts for up to 3% of the total protein constitutively secreted by cultured cells into the culture media.[11,24,25] In response to certain stimuli, its expression can be markedly increased.[25]

SPARC is expressed in multiple host tissues.[11] In the developing fetus, its expression appears to be restricted to tissues undergoing morphogenesis involving increased cell migration. In the adult, SPARC expression is evident in highly proliferating, rapid-turnover epithelia (eg, gut, lung, kidney), tissues undergoing remodeling (eg, bone), and glandular tissues, especially steroidogenic cells (eg, adrenal, testes, ovary). More relevant to the pulmonary vasculature, SPARC is expressed in EC, vascular smooth muscle cells, macrophages, fibroblasts, and the pulmonary alveolar epithelium.[11,24,26] In addition, it is also present within the intravascular compartment, both freely circulating in the plasma,[27] and in monocytes and the α-granules of platelets.[11,26,27] Monocytes and platelets both continuously traffic through the pulmonary microvasculature, where they intimately interact with the endothelial surface. It is unknown whether SPARC is presented to the pulmonary vasculature, in vivo, through an endocrine, paracrine, and/or autocrine pathway.

To better understand the physiological role of SPARC, it may be helpful to review some of the conditions under which its expression is increased. In the adult, its expression increases during tissue remodeling (eg, wound healing and angiogenesis)[26,28,29] and in response to tissue injury (eg, heat shock, heavy metal, endotoxin).[25,30–32] Other stimuli that increase SPARC expression include agents that increase cyclic adenosine monophosphate (cAMP), retinoic acid, and transforming growth factor-β.[11,33–36]

The mechanisms through which this highly conserved protein exerts its biological effects are poorly understood. SPARC is a protein in search of a physiologically relevant function(s) or a role in a disease state. Anti-SPARC antibodies induce developmental defects in *Xenopus* embryos,[37] and overexpression of SPARC in transgenic *Caenorhabditis elegans* results in an uncoordinated and morphologically abnormal phenotype.[38] Although SPARC exhibits specific binding to EC,[39] neither a SPARC receptor nor an intracellular effector mechanism has been defined. That SPARC displays multiple bioactivities for diverse cell types (eg, EC, bone, platelets) has likely added to the confusion. Of its many bioactivities, most relevant to the present discussion is its so-called counteradhesive effect for EC. The presence of SPARC permits EC attachment to the underlying substrate but inhibits EC spreading.[11,40] It labilizes FAs and induces EC shape changes, coincident with actin reorganization. Another SPARC bioactivity relevant to changes in EC shape and transendothelial flux of macromolecules is its ability to bind to other host proteins. SPARC binds to albumin, and this association can be reversed only with sodium dodecyl sulfate (SDS).[24] It also preferentially binds to specific components of the extracellular matrix (eg, collagens I, III, IV, and V, TSP-1).[11] In addition, SPARC binds to and/or antagonizes several growth factors (eg, specific dimeric forms of platelet-derived growth factor [PDGF] [PDGF-AB, PDGF-BB, but not PDGF-AA] and basic fibroblast growth factor [bFGF]).[41,42] Interestingly, SPARC antagonizes the bFGF effect on EC migration.[42] SPARC also binds Ca^{2+}, but SPARC-induced EC shape changes have not been shown to be Ca^{2+}-dependent.[43] SPARC influences the expression of several other relevant host proteins. It increases expression of collagenase, stromelysin, 92 kd gelatinase, and plasminogen activator inhibitor-1 and decreases expression of fibronectin and TSP-1.[44–46] The combined abilities of SPARC to: (1) bind to specific ECM proteins, (2) upregulate several metalloproteases for which ECM proteins can serve as substrates, and (3) influence expression of both a pro-adhesive protein (fibronectin) and another counteradhesive protein (TSP-1), suggest that the protein is operative at the cell-substrate interface.

SPARC as a Candidate Mediator of Endothelial Barrier Dysfunction

SPARC possesses features and activities that may be relevant to the pathogenesis of acute pulmonary vascular endothelial barrier dysfunction. First, SPARC is highly expressed in lung tissue[11] and is secreted constitutively by the endothelium[24,25] and vascular smooth muscle cells.[9] Further, SPARC is present in cells that circulate through the pulmonary vasculature.[11,26] Second, increased SPARC expression can be induced by injurious stimuli including endotoxin,[25] an established mediator of acute pulmonary vascular EC barrier dysfunction.[47,48] Finally, it has been demonstrated that SPARC induces actin reorganization, EC shape changes, and intercellular gap formation in tightly adherent postconfluent EC monolayers; these changes are coincident with loss of barrier function.[4,5]

Effect of SPARC on Endothelial Barrier Function

Murine SPARC was purified from the conditioned medium of mouse PYS-2 cells, a teratocarcinoma line derived from parietal yolk sac endoderm.[49] Bovine pulmonary artery EC (BPAEC) were cultured on ECM-impregnated filters mounted in modified chemotaxis chambers.[4,47,48] Endothelial barrier function was determined by measuring the movement of ^{14}C-albumin across postconfluent monolayers. Transendothelial ^{14}C-BSA flux was expressed in pmol/h. Only monolayers retaining ≥97% of the tracer were studied. This experimental system precludes hydrostatic and osmotic pressure gradients and other non-EC-derived host factors. Although this in vitro model fails to simulate in vivo conditions, it serves as a quantitative assay for homophilic EC-EC interactions.

SPARC, in the absence of serum, induced dose- and time-dependent increments in transendothelial ^{14}C-BSA flux.[4] A SPARC exposure of 6 hours increased ^{14}C-BSA flux in a dose-dependent manner (Figure 1A).

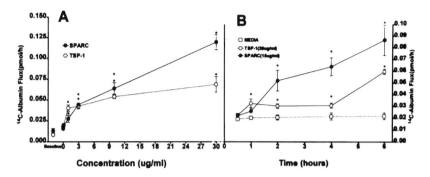

Figure 1. Effects of SPARC and TSP-1 on transendothelial flux of ^{14}C-BSA. Symbols represent mean (±SEM) transendothelial flux of ^{14}C-BSA in pmol/h. Each symbol is derived from ≥5 monolayers studied. Baseline ^{14}C-BSA flux is shown by symbols on lower left in both panel A and panel B, and each star indicates a significant increase compared with the simultaneous medium control ($P<0.05$). (A) ^{14}C-BSA flux immediately after 6-hour exposures to increasing concentrations of SPARC (—●—) or TSP-1 (—○—) in the absence of FBS, (B) ^{14}C-BSA flux immediately after increasing exposure times to fixed concentrations of either SPARC (15 μg/mL) (—●—) or TSP-1 (30 μg/mL) (—○—) and simultaneous media controls (---□---) in the absence of FBS. Modification of SPARC data from Reference 4.

The lowest SPARC concentration that increased ^{14}C-BSA flux compared with the medium control was 0.5μg/mL. At a fixed SPARC concentration (15μg/mL), SPARC exposures of ≥1h increased ^{14}C-BSA flux by 1.3-fold to 3.6-fold compared with simultaneous media controls; there were time-dependent increments throughout the 6-hour study period (Figure 1B). These studies demonstrated a SPARC stimulus-to-EC response lag time of ~1 hour. The SPARC-induced barrier dysfunction could not be blocked by prior inhibition of protein synthesis, nor could it be ascribed to loss of EC viability or EC detachment.[4] Any contribution from endotoxin or other contaminants was excluded.[4] SPARC also increased ^{14}C-BSA flux across bovine aortic and retinal microvascular EC monolayers compared with their respective controls.[4] Human pulmonary artery EC monolayers similarly responded to the SPARC stimulus (data not presented). The responsiveness of all three of these endothelia to SPARC was comparable to the response described above in BPAEC.

The effect of SPARC on EC morphology in postconfluent monolayers grown on filters was studied by scanning electron microscopy (Figure 2).[4] In control monolayers, the cells were in tight apposition with no intercellular gaps, and exhibited a cobblestone appearance (Figure 2A). In monolayers exposed to SPARC at 15μg/mL for 6 hours, cells remained attached to the substrate but retracted from each other, with resultant intercellular gaps bridged by cell processes (Figure 2B).

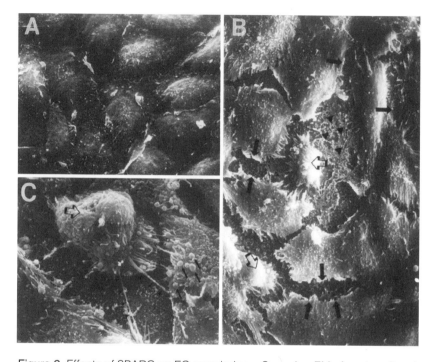

Figure 2. Effects of SPARC on EC morphology. Scanning EM of postconfluent monolayers grown on filters in assay chambers after exposure to SPARC at 15 μg/mL for 6 hours. (panels B and C) or to medium alone (panel A). (A) Control monolayers were in tight apposition and displayed the typical cobblestone appearance (× 1450). (B) Monolayers exposed to SPARC remained attached to matrix-coated filters (closed arrowheads) but exhibited extensive inter-endothelial gaps (closed arrows). Occasional cells assumed an extremely rounded phenotype (open arrows) (× 1450). Selected cells (open arrows) became rounded with marked separation from neighboring cells and displayed numerous slender processes (small arrowheads) and extensive blebs (small closed arrows) (× 2900). Reproduced from Reference 4.

Some of the cells assumed a rounded morphology, displayed numerous slender processes and extensive blebbing, and were clearly separated from neighboring cells (Figure 2C).

To determine whether the impact of SPARC on EC morphology and barrier function was mediated through EC actin reorganization, SPARC-exposed (15μg/mL, ≥2 hours) and media control monolayers were fixed, rendered permeable, stained with fluorescein-phalloidin, and examined with fluorescence microscopy (Figure 3).[4] Control EC contained continuous transcytoplasmic actin filaments and exhibited tight cell-to-cell apposition without intercellular gaps (Figure 3A). SPARC exposure induced isolated ellipsoid disruptions within the

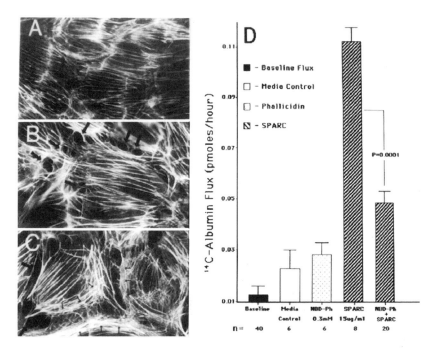

Figure 3. SPARC-Induced actin reorganization and changes in endothelial barrier function. Endothelial monolayers grown on filters were exposed to medium (panel A) or SPARC at 15 μg/mL for 2 hours or more (panels B and C). The monolayers were fixed, rendered permeable, and stained with fluorescein-phalloidin. (A) Monolayers exposed to medium alone contained continuous transcytoplasmic actin cables and exhibited tight cellular apposition without intercellular gaps. (B and C) Exposures of SPARC for 2 hours or more induced intercellular gaps (closed arrows). In panel C, note the circumferential F-actin redistribution (small closed arrows). (D) EC monolayers grown on filters pretreated with 0.3 μmol/L NBD-phallicidin (NBD-Ph) or medium alone for 3 hours prior to and throughout a 6-hour exposure to either medium with SPARC or medium alone in the absence of FBS. Vertical bars represent the mean (±SEM) transendothelial flux of ¹⁴C-BSA. Baseline (±SEM) ¹⁴C-BSA flux is shown by the closed bar. (A, B, C = × 600). Reproduced from Reference 4.

F-actin lattice restricted to the cell-cell interface (Figure 3B). In some cells, SPARC exposure increased redistribution of F-actin to the subcortical compartment, ie, to peripheral actin bands (Figure 3C). Therefore, the actin reorganization and intercellular gap formation induced by SPARC were temporally coincident with changes in barrier function. To determine whether the SPARC-induced changes in actin organization and barrier function could be causally related, EC monolayers cultured in assay chambers were preloaded with the specific F-actin stabilizing agent, phallicidin, exposed to SPARC or medium alone, and assayed for barrier function (Figure 3D). This treatment protects against depolymerization of F-actin to monomeric G-actin.[47,50] Prior F-actin stabilization protected EC monolayers against SPARC-induced barrier dysfunction, suggesting that actin depolymerization is a prerequisite to SPARC-induced opening of the paracellular pathway.

SPARC Regulates Endothelial Barrier Function Through Protein Tyrosine Phosphorylation

SPARC induces F-actin-dependent intercellular gap formation in postconfluent EC monolayers.[4] In EC, F-actin is arranged into both central transcytoplasmic cables and peripheral bands.[51] These microfilaments are linked to two types of adherens junctions, FAs and the zonula adherens (ZA).[52] Although the signal transduction pathways that regulate the state of actin assembly and integrity of either the ZA or FAs are incompletely understood, protein tyrosine phosphorylation is known to modify target proteins within all three structures.[53-55] As a first test of whether SPARC regulates endothelial barrier function through protein tyrosine phosphorylation, lysates from postconfluent EC exposed to SPARC or media were immunoblotted for phosphotyrosine-containing proteins.[5,6] Only in the presence of protein tyrosine phosphatase (PTP) inhibition with vanadate (250 µmol/L) did SPARC consistently induce tyrosine phosphorylation of a number of EC proteins. After 1 hour in the presence of vanadate, SPARC at concentrations as low as 3 µg/mL (0.09 µmol/L) increased the phosphotyrosine signal in comparison to the effect seen with vanadate alone. This increase in signal was concentration-dependent over a range of 1 µg/mL to 30 µg/mL (0.03 µmol/L to 0.9 µmol/L) SPARC. At a fixed SPARC concentration (20 µg/mL) in the presence of vanadate (250 µmol/L), exposure times as brief as 5 minutes increased protein tyrosine phosphorylation compared to the simultaneous vanadate control. Three predominant phosphotyrosine-containing bands migrated with apparent Mr of 135,000, 95,000, and 66,000; these bands were increased 2.5-fold to 12-fold over the simultaneous control. Additional phosphotyrosine-containing proteins with approximate apparent Mr of 240,000, 220,000, 185,000, and 165,000 were also increased. The concentration (~1µg/mL) and time (≥5min) requirements for SPARC-induced tyrosine phosphorylation were compatible with those previously reported for SPARC-induced changes in endothelial barrier function.[4] SPARC-induced tyrosine phosphorylation was demonstrable well within the 1-hour stimulus-to-response lag time that precedes changes in barrier function.

In order to determine whether SPARC-induced tyrosine phosphorylation of EC proteins could be causally related to changes in barrier function, two structurally and functionally dissimilar protein tyrosine kinase (PTK) inhibitors, herbimycin A and genistein, were introduced.[5,6] The concentration of each inhibitor was chosen on the basis of its activity in the barrier function assay; the maximal subthreshold concentration of each agent was used. EC monolayers were pretreated with genistein (185μmol/L) 0.5 hour prior to and throughout a 6-hour exposure to SPARC (15μg/mL, 0.75μmol/L) or media. Herbimycin A (1.0 μmol/L) was introduced ~16 hours prior to and for the duration of the SPARC exposure. ^{14}C-BSA flux across EC monolayers treated with either herbimycin A or genistein alone was not different from that of the media controls, whereas SPARC increased transendothelial ^{14}C-BSA flux. Pretreatment of monolayers with either herbimycin A or genistein protected against the SPARC-induced increment by 81% and 57%, respectively. These same two PTK inhibitors that protected against SPARC-induced endothelial barrier dysfunction clearly blocked SPARC-induced tyrosine phosphorylation of EC proteins, including the two predominant phosphotyrosine-containing bands.[5,6] Herbimycin A decreased both the 135 kd and 66 kd bands by ~87%, whereas genistein decreased the two bands by 52% and 60%, respectively. In contrast, PTP inhibition with either vanadate (2.5 μmol/L) or phenylarsine oxide (PAO) (0.1 μmol/L) enhanced the loss of barrier function in the presence of SPARC by 53% and 78%, respectively.[5,6]

Studies were then performed to determine whether the SPARC-induced loss in barrier function that appeared to be dependent on tyrosine phosphorylation could be ascribed to opening of the paracellular pathway. Accordingly, EC monolayers exposed to SPARC (15 μg/mL, 0.45 μmol/L), +/− herbimycin A (1.0 μmol/L), were stained with fluorescein-phalloidin, an F-actin-specific reagent, for fluorescence microscopy.[5,6] EC monolayers incubated with herbimycin A or media alone exhibited continuous transcytoplasmic actin filaments and cell-to-cell apposition without intercellular gaps. After exposure to SPARC for 6 hours, isolated ellipsoid disruptions within the F-actin lattice occurred, as expected, exclusively at the cell-cell interface. In EC monolayers preincubated with herbimycin A for 16 hours prior to and throughout the 6-hour exposure to SPARC, no intercellular gaps could be demonstrated. Therefore, the same PTK inhibition that protected against barrier dysfunction blocked the formation of gaps between confluent EC associated with an exogenous SPARC stimulus. To determine the cellular distribution of the phosphotyrosine-containing proteins associated with SPARC exposure, EC monolayers exposed to SPARC (20 μg/mL, 0.6 μmol/L) or media alone for 1 hour were probed with fluorescein isothiocyanate-(FITC) conjugated antiphosphotyrosine antibody for fluorescence microscopy. EC incubated with SPARC displayed a fluorescence signal that was restricted almost exclusively to intercellular boundaries.

To further assess the EC response to SPARC, Goldblum and colleagues sought to identify the phosphotyrosine-containing proteins observed in their blots. The significant increase in tyrosine phosphorylation of both the ≈95 kd and ≈68 kd bands after treatment with 20 μg/mL of SPARC for 1 hour, and their preferential decrease in phosphotyrosine signal in the presence of PTK inhibition, made these phosphoproteins logical choices to examine. Immunoscreening revealed that β-catenin and paxillin comigrated with the ≈95 kd and ≈68 kd phosphoproteins, respectively. Lysates from EC exposed for 1 hour to SPARC (0.6 μmol/L) in the presence of vanadate (250 μmol/L) or to vanadate alone were each immunoprecipitated with either anti-β-catenin or antipaxillin antibodies. The immunoprecipitates were resolved by sodium dodecyl sulfate-polyacrylamide gel electrophoresis (SDS-PAGE), and the blots were probed with biotinylated antiphosphotyrosine (4G10) antibody. As a control for any discrepancy in immunoprecipitation efficiency and/or loading of the immunoprecipitated protein, blots were stripped and reprobed with the same immunoprecipitating antibody. SPARC increased tyrosine phosphorylation of paxillin and β-catenin relative to controls, ≈2-fold and ≈4-fold, respectively. From these data, they conclude that SPARC induces tyrosine phosphorylation of both paxillin and β-catenin in EC. The lesser-fold increments in tyrosine phosphorylation seen in these experiments can be ascribed to the decreased efficiency of these antibodies to immunoprecipitate the hyperphosphorylated forms. The other phosphotyrosine-containing proteins seen in EC exposed to SPARC have not yet been identified. However, immunoscreening with antibodies raised against known ≈140 kd to ≈120 kd substrates for tyrosine phosphorylation has revealed several candidate phosphoproteins, including cadherin, p130[Cas], focal adhesion kinase (FAK), and p120[Cas]. Studies are currently under way to determine whether any of these phosphoproteins is operative during the EC response to SPARC, as well as to identify other substrates for SPARC-induced tyrosine phosphorylation.

Role of Adherens Junctions

Adherens junctions mechanically couple the actin cytoskeleton to surface receptors that either mediate cell-to-cell or cell-matrix adhesion.[52] ZA and FA integrity is, in part, determined by the state of tyrosine phosphorylation of their component proteins.[54,55] Certain features of SPARC-induced endothelial barrier dysfunction suggest involvement of the ZA. First, SPARC induces intercellular gaps at the cell-cell boundaries[4] where the ZA is located.[52,54] Second, SPARC induces EC actin reorganization, and prior F-actin stabilization with phallicidin protects against SPARC-induced barrier dysfunction.[4] Third, SPARC-induced loss of barrier function is tyrosine phosphorylation-dependent and the increased expression of phosphotyrosine-containing proteins is restricted almost exclusively to the cell-cell interface.[5,6] Finally, SPARC induces tyrosine phosphorylation of β-catenin, a key signaling and structural protein within the ZA.[56–58] These combined features suggest that SPARC may be regulating the transendothelial paracellular pathway through ZA disassembly. That SPARC also induces tyrosine phosphorylation of paxillin implicates changes in the state of FA assembly as well.[55]

Thrombospondin-1 Also Regulates Pulmonary Vascular Endothelial Barrier Function Through Protein Tyrosine Phosphorylation

Background

Thrombospondin (TSP) was first demonstrated in the releasate of thrombin-stimulated platelets in 1971.[12] Only recently has it been appreciated that there are at least five distinct but related TSP genes.[14,15,18] Platelet-derived TSP or TSP-1 is the best studied and is the TSP gene product that is addressed here. TSP-1 is a ~420 kd trimeric glycoprotein composed of three identical 145 kd polypeptide chains held together by disulfide bonds in a bola-shaped structure.[12,14] Each multidomain chain contains an NH_2-terminal globular domain, an interchain disulfide bond, a procollagen homology sequence, three repeats homologous to both properdin and a malarial coat protein, three epidermal growth factor- (EGF) like repeats, seven Ca^{2+}-binding repeats, the last of which contains an RGD-containing sequence, and the COOH-terminus. Like SPARC, TSP-1 is secreted by numerous host cells including EC, type II alveolar epithelial cells, fetal lung fibroblasts, platelets, and cells of monocyte/macrophage lineage.[12–19] TSP-1 expression is increased in blood vessels[59] as well as in cultured EC[60] in response to injurious stimuli. TSP-1 recognizes multiple EC receptors and induces multiple, and sometimes conflicting, biological responses.[12–19] It contains an NH_2-terminal heparin-binding domain that recognizes heparan sulfate proteoglycans on the EC surface, an RGD-containing sequence that binds to the $\alpha_v\beta_3$ integrin, and two repeats of the CSVTCG motif that recognize CD36.[12–19,59] Interestingly, CD36 is physically and functionally associated with src-related PTKs in EC. TSP also interacts with other endogenous proteins including transforming growth factor-β (TGF-β)[61,62] and SPARC,[63] both platelet-α-granule products. TSP influences multiple EC functions including cell attachment to and spreading on substrates,[12-19,64,65] cell motility in response to a TSP gradient,[12-19,65,66] and angiogenesis.[65,67] TSP redistributes F-actin to the peripheral EC subcortical compartment temporally coincident with FA disassembly.[68] That TSP is found in lung tissue,[12-19] is secreted by EC,[12-19] increases in response to injurious stimuli,[59,60] and induces EC F-actin reorganization[68] is compatible with a role for TSP in the loss of pulmonary vascular endothelial barrier function in response to injury.

Effect of Thrombospondin-1 on Endothelial Barrier Function

TSP-1 was purified from the releasate obtained from thrombin-stimulated human platelets.[68] TSP increased transendothelial ^{14}C-BSA flux in a dose-dependent manner (Figure 1A).[7,9] The lowest TSP concentration that induced a significant increment in ^{14}C-BSA flux compared to the media control was 1.0 µg/mL. The maximum mean (±SE) ^{14}C-BSA flux was seen with TSP 30 µg/mL, at which point the TSP-induced effect had begun to plateau or saturate. On the basis of this dose-response relationship, the EC_{50} for TSP in the barrier function assay was ~3.63 µg/mL or ~8.64 nmol/L. The effect of TSP on endothelial barrier function was also time-dependent (Figure 1B). TSP (30 µg/mL) induced significant increments in ^{14}C-BSA flux compared to the simultaneous media control after ≥0.5-hour exposures with maximum flux at 6 hours. These studies demonstrated a biphasic EC response to TSP with an initial response observed at 0.5 hour, followed by a more robust response after 4 hours. The TSP-induced barrier dysfunction could not be blocked by prior inhibition of protein synthesis, nor could it be ascribed to loss of EC viability.

Thrombospondin-1-Induced Protein Tyrosine Phosphorylation and Barrier Dysfunction

When TSP-induced tyrosine phosphorylation of EC proteins was sought by immunoblotting for phosphotyrosine-containing proteins, increased protein tyrosine phosphorylation was only evident in the simultaneous presence of two PTP inhibitors, vanadate (200 µmol/L) and PAO (1.0 µmol/L).[8,9] This effect was both concentration- and time-dependent. After an exposure of 1 hour in the presence of fixed concentrations of both vanadate (200 µmol/L) and PAO (1.0 µmol/L), TSP concentrations as low as 1.0 µg/mL increased the phosphotyrosine signal compared to the effect seen with vanadate and PAO alone; over a

TSP range of 1μg/mL to 30μg/mL, this increase in signal was concentration-dependent. TSP (30 μg/mL) in the presence of fixed concentrations of both vanadate (200 μM) and PAO (1.0 μM), increased the phosphotyrosine signal compared to the simultaneous vanadate/PAO control with exposure times as brief as 0.5 hour.

To determine whether the state of EC protein tyrosine phosphorylation mediated TSP-induced changes in barrier function, TSP was presented to monolayers in the presence of one of two PTK inhibitors.[8,9] Pretreatment of monolayers with either herbimycin A or genistein protected against the TSP-induced increment by >80% and >50%, respectively. In contrast, PTP inhibition with either vanadate or PAO enhanced the loss of barrier function in the presence of TSP by 23% and 45%, respectively.[8,9] Pretreatment of monolayers with herbimycin A also protected against TSP-induced intercellular gap formation. When TSP-exposed EC were probed with FITC-conjugated antiphosphotyrosine antibody, the fluorescence signal was almost exclusively restricted to intercellular boundaries in plaque-like structures. Therefore, TSP-1 was shown to induce both increments of transendothelial ^{14}C-BSA flux and tyrosine phosphorylation of EC proteins, and PTK inhibition blocked both TSP-induced intercellular gap formation and loss of endothelial barrier function.[7–9]

Conclusion

The fact that SPARC and TSP-1 each induces EC protein tyrosine phosphorylation and that PTK inhibition protects against the SPARC/TSP-induced EC response implicates activation of one or more EC PTKs. That SPARC/TSP-induced tyrosine phosphorylation of EC proteins was apparent only in the presence of rigorous PTP inhibition, and that PTP inhibition enhanced SPARC/TSP-induced barrier dysfunction implicates involvement of one or more PTPs. Goldblum and colleagues hypothesize that the counteradhesive proteins, SPARC and TSP-1, activate receptor and/or nonreceptor PTKs that tyrosine phosphorylate multiple EC proteins. In the case of SPARC, for which there are more data, at least one of these PTKs phosphorylates β-catenin on tyrosine, which may promote ZA disassembly with diminished EC homophilic adhesion and disruption of the ZA-actin cytoskeletal linkage.[56–58]

Either src and/or FAK might also tyrosine phosphorylate paxillin, an established component of FAs. Whether changes in the state of assembly of FAs are involved and/or whether paxillin functions as a signaling molecule, independent of FA physiology, is unclear. Certainly, changes in FA integrity influence actin organization, EC shape, and EC-

EC orientation. Adherens junction integrity may also contribute to competence of other specialized intercellular junctions (eg, zonula occludins). The ability of counteradhesive proteins to regulate the paracellular pathway may have implications for more than the transendothelial flux of macromolecules. This same paracellular pathway may also be used for transendothelial migration of leukocytes and/or tumor cell metastasis.

References

1. Sage EH, Bornstein P. Extracellular proteins that modulate cell-matrix interactions. *J Biol Chem* 1991;266:14831–14834.
2. Chiquet-Ehrismann R. Anti-adhesive molecules of the extracellular matrix. *Curr Opin Cell Biol* 1991;3:800–804.
3. Chiquet-Ehrismann R. Inhibition of cell adhesion by anti-adhesive molecules. *Curr Opin Cell Biol* 1995;7:715–719.
4. Goldblum SE, Ding X, Funk S, et al. SPARC regulates cell shape and endothelial barrier function. *Proc Natl Acad Sci U S A* 1994;91:3448–3452.
5. Young BA, Ding X, Wang P, et al. SPARC regulates endothelial barrier function through a tyrosine phosphorylation-dependent pathway. *Mol Biol Cell* 1995;6(suppl):50a.
6. Young BA, Wang P, Gustafson TA, et al. The counteradhesive protein SPARC induces tyrosine phosphorylation of β-catenin and paxillin and regulates an endothelial paracellular pathway through protein tyrosine phosphorylation. (Manuscript submitted.)
7. Goldblum SE, Wang P, Ding X, et al. Thrombospondin regulates endothelial barrier function. *Fed Proc* 1995;9:A962.
8. Goldblum SE, Wang P, Ding X, et al. Thrombospondin-1 regulates endothelial barrier function through protein tyrosine phosphorylation. Presented at "The Thrombospondin Gene Family and its Functional Relatives: Tenascins, Osteopontin, and SPARC." Seattle, WA: June 19–22, 1996.
9. Goldblum SE, Wang P, Young BA, et al. Thrombospondin-1 regulates an endothelial paracellular pathway through protein tyrosine phosphorylation in vitro. (Manuscript submitted.)
10. Clezardin P, Malaval L, Morel M-C, et al. Osteonectin is an α-granule component involved with thrombospondin in platelet aggregation. *J Bone Miner Res* 1991;6:1059–1070.
11. Lane T, Sage EH. The biology of SPARC, protein that modulates cell-matrix interactions. *FASEB J* 1994;8:163–173.
12. Lawler J. The structural and functional properties of thrombospondin. *Blood* 1986;67:1197–1209.
13. Mosher DF. Physiology of thrombospondin. *Annu Rev Med* 1990;41:85–97.
14. Bornstein P. Thrombospondins: structure and regulation of expression. *FASEB J* 1992;6:3290–3299.
15. Adams J, Lawler J. The thrombospondin family. *Curr Biol* 1993;3:188–190.
16. Lahav J. The functions of thrombospondin and its involvement in physiology and pathophysiology. *Biochim Biophys Acta* 1993;1182:1–14.
17. Frazier WA. Thrombospondin: A modular adhesive glycoprotein of platelets and nucleated cells. *J Cell Biol* 1987;105:625–632.

18. Bornstein P, Sage EH. Thrombospondins. *Methods Enzymol* 1994;245: 62–85.
19. Bornstein P. Diversity of function is inherent in matricellular proteins: An appraisal of Thrombospondin 1. *J Cell Biol* 1995;130:503–506.
20. Erickson HP, Bourdon MA. Tenascin: An extracellular matrix protein prominent in specialized embryonic tissues and tumors. *Annu Rev Cell Biol* 1989;5:71–92.
21. Erickson HP. Tenascin-C, tenascin-R and tenascin-X: A family of talented proteins in search of functions. *Curr Opin Cell Biol* 1993;5:869–876.
22. Lane TF, Sage EH. Functional mapping of SPARC: Peptides from two distinct Ca^{++}-binding sites modulate cell shape. *J Cell Biol* 1990;111:3065–3076.
23. Schnitzer JE, Oh P. Antibodies to SPARC inhibit albumin binding to SPARC, gp60, and microvascular endothelium. *Am J Physiol* 1992;263: H1872–H1879.
24. Sage H, Johnson C, Bornstein P. Characterization of a novel serum albumin-binding glycoprotein secreted by endothelial cells in culture. *J Biol Chem* 1984;259:3993–4007.
25. Sage H, Tupper J, Bramson R. Endothelial cell injury in vitro is associated with increased secretion of an M_r 43,000 glycoprotein ligand. *J Cell Physiol* 1986;127:373–387.
26. Reed MJ, Puolakkainen P, Lane TF, et al. Differential expression of SPARC and thrombospondin 1 in wound repair: Immunolocalization and in situ hybridization. *J Histochem Cytochem* 1993;41:1467–1477.
27. Stenner DD, Tracy RP, Riggs BVL, et al. Human platelets contain and secrete osteonectin, a major protein of mineralized bone. *Proc Natl Acad Sci U S A* 1986;83:6892–6896.
28. Iruela-Arispe ML, Hasselaar P, Sage H. Differential expression of extracellular proteins is correlated with angiogenesis in vitro. *Lab Invest* 1991; 64:174–186.
29. Iruela-Arispe ML, Diglio CA, Sage EH, et al. Modulation of extracellular matrix proteins by endothelial cells undergoing angiogenesis in vitro. *Arterioscler Thromb* 1991;11:805–815.
30. Sage H, Decker J, Funk S, et al. SPARC: A Ca^{2+}-binding extracellular protein associated with endothelial cell injury and proliferation. *J Mol Cell Cardiol* 1989;21(suppl I):13–22.
31. Neri M, Descalzi-Cancedda F, Cancedda R. Heat-shock response in cultured chick embryo chondrocytes. Osteonectin is a secreted heat-shock protein. *Eur J Biochem* 1992;205:569–574.
32. Sauk JJ, Norris K, Kerr JM, et al. Diverse forms of stress result in changes in cellular levels of osteonectin/SPARC without altering mRNA levels in osteoligament cells. *Calcif Tissue Int* 1991;49:58–62.
33. Wrana JL, Kubota T, Zhang Q, et al. Regulation of transformation-sensitive secreted phosphoprotein (SPPI/osteopontin) expression by transforming growth factor-β. Comparisons with expression of SPARC (secreted acidic cysteine-rich protein). *Biochem J* 1991;273:523–531.
34. Wrana JL, Overall, CM, Sodek J, et al. Regulation of the expression of a secreted acidic protein rich in cysteine (SPARC) in human fibroblasts by transforming growth factor β. *Eur J Biochem* 1991;197:519–528.
35. Ford R, Wang G, Jannati P, et al. Modulation of SPARC expression during butyrate-induced terminal differentiation of cultured human keratinocytes: Regulation via a TGF-β-dependent pathway. *Exp Cell Res* 1993;206:261–275.

36. Kopp JB, Bianco P, Young MF, et al. Renal tubular epithelial cells express osteonectin in vivo and in vitro. *Kidney Intl* 1992;41:56–64.

37. Purcell L, Gruia-Gray J, Scanga S, et al. Developmental anomalies of *Xenopus* embryos following microinjection of SPARC antibodies. *J Exp Zool* 1993;265:153–164.

38. Schwarzbauer J, Spencer CS. The *Caenorhabditis elegans* homolog of the extracellular calcium binding protein SPARC/osteonectin affects nematode body morphology and mobility. *Mol Biol Cell* 1993;4:941–952.

39. Yost JC, Sage EH. Specific interaction of SPARC with endothelial cells is mediated through a carboxyl-terminal sequence containing a calcium-binding EF hand. *J Biol Chem* 1993;268:25790–25796.

40. Sage H, Vernon RB, Funk SE, et al. SPARC, a secreted protein associated with cellular proliferation, inhibits cell spreading in vitro and exhibits Ca^{2+}-dependent binding to the extracellular matrix. *J Cell Biol* 1989;109: 341–356.

41. Raines EW, Lane TF, Isruela-Arispe ML, et al. The extracellular glycoprotein SPARC interacts with platelet-derived growth factor (PDGF)-AB and -BB and inhibits the binding of PDGF to its receptors. *Proc Natl Acad Sci U S A* 1992;89:1281–1285.

42. Hasselaar P, Sage EH. SPARC antagonizes the effect of basic fibroblast growth factor on the migration of bovine aortic endothelial cells. *J Cell Biochem* 1992;49:272–283.

43. Sage EH. Modulation of endothelial cell shape by SPARC does not involve chelation of extracellular Ca^{2+} and Mg^{2+}. *Biochem Cell Biol* 1992;70:56–62.

44. Hasselaar P, Loskutoff DJ, Sawdey M, et al. SPARC induces the expression of type 1 plasminogen activator inhibitor in cultured bovine aortic endothelial cells. *J Biol Chem* 1991;266:13178–13184.

45. Lane TF, Iruela-Arispe ML, Sage EH. Regulation of gene expression by SPARC during angiogenesis in vitro. Changes in fibronectin, thrombospondin-1, and plasminogen activator inhibitor-1. J Biol Chem 1992;267: 16736–16745.

46. Tremble PM, Lane TF, Sage EH, et al. SPARC, a secreted protein associated with morphogenesis and tissue remodeling, induces expression of metalloproteinases in fibroblasts through a novel extracellular matrix-dependent pathway. *J Cell Biol* 1993;121:1433–1444.

47. Goldblum SE, Ding X, Brann TW, et al. Bacterial lipopolysaccharide induces actin reorganization, intercellular gap formation and endothelial barrier dysfunction in pulmonary vascular endothelial cells Concurrent F-actin depolymerization and new actin synthesis. *J Cell Physiol* 1993;157:13–23.

48. Goldblum SE, Brann TW, Ding X, et al. Lipopolysaccharide (LPS)-binding protein (LBP) and soluble CD14 function as accessory molecules for LPS-induced changes in endothelial barrier function. *J Clin Invest* 1994;93: 692–702.

49. Sage H, Vernon RB, Decker J, et al. Distribution of calcium-binding protein SPARC in tissues of embryonic and adult mice. *J Histochem Cytochem* 1989;37:819–829.

50. Goldblum SE, Ding X, Campbell-Washington, J. Tumor Necrosis factorα induces endothelial cell F-actin depolymerization, new actin synthesis, and barrier dysfunction. *Am J Physiol* 1993;264:C894–C905.

51. Wong MKK, Gotlieb AI. Endothelial cell monolayer integrity. I. Characterization of dense peripheral band of microfilaments. *Arteriosclerosis* 1986;6:212–219.

52. Geiger B, Ginsberg D, Salomon D, et al. The molecular basis for the assembly and modulation of adherens-type junctions. *Cell Diff Dev* 1990;32: 343–354.
53. Howard PK, Sefton BM, Firtel RA. Tyrosine phosphorylation of actin in *dictyostelium* associated with cell-shape changes. *Science* 1993;259:241–244.
54. Matsuyoshi N, Hamaguchi M, Taniguchi S, et al. Cadherin-mediated cell-cell adhesion is perturbed by v-*src* tyrosine phosphorylation in metastatic fibroblasts. *J Cell Biol* 1992;118:703–714.
55. Turner CE. Paxillin: A cytoskeletal target for tyrosine kinases. *BioEssays* 1994;16:47–52.
56. Kemler R. From cadherins to catenins: cytoplasmic protein interactions and regulation of cell adhesion. *Trends Genetics* 1993;9:317–321.
57. Gumbiner BM. Signal transduction by β-catenin. *Curr Opin Cell Biol* 1995; 7:634–640.
58. Yamada KM and Geiger B. Molecular interactions in cell adhesion complexes. *Curr Opin Cell Biol* 1997;9:76–85.
59. Wight TN, Raugi GJ, Mumby SM, et al. Light microscopic immunolocation of thrombospondin in human tissues. *J Histochem Cytochem* 1985;33: 295–302.
60. Ketis NV, Lawler J, Hoover RL, et al. Effects of heat shock on the expression of thrombospondin by endothelial cells in culture. *J Cell Biol* 1988;106: 893–904.
61. Murphy-Ullrich JE, Schultz-Cherry S, Höök, M, et al. Transforming growth factor-β complexes with thrombospondin. *Mol Biol Cell.* 1992;3: 181–188.
62. Schultz-Cherry S, Murphy-Ullrich JE. Thrombospondin causes activation of latent transforming growth factor-β secreted by endothelial cells by a novel mechanism. *J Cell Biol* 1993;122:923–932.
63. Clezardin P, Malaval L, Ehrensperger A-S, et al. Complex formation of human thrombospondin with osteonectin. *Eur J Biochem* 1988;175: 275–284.
64. Lawler J, Weinstein R, Hynes RO. Cell attachment to thrombospondin: The role of ARG-GLY-ASP, calcium, and integrin receptors. *J Cell Biol* 1988;107:2351–2361.
65. Taraboletti G, Roberts D, Liotta LA, et al. Platelet thrombospondin modulates endothelial cell adhesion, motility, and growth: A potential angiogenesis regulatory factor. *J Cell Biol* 1990;111:765–772.
66. Mansfield PJ, Boxer LA, Suchard SJ. Thrombospondin stimulates motility of human neutrophils. *J Cell Biol* 1990;111:3077–3086.
67. Iruela-Arispe ML, Bornstein P, Sage H. Thrombospondin exerts an antiangiogenic effect on cord formation by endothelial cells in vitro. *Proc Natl Acad Sci U S A* 1991;88:5026–5030.
68. Murphy-Ullrich JE, Hüük, M. Thrombospondin modulates focal adhesions in endothelial cells. *J Cell Biol* 1989;109:1309–1319.

Chapter 20

Oxidants and Endotoxin-Induced Endothelial Injury

Barbara Meyrick, PhD

Injury to the lung's endothelium is of prime importance in the pathogenesis of the adult respiratory distress syndrome (ARDS). The most common clinical setting for this syndrome is gram-negative bacterial sepsis or endotoxemia.[1] This syndrome can be mimicked in animals and in endothelial cells in culture.[2] For example, a single infusion of *E. coli* endotoxin into sheep results in alterations in pulmonary function including an increase in microvascular permeability, increased prostanoid release (mainly those known to be produced by endothelial cells), and endothelial damage. The latter is seen as early as 30 minutes following the beginning of endotoxin infusion as a widened edematous interstitial space in the alveolar wall.

The endothelial changes can also be mimicked in cultured endothelial cells where exposure to endotoxin results in a reduction in barrier function, increased prostanoid and lactate dehydrogenase release, and eventual cell death.[3] Thus, both in vitro and in vivo methods demonstrate that endotoxin causes endothelial retraction and injury, alterations in prostanoid release, and an increase in pulmonary vascular permeability.

While serum factors such as lipopolysaccharide-binding protein and CD14[4] are important to the initiation of endotoxin-induced endothelial changes, the mechanism responsible for the perturbations is still not certain. The mechanism is very complex, and evidence suggests that cyclic nucleotides, proteases, and intracellular generation of reactive oxygen species contribute to the changes.[5–7] This chapter briefly presents the evidence indicating that reactive oxygen species, includ-

Supported by a grant from the National Heart, Lung and Blood Institute, HL 34208.

From: Weir EK, Reeves JT (eds). *Pulmonary Edema.* Armonk, NY: Futura Publishing Company, Inc.; ©1998.

ing nitric oxide ($^{.}$NO) and peroxynitrite (ONOO$^-$), and the antioxidant enzyme, mangano superoxide dismutase (MnSOD) contribute to the endothelial changes.

Endotoxin and Intracellular Generation of Reactive Oxygen Species

In an earlier study, Brigham and colleagues[7] found that 30 minutes preincubation with either dimethylsulfoxide (DMSO), a free radical scavenger with its most profound effect on the hydroxyl radical, and the xanthine oxidase inhibitor allopurinol, attenuated the endotoxin-induced cytotoxicity in cultured bovine pulmonary artery endothelial cells (BPAEC). The iron chelator, deferoxamine, also had a

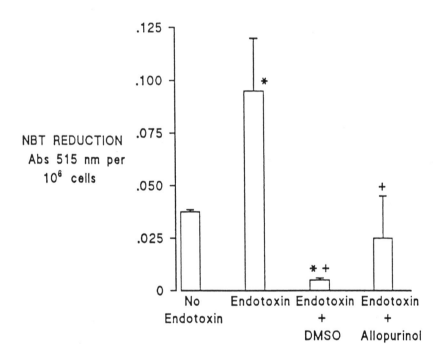

Figure 1. Attenuation of endotoxin-stimulated intracellular free radical generation in BPAEC by the free radical scavenger dimethyl sulfoxide and the xanthine oxidase inhibitor allopurinol. The endothelial cells were exposed to endotoxin (0.1 µg/mL) for 15 minutes and the data are presented as reduction of nitroblue tetrazolium per 10^6 cells. Data are presented as mean±SEM; n=6; $^*P<0.05$ compared to controls; $^+P<0.05$ compared to endotoxin. Data reprinted with permission from References 2 and 7.

similar protective effect.[8] Further, DMSO, but not allopurinol, reduced endotoxin-stimulated prostacyclin and prostaglandin E_2 (PGE_2) release. DMTU had a similar effect to DMSO.[2] These data indicate that intracellular generation of reactive oxygen species may contribute to endotoxin-induced endothelial injury and that prostaglandin production and release is likely to occur through a xanthine-independent mechanism.

In confirmation of the idea that endotoxin causes generation of reactive oxygen species, it was established that BPAEC reduced nitroblue tetrazolium within 15 minutes of endotoxin treatment, and that this reduction was inhibited by both DMSO and allopurinol (Figure 1).[7] Increased release of lipid peroxidation products, conjugated dienes, in culture medium 30 minutes following exposure of endothelium to endotoxin and oxidation of dichlorofluoroscein diacetate to its fluorescent by-product was also observed. Each of these endpoints were suppressed in the presence of either DMSO or allopurinol.[7]

Such measures, although not specific for assessment of reactive oxygen species, when taken together, begin to make the argument that early intracellular generation of reactive oxygen species may accompany exposure to endotoxin, and that these species may contribute to the endothelial perturbations. Other studies[9–11] have confirmed that alterations in intracellular generation of reactive oxygen species accompany endothelial injury, and more recently the strong oxidants ·NO and $ONOO^-$ have also been implicated in these perturbations.

Endotoxin and Intracellular Antioxidants

If intracellular generation of reactive oxygen species is involved in endotoxin-induced endothelial changes, it might also be expected that intracellular concentrations of antioxidants are also increased. Measurement of a number of antioxidants in bovine endothelial cells failed to detect any alterations in levels of fumarase, cytochrome c oxidase, catalase, glutathione peroxidase, and the cytosolic, copper/zinc (CuZn) superoxide dismutase (SOD), with exposure to endotoxin.[12] The most striking finding was that endotoxin caused a specific and time-dependent increase in the mitochondrial antioxidant enzyme, MnSOD (Figure 2). The increase was significant by 4 hours of endotoxin and continued to rise over the 24 hours of the study. The SODs are the first line of antioxidant defense, and they catalyze the dismutation of two superoxide radicals to yield H_2O_2 and O_2.

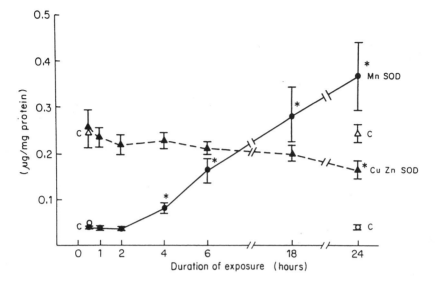

Figure 2. Manganous (Mn) and copper zinc (CuZn) superoxide dismutase (SODs) concentrations in pulmonary arterial endothelial cells with and without exposure to endotoxin (0.1 μg/mL). Closed circles = MnSOD with endotoxin; open circles = Mn SOD without endotoxin; closed triangles = CuZn with endotoxin; open triangle = CuZn SOD with endotoxin; bars = mean±SEM; n=5. For MnSOD, *values are significantly *(P*<0.05) different from preceding values; 24 h value is also significantly different from time-matched control. For CuZn SOD, 24 h value is significantly lower than time-matched control (*P*<0.05). Reprinted with permission from Reference 12.

Mangano Superoxide Dismutase Gene Expression

Northern analysis of total RNA isolated from pulmonary artery endothelial cells exposed to endotoxin showed a gradual increase in the three isoforms of bovine MnSOD mRNA, 3.4, 1.7, and 1.4 kb in size. The increase in MnSOD mRNA paralleled the temporal increase in protein. Induction of MnSOD mRNA was seen as early as 2 hours of endotoxin exposure, peaked by 8 hours, and was declining by 24 hours.[13] Mitchell and colleagues[14] have also shown that the MnSOD gene is regulated at the pretranscriptional level and that DMSO attenuates the endotoxin-stimulated increase in MnSOD mRNA (Figure 3), whereas allopurinol has no effect on modulation of this gene.

These data indicate that the protective effect of DMSO on the endotoxin-induced endothelial changes is accompanied by a reduction in MnSOD mRNA. The failure of allopurinol to inhibit the endotoxin-induced increase in MnSOD gene expression suggests that this antioxidant enzyme is unlikely to mediate the cytotoxic effects of endotoxin.

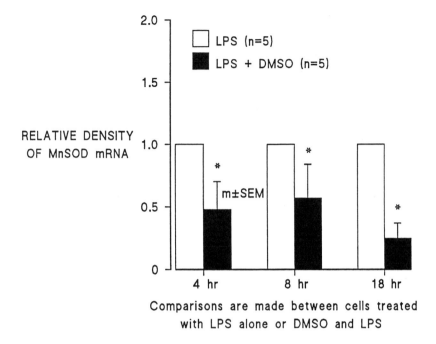

Figure 3. Laser densitometer reading of Northern blot analysis. Endothelial cells were treated with DMSO (solid bars) and/or endotoxin (open bars) for 4, 8, and 18 hours. DMSO significantly inhibited the endotoxin-induced increase in MnSOD mRNA. For each time point, intensitiy of the major band of mRNA for MnSOD in LPS-stimulated cells was assigned to be equal to 1.0. Relative intensities represent mean±SEM; n=5; $P<0.05$. Adapted with permission from Reference 14.

Inhibition of the endotoxin-induced increase in MnSOD mRNA by DMSO, on the other hand, perhaps suggests that the hydroxyl radical contributes to regulation of the MnSOD gene and that either the Mn-SOD gene or the hydroxyl radical, or both, contribute to the increased prostaglandin synthesis.

An interest in the mechanism of endotoxin-induced endothelial injury and the role of MnSOD caused Meyrick and Magnuson[13] to initiate studies that examine the molecular mechanisms that regulate Mn-SOD gene expression in lung endothelial cells. The 5' flanking region of the MnSOD gene was isolated from a bovine liver genomic library using a cDNA for human MnSOD (generously supplied by Dr. Yen-Shi Ho). Restriction mapping and Southern analysis of the fragment of genomic MnSOD revealed a 2.8 kb fragment that contained Exons 1 and 2 and a 1 kb fragment of the 5' flanking region. Sequencing of the 5' flanking region of this gene revealed that the promoter was GC rich and lacked a CAAT and TATA box. Consensus sequences for 7 SP-1 enhancer sites and one AP-2 site were found in the 5' flanking region.[13]

Deletion fusion gene constructs of the 5' flanking regions linked to the firefly luciferase reporter gene and a construct containing β-galactosidase were cotransfected into both BPAEC and HIT (hamster insulinoma tumor) cells, and demonstrated promoter activity in the region from −980 to +30 bases. The largest construct showed approximately 20% of that observed under the same conditions for the respiratory syncytial virus (RSV) promoter. The three shorter constructs showed less activity than the largest, showing a significant reduction in relative transcription activity between 955 and 318 and an increase from 318 to 176, suggesting the presence of a repressor or silencer within this region. The smallest construct showed a further fall in transcriptional activity to approximately 25% of the value for the largest construct. Transfection of the deletion constructs into HIT cells gave a slightly different picture with a gradual size-related reduction in transcription, indicating intercellular differences in the regulation of this gene.[15] Further studies with constructs containing up to the first 5 kb of the 5' flanking region also failed to reveal an endotoxin response element (B. Meyrick and H. Jiang, unpublished data, 1996).

Endotoxin and Human Pulmonary Artery Endothelial Cells

Recent studies have shown that human pulmonary artery cells behave similarly to bovine cells in response to endotoxin. Human cells show increased PGE_2 (Figure 4) and prostacyclin release, increased lactate dehydrogenase release and apoptosis,[15] and an increase in MnSOD gene expression (B. Meyrick, unpublished observations, 1996) in response to endotoxin, as do the bovine cells. The response in the cultured human cells is, however, not as severe as in the bovine endothelial cells.

Nitric Oxide and Peroxynitrite and Endotoxin-Stimulated Prostaglandin Release

As mentioned above, exposure of bovine and human pulmonary artery endothelial cells to endotoxin results in a striking increase in prostanoid release. Several papers have demonstrated a link between ·NO and regulation of prostaglandin production,[16] but results from these studies are not consistent. For example, ·NO has been shown to stimulate cyclooxygenase activity in a rabbit model of renal inflammation,[17] in murine islets of Langerhans,[18] and in bovine coronary mi-

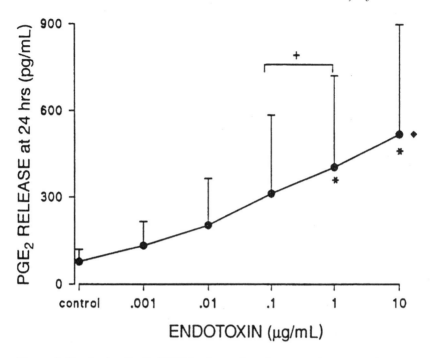

Figure 4. Prostaglandin E$_2$ (PGE$_2$) release from human pulmonary artery endothelial cells after a 24-hour exposure to various concentrations of endotoxin.
Values are the mean ±SEM; n=7. Significantly different (*P*<0.05) by analysis
of variance (ANOVA): *compared with control; –compared with all other
groups; +between groups as indicated. Reprinted with permission from Reference 15.

crovascular cells.[19] However, ·NO has also been shown to downregulate prostanoid production in rat Kupffer cells,[20] and further, PGE$_2$ has
been shown to depress interleukin-1-stimulated induction of nitric
oxide synthase (NOS).[21] Upregulation of NOS and cyclooxygenase-2
(COX-2) gene expression and activity has been suggested to occur in
parallel.[16] Such data have led to the notion that modulation of both of
these genes may be tissue- and species-dependent.

While the original descriptions of the effect of both the strong oxidants ·NO and ONOO$^-$ demonstrated deleterious effects on cultured
cells,[9–11] more recent studies indicate that both of these agents may also
provide an antioxidant effect. For example, inhaled ·NO has been shown
to attenuate the oxidant-induced increases in lung capillary permeability,[22,23] and exogenous generation of ·NO has been shown to inhibit peroxide-induced injury of rat lung microvascular cells.[24] In addition,
ONOO$^-$ may function as a vasodilator through nitrosylation of
gluthathione (GSH) or other protein thiols and its later release of ·NO.[25]

Meyrick and colleagues recently examined the effect of endogenous and exogenous generation of ·NO and ONOO⁻ on endotoxin-stimulated prostaglandin release in BPAEC. To date, these studies demonstrate that the endotoxin-induced increase in prostacyclin and PGE_2 synthesis and release is accompanied by upregulation of COX-2 mRNA. The increase in COX-2 mRNA is striking by 3 hours of endotoxin, and remains elevated over an 18-hour period.[26] Endotoxin also causes an increase in ecNOS mRNA[27], although as mentioned in other reports, this occurs without a detectable increase in intracellular ·NO.[28]

In order to examine the notion that increased levels of intracellular ·NO and ONOO⁻ may provide a protective effect on endotoxin-induced endothelial prostaglandin release, endothelial cells were pretreated with either the ·NO donor 1 mmol/L S-nitroso-N-acetylpenicillamine (SNAP) or 0.5 mmol/L sodium nitroprusside (SNP), the ONOO⁻ donor 1 mmol/L 3-morpholinosynonimine (SIN-1), and the nitric oxide synthase inhibitor 0.1 mmol/L N^G-nitro-L-arginine methyl ester (L-NAME).[26] Both SNAP and SIN-1 resulted in inhibition of both prostacyclin and PGE_2 release. SNP provided a less marked protection than SIN-1 and SNAP, and L-NAME showed no protective effect. The protective effect of SIN-1 and SNAP were accompanied by marked reductions in the endotoxin-induced increase in COX-2 mRNA. Further, the protective effects occurred in conjunction with four- and 11-fold increases in intracellular nitrite concentrations, indicating that the exogenously generated ·NO and ONOO⁻ entered the cell.[26] Such data are consistent with the idea that strikingly increased concentrations of intracellular ·NO and ONOO⁻ may protect against endotoxin-stimulated prostaglandin release.

In summary, it seems that intracellular generation of reactive oxygen species may contribute to endotoxin-induced endothelial perturbations; endotoxin-stimulated increases in MnSOD are not associated with endotoxin-stimulated cytotoxicity but may play a role in regulation of prostaglandin production, which is perhaps modulated by the hydroxyl radical; the first 5 kb of the 5' flanking region of the bovine MnSOD gene does not contain an endotoxin-responsive element; and supranormal intracellular concentrations of ·NO and ONOO⁻ inhibit endotoxin-stimulated prostanoid release and thus may invoke an antioxidant effect.

References

1. Brigham KL, Meyrick BO. Endotoxin and lung injury. *Am Rev Respir Dis* 1989;133:913–927.
2. Read MA, Meyrick B. Effects of endotoxin on lung endothelium. In:

Brigham KL (ed): *Endotoxin and the Lungs.* New York: Marcel Decker, Inc.; 1994;83–110.

3. Meyrick B, Ryan US, Brigham KL. Direct effects of *E. coli* endotoxin on structure and permeability of pulmonary endothelial monolayers and the endothelial layer of intimal explants. *Am J Pathol* 1986;122:140–151.
4. Tobias PS, Mathison J, Mintz D, et al. Participation of lipopolysaccharide-binding protein in lipopolysaccharide-dependent macrophage activation. *Am J Respir Cell Mol Biol* 1992;7:239–245.
5. Hussein A, Meyrick B, Graber S, et al. Inhibition of endotoxin induced cytotoxicity and prostacyclin production in cultured bovine pulmonary artery endothelial cells by phosphodiesterase inhibition. *Exp Lung Res* 1988;14:637–654.
6. Tumen J, Meyrick B, Berry L, et al. Antiproteinases protect cultured lung endothelial cells from endotoxin injury. *J Appl Physiol* 1988;65:835–843.
7. Brigham KL, Meyrick B, Berry LC, et al. Antioxidants protect cultured bovine lung endothelial cells from injury by endotoxin. *J Appl Physiol* 1987;63:840–850.
8. Rinaldo JE, Gorry M. Protection by deferoxamine from endothelial injury: A possible link with inhibition of intracellular xanthine oxidase. *Am J Respir Cell Mol Biol* 1990;3:525–533.
9. Freeman B. Free radical chemistry of nitric oxide. *Chest* 1994;105(suppl): 79S–84S.
10. Beckman JS, Beckman TW, Chen J, et al. Apparent hydroxyl radical production by peroxynitrite: Implications for endothelial injury from nitric oxide and superoxide. *Proc Natl Acad Sci U S A* 1990;87:1620–1624.
11. Kooy NW, Royall JA. Agonist-induced peroxynitrite production from endothelial cells. *Arch Biochem Biophys* 1994;310:352–359.
12. Shiki Y, Meyrick B, Brigham KL, et al. Endotoxin increases superoxide dismutase in cultured bovine pulmonary artery endothelial cells. *Am J Physiol* 1987;252:C436–C440.
13. Meyrick B, Magnuson MA. Identification and functional characterization of the bovine manganous superoxide dismutase promoter. *Am J Respir Cell Mol Biol* 1994;10:113–121.
14. Mitchell J, Jiang H, Berry L, et al. Effects of antioxidants on lipopolysaccharide-stimulated induction of mangano superoxide dismutase mRNA in bovine pulmonary artery endothelial cells. *J Cell Physiol* 1996;169: 333–340.
15. Meyrick B, Berry LC, Christman B. Response of cultured human pulmonary artery endothelial cells to endotoxin. *Am J Physiol* 1995;268: L239–L244.
16. Vane JR, Mitchell JA, Appleton I, et al. Inducible isoforms of cyclooxygenase and nitric oxide synthase in inflammation. *Proc Natl Acad Sci U S A* 1994;91:2046–2050.
17. Salvemini D, Seibert K, Masferrer JL, et al. Endogenous nitric oxide enhances prostaglandin production in a model of renal inflammation. *J Clin Invest* 1994;93:1940–1947.
18. Corbett JA, Lancaster JR Jr, Sweetlan MA, et al. Interleukin-1-β-induced formation of EPR-detectable iron-nitrosyl complexes in islets of Langerhans: Role of nitric oxide and interleukin-1-β-induced inhibition of insulin secretion. *J Biol Chem* 1991;266:21351–21354.
19. Davidge ST, Baker ST, McLaughlin MK, et al. Nitric oxide produced by endothelial cells increases production of eicosanoids through activation of prostaglandin H synthase. *Circ Res* 1995;77:274–283.

20. Stadler J, Harbredtch BG, Di Silvio M, et al. Endogenous nitric oxide inhibits the synthesis of cyclooxygenase products and interleukin-6 by rat Kupffer cells. *J Leuk Biol* 1993;53:165–172.

21. Tetsuka T, Daphna-Iken D, Srivastava SK, et al. Cross-talk between cyclooxygenase and nitric oxide pathways: Prostaglandin E_2 negatively modulates induction of nitric oxide synthase by interleukin-1. *Proc Natl Acad Sci U S A* 1994;91:12168–12172.

22. Poss WB, Timmons OD, Farrukh IS, et al. Inhaled nitric oxide prevents the increase in pulmonary vascular permeability cause by hydrogen peroxide. *J Appl Physiol* 1995;79:886–891.

23. Wu M, Pritchard KA Jr, Kaminski PM, et al. Involvement of nitric oxide and nitrosthiols in relaxation of pulmonary arteries to peroxynitrite. *Am J Physiol* 1994;266:H2108–H2113.

24. Chang J, Raoo NV, Markewitz BA, et al. Nitric oxide donor prevents hydrogen peroxide-mediated endothelial cell injury. *Am J Physiol* 1996;270: L931–L940.

25. Liu S, Beckman JS, Ku DD. Peroxynitrite, a product of superoxide and nitric oxide produces coronary artery vasorelaxation in dogs. *J Pharmacol Exp Ther* 1994;268:1114–1121.

26. Watson PL, Christman B, Berry L, et al. Exogenous nitric oxide and peroxynitrite inhibit endotoxin-induced prostanoid formation in bovine pulmonary artery endothelial cells (BPAEC). *Am J Respir Crit Care Med* 1996; 153:A571.

27. Meyrick B, Berry LC, Christman B. Increased nitric oxide generation inhibits endotoxin-stimulated cytotoxicity and prostacyclin release from bovine pulmonary artery endothelial cells. *Am J Respir Crit Care Med* 1995;151:A630.

28. Myers PR, Wright TF, Tanner MA, et al. EDRF and nitric oxide production in cultured endothelial cells: Direct inhibition by *E. coli* endotoxin. *Am J Physiol* 1992;262:H710–H718.

Chapter 21

Effects of Extracellular Nucleotides on Lung Vascular Endothelial Cells

Sharon Rounds, MD, Doloretta D. Dawicki, PhD, Annie Lin Parker, MD, and Laura L. Likar, MD

Introduction

Increased permeability pulmonary edema, also called the adult respiratory distress syndrome (ARDS), is a devastating illness that results in high mortality despite advances in supportive care.[1] ARDS frequently occurs in the setting of multiple organ dysfunction syndrome (MODS), in which injury to multiple organs further enhances mortality. Studies of ARDS and MODS indicate a pathogenetic role of injury to vascular endothelium by inflammatory cells, especially polymorphonuclear neutrophilic leukocytes (PMNs).[2] However, although PMNs and their activation are likely to play roles in the pathogenesis of the vascular injury that results in ARDS or MODS, their accumulation alone is not sufficient.[3] It is likely that additional changes in endothelium are necessary for vascular injury to occur. Multiple investigators, including the authors, have demonstrated mechanisms by which endothelial cells enhance[4,5] or inhibit[6] PMN function. It has also been found that extracellular nucleotides enhance PMN adherence to endothelium and directly injure endothelial cells via apoptosis.

Circulating adenine nucleotides have been measured after vascular injury in the range of 10 to 20 μmol/L.[7] Potential sources include ex-

Supported by grants from VA Merit Review, HL34009 from the NIH, Cystic Fibrosis Foundation, and Glaxo-Wellcome.

From: Weir EK, Reeves JT (eds). *Pulmonary Edema*. Armonk, NY: Futura Publishing Company, Inc.; ©1998.

ocytotic release from platelets, endothelial cells, nerves, and adrenal medulla.[8] Platelet release of nucleotides is of particular interest in acute vascular injury because of close associations between platelets and PMN in the circulation and at sites of thrombus formation and tissue damage. In addition, nucleotides may be released from cells undergoing necrosis, such as during hemolysis or rhabdomyolysis. This is likely a rich source of nucleotides, since intracellular concentrations are in the range of 1 to 3 mmol/L.[8] It has been estimated that circulating concentrations of adenosine triphosphate (ATP) up to 100 μmol/L are possible after traumatic injuries.[8] Finally, nucleotides may be secreted from endothelial and other cells via intrinsic membrane transporters.[8]

Extracellular nucleotides have significant effects on a variety of physiological functions such as vascular tone, platelet aggregation, neural transmission, and immunomodulation.[9] Physiological effects of extracellular nucleotides in vivo are likely modulated by hydrolysis by ectonucleotidases (eg, on endothelial cells)[10,11] and by complexing to divalent cations, limiting the availability of active tetrabasic forms.[12]

Extracellular Nucleotides and PMN-Endothelial Cell Adhesion

Extracellular adenine nucleotides modulate both endothelial and PMN function. Physiological effects of extracellular nucleotides on neutrophils and endothelial cells appear to be receptor mediated. It should be noted that the classification system for purinoceptors is undergoing revision in view of the recently reported cloning of P2y, P2u, P2x, and P2z receptors.[13] Purinoceptor terminology based on agonist specificity is used in this chapter because the endothelial cell and PMN receptors involved in ATP-induced cell-to-cell interaction have not yet been cloned. Analysis of purinoceptor subtype has been difficult due to lack of specific antagonists, but it appears that both cell types respond in a fashion consistent with both P2y and/or P2u receptors, as defined by agonist specificity.[14] Extracellular ATP and uridine triphosphate (UTP) have been found to act directly on vascular endothelial cells by P2y and P2u receptors, causing inositol phosphate hydrolysis and increased intracellular calcium via a G-protein linked mechanism.[14] Adenine nucleotides also act directly on PMNs, increasing intracellular calcium concentration,[15] superoxide release,[16] aggregation,[17] expression of the adhesion molecule CD11b/CD18,[18] and degranulation.[19,20] The tetrabasic form of nucleotides (uncomplexed to cations, ie, ATP^{-4}, UTP^{-4}) appears to be a physiologically significant ligand for endothelial cells[21] and for PMNs.[22] Other purinergic receptors have been described on other cell types: the P2t receptor on platelets, which mediates cation influx; the P2x receptor on excitable tissues, such as smooth muscle, which mediates cation influx and rapid depolarization[9]; and the P2z receptor on fibroblasts,[23] mast cells,[24] and macrophages,[25] which mediates permeabilization via formation of nonselective membrane pores.

Using cultured human pulmonary arterial endothelial cells (HPAECs), the authors found that extracellular ATP and UTP stimulate PMN adhesion in a dose-dependent fashion (Figure 1).[26,32] Using cultured bovine pulmonary arterial endothelial cells and the myeloid progenitor cell, HL-60 cells, they found that the rank order of agonist specificity is characteristic of P2y/P2u purinoceptors.[26] Photoaffinity labeling of endothelial cells with the purinoceptor agonist, 8-Az-[α-^{32}P]ATP showed the presence of two ATP-binding proteins of molecular weight 48 kd and 87 kd. Patterns of inhibition of photoaffinity binding showed that the 48 kd protein is likely a P2u purinoceptor.[26]

The time course of nucleotide-induced PMN adhesion to endothelial cells was rapid, with peak adherence reached within 15 minutes, similar to the time course of thrombin-induced adhesion reported by Zimmerman and colleagues.[27] Adherence of activated PMN to endothelial cells is the initial event in a multistep inflammatory process, leading to changes in vascular permeability and emigration of PMN into tissues.[27] The adhesion of PMN to endothelial cells entails regulated expression of molecules on both endothelial cells and leukocytes. These adhesion molecules have different structures and mechanisms of expression, and it appears that combinations of molecules, rather than single pairs of ligands and receptors, regulate PMN adhesion and activation at the endothelial cell surface.[27]

A well-studied model of the adhesive interaction between PMN and endothelial cells is the adherence of PMN to endothelium activated with thrombin.[28] The time course of thrombin-induced adherence is rapid, with maximal adherence occurring within 15 minutes.[28] This is in contrast to the more delayed adhesive interaction induced by interleukin-1,[29] tumor necrosis factor (TNF),[30] and endotoxin lipopolysaccharide (LPS).[31] Since the time course of nucleotide-induced PMN adhesion is similar to that reported for thrombin, the authors investigated to see whether similar mechanisms were involved.[32] They found that blocking antibody to P-selectin and intracellular adhesion molecule−1 (ICAM−1) did not inhibit ATP-induced PMN adhesion to cultured human endothelial cells (Figure 2), although the antibodies did inhibit thrombin-induced PMN adhesion, as described by others.[28] In addition, blocking antibodies to β subunit of the CD11/CD18 integrin complex also did not inhibit ATP-induced PMN adhesion.[26] On the other hand, the platelet activating factor (PAF) receptor antagonists, WEB-2086 and L-659,989, did inhibit ATP-induced PMN adhesion (Figure 3).

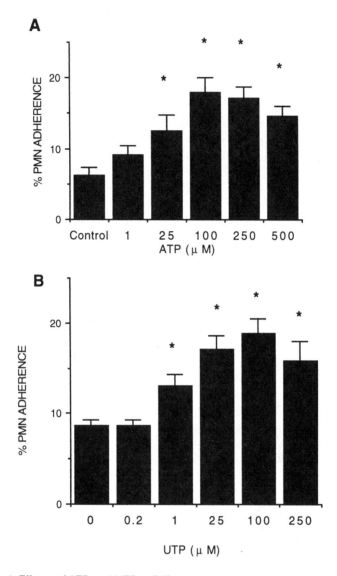

Figure 1. Effects of ATP and UTP at Different concentrations on adherence between human neutrophils (PMNs) and human pulmonary artery endothelial cells (HPAEC). Confluent cultures of HPAEC in 24 well plates were incubated for 15 minutes with different concentrations of ATP (panel A) or UTP (panel B) and 5×10^5 ^{51}Cr-labeled human PMNs in MEM/0.1% BSA at 37°C in 95% air, 5% CO_2. Neutrophil adherence was assessed by the adherent radioactivity after removal of nonadherent ^{51}Cr-labeled PMN. n=12; *P<0.05 compared to control.

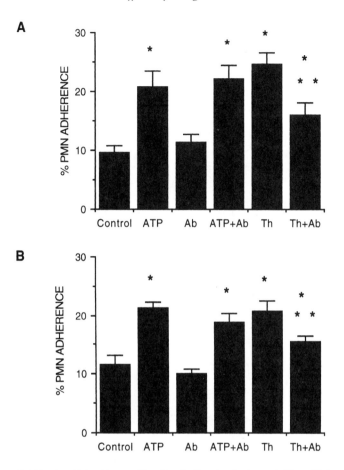

Figure 2. Effects of blocking antibodies to P-selectin (panel A) and intercellular adhesion molecule-1 (ICAM-1) (panel B) on ATP-induced adherence between human neutrophils and human pulmonary artery endothelial cells (HPAEC). Confluent cultures of HPAEC in 24 well plates were incubated for 15 minutes with 100 μmol/L ATP or 2 U/mL thrombin (Th), 10 μg/mL blocking antibodies (Ab) and 5×10^5 ^{51}Cr-labeled human PMNs in MEM/0.1% BSA at 37°C in 95% air, 5% CO_2. Neutrophil adherence was assessed by adherent radioactivity after removal of nonadherent ^{51}Cr-labeled PMN. P-selectin Ab: n=24; ICAM-1 Ab: n=12; *P<0.05 compared to control; **P<0.05 compared to thrombin.

Similar effects were observed with UTP-induced PMN adhesion.[26] Preincubation of both endothelial cells and PMN with ATP or UTP stimulated the adhesive interaction, effects that were inhibited by PAF receptor blockers.[26] These results suggest that PAF or a PAF-like substance are important mediators of nucleotide-induced PMN adhesion to endothelial cells. This effect of nucleotides is mediated via effects on both PMN and endothelial cells.

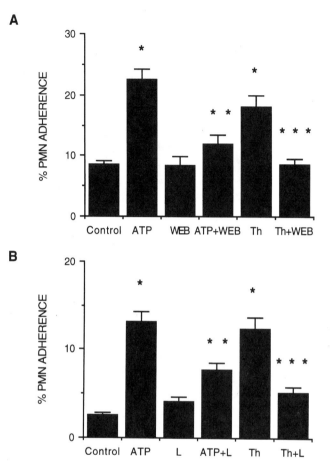

Figure 3. Effects of platelet activating factor (PAF) receptor antagonists WEB 2086 (panel A) and L-659,989 (panel B) on ATP-induced adherence between human neutrophils and human pulmonary artery endothelial cells (HPAEC). Confluent cultures of HPAEC in 24 well plates were incubated for 15 minutes with 100 μmol/L ATP or 2 U/mL thrombin (Th), PAF receptor antagonist (25 μmol/L WEB 2086 or 0.25 μmol/L L-659,989), and 5×10^5 ^{51}Cr-labeled human PMNs in MEM/0.1% BSA at 37°C in 95% air, 5% CO_2. Neutrophil adherence was determined by adherent radioactivity after removal of nonadherent ^{51}Cr-labeled PMN. WEB 2086 (WEB): n=16; L-659,989(L): n=20; *$P<0.05$ compared to control; **$P<0.05$ compared to ATP; ***$P<0.05$ compared to thrombin.

PAF is a biologically active phospholipid, not constitutively present in resting endothelial cells. It is synthesized within minutes of stimulation by a number of substances including thrombin, bradykinin, histamine, and ATP.[33] The juxtacrine interaction of thrombin-stimulated endothelial cells and PMN has been elegantly reviewed by Zimmerman et al.[27] PAF is synthesized and coexpressed with P-selectin on thrombin-activated endothelial cells.[28] PAF binds to a receptor on the neutrophil that is a member of the G-protein-linked family.[34] PAF receptor activation induces upregulation of CD11/CD18 integrin complex constitutively present on the neutrophil plasma membrane.[35] Activated CD11/CD18 integrin may then bind to its counter-receptors, including ICAM-1 on endothelial cells, leading to enhanced adhesion. Binding of CD11/CD18 integrins on activated neutrophils to ICAM-1 on endothelial cells has been shown to facilitate transendothelial migration.[36]

The authors' negative studies with anti-P-selectin Ab argue against a P-selectin-mediated mechanism. The process could be mediated by another lectin-like adhesion molecule that is yet to be characterized. Their concurrent control experiments demonstrate that the P-selectin-blocking Ab G1 successfully inhibited thrombin-stimulated PMN adherence HPAECs, therefore the failure of these antibodies to inhibit ATP-induced adherence is not due to problems in experimental design. On the other hand, successful inhibition of the ATP effect by PAF receptor antagonists supports the conclusion that PAF is a mediator of ATP-induced leukocyte adherence to endothelial cells. The inability of anti-ICAM-1 and anti-β subunit antibodies to inhibit ATP-induced adherence can be interpreted several ways. One possibility is that even though PAF is a mediator of the ATP effect, it does not activate leukocyte CD11/CD18 integrin to enhance adhesion, as in the thrombin system. Another possible interpretation is that this is a multistep process, and that inhibition of the β-integrin contribution is not enough to abrogate stimulated adherence. It is also possible that PAF may have the ability to activate an alternative pathway despite inhibition of CD11/CD18 integrin complex.

These results are similar to those reported by Sellak et al[37] on the mechanism of leukocyte adherence stimulated by reactive oxygen species. Those investigators found that sialic acid, but not P-selectin-blocking Ab, inhibited PMN adhesion to HUVECs after incubation with hypoxanthine/xanthine oxidase. This supports the contention that other lectin mechanisms are involved with enhanced leukocyte-endothelial cell adherence.

The authors conclude that ATP and UTP stimulate PMN adherence to endothelium through a mechanism mediated via PAF or a PAF-like substance associated with both cell types. This interaction is summarized in Figure 4. Unlike thrombin-stimulated adherence, this mechanism is not sensitive to P-selectin, ICAM-1, and β-integrin-blocking antibodies. This suggests that there may be other PAF-mediated mechanisms for neutrophil adherence to endothelium.

Summary: Mechanism of Adhesion

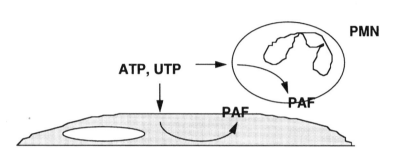

Endothelial Cell

Figure 4. Summary of studies of the mechanism of nucleotide-induced adhesion of PMN to endothelial cells.

Endothelial Cell Metabolism of Nucleotides

In addition to nucleotide interactions with purinceptors on endothelial cells, endothelial cells are also capable of metabolizing circulating nucleotides. These metabolic pathways are illustrated in Figure 5.

ATP is hydrolyzed to adenosine by endothelial cells via surface ectonucleotidases.[11] It has been demonstrated that 5'-nucleotidase activity of intact pulmonary artery endothelial cells can be stimulated by endotoxin.[10] This suggests that under conditions that could cause vascular injury, potentially injurious nucleotides could be more effectively hydrolyzed to adenosine.

In most circumstances, extracellular ATP (exATP) is the most important source of extracellular adenosine.[8] Adenosine can interact with endothelial cell P1 purinoceptors of the A2 type, stimulating adenyl cyclase. Adenosine is also taken up into cells by passive and facilitated diffusion, the latter inhibitable by dipyridamole.[38] Once intracellular, adenosine is incorporated into adenine nucleotides via adenosine kinase and is metabolized to inosine and hypoxanthine via adenosine deaminase.[39] Another pathway of intracellular adenosine metabolism relates to homocysteine metabolism. The enzyme, S-adenosylhomocysteine hydrolase (SAH) catalyzes the hydrolysis of S-adenosylhomocysteine to adenosine and homocysteine with a Km of 10^{-6} μmol/L.[40]

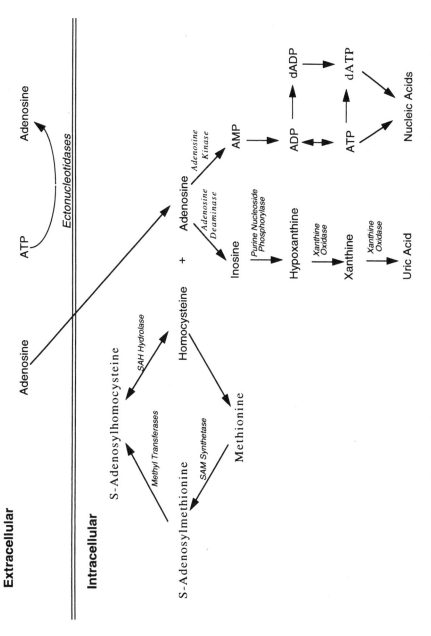

Figure 5. Illustration of the pathways for hydrolysis, uptake, and intracellular metabolism of extracellular nucleotides by endothelial cells.

The authors used cultured main pulmonary artery endothelial cells to study the effects of endotoxin-induced injury on adenosine metabolism.[39] They found that endotoxin did not alter uptake of ^{3}H-adenosine into endothelial cells or incorporation into nucleotides and hypoxanthine. However, endotoxin did enhance release of radiolabeled adenosine metabolites. Analysis of patterns of release indicated that hypoxanthine and inosine were secreted into culture media in greater quantities after endotoxin injury.[39] It is possible that the adenosine deaminase pathway of adenosine metabolism may act to amplify and exacerbate endotoxin-induced endothelial cell injury, since both hypoxanthine and inosine can act as substrates for xanthine oxidase, resulting in production of hydrogen peroxide (see Figure 5).

Direct Injurious Effects of Extracellular Nucleotides

A spectrum of endothelial cell injury appears to be associated with the endothelial cell dysfunction that results in increased permeability pulmonary edema. Dysfunction, without morphological change, is evident from studies of metabolic functions of the endothelium.[41] At the other end of the spectrum is frank necrosis with endothelial cell lysis and denudation of the vasculature.

In other cell types, such as immunocompetent cells, ATP has been demonstrated to cause cytotoxicity by three distinct means: cell lysis, apoptosis, and by sustained opening of P2z receptor-mediated pores.[42] The effects of ATP on cell permeability appear to be specific for that nucleotide and are mediated by the tetrabasic form of ATP (ATP^{-4}). ATP causes ligand-gated cation influx into lymphocytes[43] and hepatocytes[44] via a P2x receptor. The P2z response is that of sustained opening of pores which are permeant to larger molecules of molecular weight up to 1000 kd.[25] Of interest, the cytolytic P2z receptor recently cloned from rat brain was homologous to P2x ATP-gated ion channels.[45] Thus, the same receptor (P2X$_7$) appears to be capable of both transient cation currents and cytolysis. Effects of ATP vary among cell types. DNA fragmentation, characteristic of apoptosis, occurs in some cells,[46] while membrane lysis is the predominant effect in others.[43] It has been postulated that P2x and/or P2z receptors are responsible for ATP-mediated cell lysis and that ATP-mediated cell lysis may be an important mechanism of cell-mediated cytotoxicity.[42] It is also possible that P2z-mediated pores are important in cell-to-cell communication, allowing intercellular passage of larger-molecular-weight substances.[47] At this time, P2x and P2z receptors have not been identified on endothelial cells.

Another form of endothelial cell loss is that due to apoptosis, or "programmed" or "physiological" cell death. Evidence for apoptosis in lungs from patients with ARDS has been reported by Polunovsky et al.[48] Apoptotic cell death is morphologically distinct from necrosis or lysis and is characterized by cell shrinkage and nuclear condensation, followed by formation of apoptotic bodies and phagocytosis by other cells.[49,50] The process of apoptosis consists of "controlled autodigestion" of the cell. In contrast, cell death by necrosis is a more acute form of injury, characterized by cell swelling and lysis.

Apoptosis is important in a number of physiological processes including embryonic development and immune system control.[49,50] Apoptosis may also play a role in a number of diseases in which there is imbalance between cell division and cell death, such as carcinogenesis, degenerative disorders, and ischemia/reperfusion injury.[51] There has been an explosion of research into mechanisms of apoptosis because of the potential importance of controlled cell loss. Apoptosis is initiated by signals which may differ among cell types, such as growth factor withdrawal,[52] cytokines,[53] or toxins.[54] This results in activation of a poorly defined "central death signal" with activation of genes that promote death or inhibition of genes that are protective. Very little is known about the mediators of the process between initiation of apoptosis and gene activation. Indeed, in some cell-free systems gene activation does not appear to be necessary.[50] As apoptosis proceeds, endonucleases which fragment DNA are activated, cell cytoskeletal organization changes, and ion homeostasis is altered, resulting in the characteristic morphology of shrunken cells with pycnotic nuclei.[49,50]

Studies of apoptosis in development of *Drosophila melanogaster* and *Caenorhabditis elegans* have provided seminal information regarding genetic regulation of apoptosis.[50] As research has progressed in mammalian systems, it has become apparent that the physiological stimuli and conditions for progression differ among cell types.[49] It is believed that there is a common pathway for genetic regulation, however, which may involve activation of a gene analogous to the *reaper* gene in *Drosophila*, which in turn regulates the function of death-promoting genes, such as that responsible for production of interleukin-1β-converting enzyme (ICE), and protective genes such as that responsible for production of Bcl-2.[50] Apoptosis is thought to be due to a disruption of balance between death-promoting processes and protective processes.

Very little is known about apoptosis in acute lung injury. Because of the potential importance of this process in both lung injury and repair, the National Heart, Lung, and Blood Institute-(NHLBI) sponsored Task Force for Cardiopulmonary Research in Critical Care Medicine has recommended increased research into mechanisms of apoptosis and lung repair.[55] Polunovsky and colleagues[48] have described apoptotic cells in lungs from patients in the fibroproliferative phase of ARDS and have reported the existence of a substance obtained by bronchoalveolar lavage done during the repair phase, which stimulated apoptosis of cultured endothelial cells.

With regard to endothelial cells, several agents and conditions have been reported to cause apoptosis of cultured cells, including tumor necrosis factor-α (TNFα),[53] cycloheximide,[53] withdrawal of basic fibroblast growth factor (bFGF),[52] loss of cell adhesion and the acquisition of a rounded shape,[56] and LPS.[57]

In 1991, Zheng and colleagues[46] reported that exATP caused apoptosis of lymphocytes, a process associated with increased Ca^{2+} influx and prevented by coincubation with cycloheximide. Adenosine, a product of ectonucleotidase hydrolysis of exATP, caused apoptosis of HL-60 cells[58] and T lymphocytes.[59]

The authors assessed the effects of extracellular ATP on endothelial cell apoptosis and found that extracellular ATP, in concentrations similar to those feasible under pathophysiological conditions in vivo, caused apoptosis of cultured pulmonary artery endothelial cells. Apoptosis was assessed by the formation of DNA fragments characteristic of endonuclease activity, by use of agarose gel electrophoresis of DNA extracted from pulmonary artery endothelial cells incubated with ATP. In other studies they found that 24 hours of incubation with ATP and adenosine caused release of soluble DNA and morphological changes characteristic of apoptosis.[60] Thus, extracellular ATP and adenosine cause apoptosis of pulmonary endothelial cells. This effect of extracellular nucleotides may be important in the perpetuation of endothelial cell injury and increased permeability pulmonary edema.

Summary

Extracellular purine and pyrimidine nucleotides are released under conditions of cell lysis and are capable of interacting with endothelial cells via purinoceptor mediated actions. Nucleotide-induced enhancement of PMN adhesion to endothelial cells is an example of purinoceptor-mediated action. In addition, endothelial cells are capable of hydrolysis, uptake, and intracellular metabolism of extracellular nucleotides. Agents capable of causing endothelial cell injury, such as endotoxin, can modulate nucleotide hydrolysis and metabolism. Finally, extracellular ATP and adenosine can cause direct endothelial cell injury by the process of "programmed cell death" or apoptosis.

Acknowledgements   We thank our collaborators, Drs. Alice Bonitati, Kailash Agarwal, James Wyche, and Devasis Chatterjee, for their important contributions to these studies. The authors thank Nancy Parks, Jean McGowan-Jordan, Steven Bullard, Lily Hsieh, and Soneath Pond for excellent technical assistance. We also thank Boehringer-Ingelheim, Merck, and Centocor for the contribution of reagents used in these studies.

References

1. Fowler AA, Hammon RF, Good JT, et al. Adult respiratory distress syndrome: Risks and common predispositions. *Ann Intern Med* 1983;98: 593–597.
2. Tate RM, Repine JE. Neutrophils and the adult respiratory distress syndrome. *Am Rev Respir Dis* 1983;128:552–559.
3. Meyrick BP, Brigham KL. The effects of a single infusion of zymosan-activated plasma on the pulmonary microcirculation of sheep. *Am J Pathol* 1984;114:32–45.
4. Farber HW, Weller PF, Rounds S, et al. Generation of lipid neutrophil chemoattractant activity by histamine-stimulated cultured endothelial cells. *J Immunol* 1986;137:2918–2924.
5. Farber HW, Center DM, Rounds S. Effect of ambient oxygen on cultured endothelial cells from different vascular beds. *Am J Physiol* 1987;253: H878–H883.
6. Render ML, Rounds S. Studies on the mechanism of decreased polymorphonuclear neutrophil adherence to post-confluent cultured endothelial cells. *Am Rev Respir Dis* 1988;138:1115–1123.
7. Born GVR, Kratzer MAA. Source and concentration of extracellular adenosine triphosphate during haemostasis in rats, rabbits and man. *J Physiol (Lond)* 1984;354:419–429.
8. Gordon JL. Extracellular ATP: Effects, sources and fate. *Biochem J* 1986;233: 309–319.
9. Dubyak GR, El-Moatassim C. Signal transduction via P_2-purinergic receptors for extracellular ATP and other nucleotides. *Am J Physiol* 1993;265: C577-C606.
10. Bonitati AE, Agarwal KC, Rounds S. A simple assay for ecto-5'-nucleotidase using intact pulmonary artery endothelial cells: Effect of endotoxin-induced cell injury. *Biochem Pharmacol* 1993;46:1467–1473.
11. Gordon EL, Pearson JD, Slakey LL. The hydrolysis of extracellular adenine nucleotides by cultured endothelial cells from pig aorta: Feed-forward inhibition of adenosine production at the cell surface. *J Biol Chem* 1986;261:15496–15504.
12. Dahlquist R, Diamant B. Interaction of ATP and calcium on the rat mast cell: Effect on histamine release. *Acta Pharmacol et Toxicol* 1974;34:368–384.
13. Fredholm BB, Abbracchio MP, Burnstock G, et al. VI. Nomenclature and classification of purinoceptors. *Pharmacol Rev* 1994;46:143–156.
14. Pirotton S, Motte S, Côte S, Boeynaems J-M. Control of endothelial function by nucleotides: Multiple receptors and transduction mechanisms. *Cell Signal* 1993;5:1–8.
15. Kuhns DB, Wright DG, Nath J, et al. ATP induces transient elevations of $[Ca^{2+}]_i$ in human neutrophils and primes these cells for enhanced O_2- generation. *Lab Invest* 1988;58:448–453.
16. Walker BAM, Hagenlocker BE, Douglas VK, Tarapchak SJ, Ward PA. Nucleotide responses of human neutrophils. *Lab Invest* 1991;64:105–112.
17. Ford-Hutchinson AW. Aggregation of rat neutrophils by nucleotide triphosphates. *Br J Pharmacol* 1982;76:367–371.
18. Freyer DR, Boxer LA, Axtell RA, Todd RF III. Stimulation of human neutrophil adhesive properties by adenine nucleotides. *J Immunol* 1988;141: 580–586.
19. Cockcroft S, Stutchfield J. ATP stimulates secretion in human neutrophils

and HL60 cells via a pertussis toxin-sensitive guanine nucleotide-binding protein coupled to phospholipase C. *FEBS Lett* 1989;245:25–29.

20. Wenzel-Seifert K, Seifert R. Nucleotide-, chemotactic peptide- and phorbol ester-induced exocytosis in HL-60 leukemic cells. *Immunobiology* 1990; 181:298–316.

21. Motte S, Pirotton S, Boeynaems JM. Evidence that a form of ATP uncomplexed with divalent cations is the ligand of P2y and nucleotide P2u receptors on aortic endothelial cells. *Br J Pharmacol* 1993;109:967–971.

22. Yu GH, Ward PA. Structural requirements for binding of adenosine-5'-O-(3-thiotriphosphate) (ATPγS) to human neutrophils. *Immunopharmacology* 1990;20:175–182.

23. Saribas AS, Lustig KD, Zhang X, Weisman GA. Extracellular ATP reversibly increases the plasma membrane permeability of transformed mouse fibroblasts to large macromolecules. *Anal Biochem* 1993;209:45–52.

24. Cockcroft S, Gomperts BD. The ATP^{-4} receptor of rat mast cells. *Biochem J* 1980;188:789–798.

25. Steinberg TH, Newman AS, Swanson JA, Silverstein SC. ATP permeabilizes the plasma membrane of mouse macrophages to fluorescent dyes. *J Biol Chem* 1987;262:8884–8888.

26. Dawicki DD, McGowan-Jordan J, Bullard S, et al. Extracellular nucleotides stimulate leukocyte adherence to cultured pulmonary artery endothelial cells. *Am J Physiol* 1995;268:L666-L673.

27. Zimmerman GA, Prescott SM, McIntyre TM. Endothelial cell interaction with granulocytes: Tethering and signaling molecules. *Immunol Today* 1992;13:93–100.

28. Lorant DE, Patel KD, McIntyre TM, et al. Coexpression of GMP-140 and PAF by endothelium stimulated by histamine or thrombin: A juxtacrine system for adhesion and activation of neutrophils. *J Cell Biol* 1991;115: 223–234.

29. Bevilacqua MP, Pober JS, Wheeler ME, et al. Interleukin 1 acts on cultured human vascular endothelium to increase the adhesion of polymorphonuclear leukocytes, monocytes and related leukocyte lines. *J Clin Invest* 1985;76:2003–2011.

30. Bevilacqua MP, Pober JS, Mendrick DS, et al. Identification of an inducible endothelial-leukocyte adhesion molecule. *Proc Natl Acad Sci U S A* 1987; 84:9238–9242.

31. Pohlman TH, Stanness KH, Beatty PG, et al. An endothelial cell surface factor(s) induced in vitro by lipopolysaccharide, interleukin 1, and tumor necrosis factor-α increases neutrophil adherence by CD_w18-dependent mechanism. *J Immunol* 1986;136:4548–4553.

32. Parker AL, Likar LL, Dawicki DD, Rounds S. Mechanism of ATP-induced leukocyte adherence to cultured pulmonary artery endothelial cells. *Am J Physiol* 1996;270:L695-L703.

33. McIntyre TM, Zimmerman GA, Satoh K, Prescott SM. Cultured endothelial cells synthesize both platelet-activating factor and prostacyclin in response to histamine, bradykinin, and adenosine triphosphate. *J Clin Invest* 1985;76:271–180.

34. Honda Z, Nakamura M, Miki I, et al. Cloning by functional expression of platelet-activating factor receptor from guinea pig lung. *Nature (Lond)* 1991;349:342–346.

35. Zimmerman GA, McIntyre TM, Mehra M, Prescott SM. Endothelial cell-associated platelet-activating factor: A novel mechanism for signaling intercellular adhesion. *J Cell Biol* 1990;110:529–540.

36. Smith CW, Marlin SD, Rothlein R, et al. Cooperative interactions of LFA-1 and Mac-1 with intercellular adhesion molecule-1 in facilitating adherence and transendothelial migration of human neutrophils in vitro. *J Clin Invest* 1989;83:2008–2017.

37. Sellak H, Franzini E, Hakim J, Pasquire C. Reactive oxygen species rapidly increase endothelial ICAM-1 ability to bind neutrophils without detectable upregulation. *Blood* 1994;83: 2669–2677.

38. Dawicki DD, Agarwal K, Parks RE. Role of adenosine uptake and metabolism by blood cells in the antiplatelet actions of dipyridamole, dilazep, and nitrobenzylthioinosine. *Biochem Pharmacol* 1986;34:3965–3972.

39. Rounds S, Hsieh L, Agarwal KC. Effects of endotoxin injury on endothelial cell adenosine metabolism. *J Lab Clin Med* 1994;123:309–317.

40. Ueland PM. Pharmacological and biochemical aspects of S-adenosylhomocysteine and S-adenosylhomocysteine hydrolase. *Pharmacol Rev* 1982; 34:223–253.

41. O'Brien RF, Makarski JS, Rounds S. Studies on the mechanism of decreased angiotensin I conversion in rat lungs injured with alpha-naphthylthiourea. *Exp Lung Res* 1985;8:243–259.

42. Steinberg TH, DiVirgilio F. Cell-mediated cytotoxicity: ATP as an effector and the role of target cells. *Curr Opin Immunol* 1991;3:71–75.

43. Pizzo P, Zanovello P, Bronte V, DiVirgilio F. Extracellular ATP causes lysis of mouse thymocytes and activates a plasma ion channel. *Biochem J* 1991;274:139–144.

44. Tinton SA, Lefebvre VH, Cousin OC, Buc-Calderon PM. Cytolytic effects and biochemical changes induced by extracellular ATP to isolated hepatocytes. *Biochim Biophys Acta* 1993;1176:1–6.

45. Surprenant A, Rassendren F, Kawashima E, et al. The cytolytic P2Z receptor for extracellular ATP identified as a P2x receptor (P2X$_7$). *Science* 1996;272:735–738.

46. Zheng LM, Zychlinsky A, Liu C-C, et al. Extracellular ATP as a trigger for apoptosis or programmed cell death. *J Cell Biol* 1991;112:279–288.

47. Beyer EC, Steinberg TH. Evidence that the gap junction protein connexin-43 is the ATP-induced pore of mouse macrophages. *J Biol Chem* 1991; 266:7971–7974.

48. Polunovsky VA, Chen B, Henke C, et al. Role of mesenchymal cell death in lung remodelling after injury. *J Clin Invest* 1993;92:388–397.

49. Schwartzman RA, Cidlowski JA. Apoptosis: The biochemistry and molecular biology of programmed cell death. *Endocr Rev* 1993;14:133–151.

50. Steller H. Mechanisms and genes of cellular suicide. *Science* 1995;267: 1445–1449.

51. Thompson CB. Apoptosis in the pathogenesis and treatment of disease. *Science* 1995;267:1456–1462.

52. Kondo S, Yin D, Aoki T, et al. bcl-2 Gene prevents apoptosis of basic fibroblast growth factor-deprived murine aortic endothelial cells. *Exp Cell Res* 1994;213:428–432.

53. Polunovsky VA, Wendt CH, Ingbar DH, et al. Induction of endothelial cell apoptosis by TNFα: Modulation by inhibitors of protein synthesis. *Exp Cell Res* 1994;214:584–594.

54. Araki S, Ishida T, Yamamoto T, et al. Induction of apoptosis by hemorrhagic snake venom in vascular endothelial cells. *Biochem Biophys Res Commun* 1993;190:148–153.

55. Lenfant C. Task force on research in cardiopulmonary dysfunction in critical care medicine. *Am J Respir Crit Care Med* 1995;151:243–248.

Chapter 22

Promotion of Regeneration and Repair After Acute Lung Injury

Peter B. Bitterman, MD and
Vitaly Polunovsky, PhD

Introduction

Following acute diffuse lung injury from any cause, microvascular and alveolar damage results in intravascular and intra-alveolar coagulation. Among the structural changes observed as lung repair ensues, is a large-scale relocation and expansion of the mesenchymal cell population. In the microcirculation, there is an increase in circulatory resistance due to muscularization of nonmuscular vessels, and an increased wall thickness in already muscularized vessels. In the alveolar airspace, shunt results as myofibroblast egress from the interstitium into the airspace leads to effacement of the gas exchange surface. Central to effective repair is regression of these mesenchymal cell changes coordinated with reendothelialization of the blood-lung interface and reepithelialization of the air-lung interface. When patients die with acute lung injury, elimination of excess mesenchymal cells does not occur; this fact focuses attention on the molecular regulation of mesenchymal cell viability as a potential determinant of patient survival. This chapter reviews selected aspects of viability regulation, with focus on the role of translational control in fibroblast apoptosis.

This work was supported by the following grant: National Institutes of Health (NIH)SCOR in Acute Lung Injury 1P50 HL 50152.

Apoptosis and the Regulation
of Cell Population Size

Physiological control of cell population size in multicellular organisms represents a balance between proliferation, quiescence, and death. During ontogeny and tissue repair, only selected cells survive to constitute the cellular pool in tissues and organs.[1,2] Most animal cells are capable of undergoing apoptosis, an intrinsic latent suicide program which triggers a characteristic set of metabolic and morphological alterations.[3-5] This highly conserved process not only leads to removal of defective and damaged cells, but also eliminates healthy cells in order to maintain tissue homeostasis. Substantial evidence now exists that proliferating cells in somatic tissue exhibit appreciable apoptosis during normal development and in the process of regeneration following injury, suggesting that cell death may be intimately linked to cell cycle transit.

This chapter presents potential mechanisms that couple cell proliferation and survival in mammalian fibroblasts in an effort to understand the control of fibroblast population size in fibroproliferative lung disorders (reviewed in Reference 6). The authors have previously implicated fibroblast apoptosis in the fibroproliferative response following acute lung injury.[7] They have also demonstrated that manipulation of the rate of protein synthesis can change the dynamic balance between positive and negative regulators of apoptosis.[8] Based on their data and an extensive body of knowledge about the relationship between cell cycle events and the regulation of programmed cell death, the authors propose that translational control might be involved in coupling cell cycle transit to survival in mammalian fibroblasts. To examine this possibility, they have modulated the rate-limiting protein in this process, eukaryotic initiation factor 4E (eIF4E), which is known to selectively influence regulators of cell cycle transit such as Ras and cyclin D1. Data are presented which indicates that eIF4E strongly promotes fibroblast survival.[9]

Overview of Selected Aspects of
Cell Cycle Transit Control

Coupling of extracellular proliferative signaling with the cell cycle engine is accomplished by an integrated system of cyclins, partner kinases, and kinase inhibitors that regulate critical accelerators and brakes of cell cycle transit. The cell cycle includes three tightly regulated transitions: R-point (start) transition, interphase-prophase transition, and metaphase-anaphase transition.[10–12] Unlike the second two transitions, which are autonomously controlled, R-point transit is dependent on external inputs from growth factors and extracellular matrix. The genes directly involved in the proliferative response can be grouped based on their temporal pattern of expression. The first group of genes is activated by growth factors and is responsible for transition through the R-point to autonomous cycling. This group includes a set of genes for transcription factors (eg, Myc, Jun, and the E2F family), as well as genes encoding D-type cyclins. The D-type cyclins assemble with partner kinases, Cdk4 and Cdk6, to form functional holoenzymes which hyperphosphorylate the retinoblastoma protein (Rb). This decreases the affinity of Rb for E2F, freeing up this transcription factor to activate genes whose products are necessary for S-phase entry.[13,14] A second major group of genes encodes proteins that control the transition through cell cycle checkpoints, DNA synthesis, and mitosis. This class of regulatory molecules includes cyclin E and cyclin A, which partner with Cdk2 to control S-phase entry and the S-phase transition, respectively. The Cdk member Cdc2 is mainly associated with B-type cyclins, and regulates the M-phase transition. The third group of genes encodes products that are required for DNA replication and mitosis.

Cyclin/Cdk complexes are negatively regulated by inhibitors that can bind to Cdk and suppress their kinase activity (reviewed in References 13, 15–17). Two families of Cdk inhibitors have been identified based on sequence similarities and mode of action. The Ink family of inhibitors includes p16^{Ink4A} (p16) and three related peptides: p15^{Ink4B} (p15), p18^{Ink4C} (p18), and p19^{Ink4D} (p19). A hallmark of this family is their binding specificity to monomeric Cdk4 and Cdk6, which prevents partnering with cyclin D. The second family of inhibitors, termed the "p21 family," includes three gene products: p21, p27, and p57. Unlike the Ink4s, p21 family members have a higher affinity for cyclin/Cdk complexes than to monomeric Cdk subunits, and they inhibit the activity of these complexes. The expression of p21 is induced in cells overexpressing p53 in response to DNA damage, in senescent cells, and in some terminally differentiated cells. p27 can inhibit the activity of cyclin D-, cyclin E-, and cyclin A-dependent kinases. In quiescent cells up through mid G_1, p27 is present in excess and inactivates cyclin-Cdk complexes. When cells approach the R-point in the latter portion of G_1, p27 drops in concert with translational activation of cyclin D-dependent kinases, followed by activation of kinases associated with cyclin E and cyclin A. Activation of cyclin biosynthesis by growth factors such as platelet-derived growth factor (PDGF) or basic fibroblast growth factor (bFGF) is not a sufficient condition to enter S phase. Other growth factors, such as (insulin-like growth factor-1 (IGF-1), are required to eliminate p27 and permit DNA synthesis to begin.

Summary

Cell cycle transit is driven by growth factor-activated positive regulators including specific transcription factors and cyclin/Cdk complexes. Together with a defined set of negative regulators including Cdk inhibitors and Rb, they provide an effective mechanism for cell cycle control by extracellular signals. Pertinent to the thesis of this chapter, a number of the participants in proliferative pathways not only regulate cycle transit but also regulate viability. It is this group of effectors, participating in both the proliferative and apoptotic pathways, that is suspected to provide clues to how physiological coupling of proliferation and viability is achieved.

Cell Cycle Transit Is Potentially Lethal

Apoptotic pathways may be activated each time a cell emerges from quiescence. The following are five lines of evidence to support this idea: (1) Cells committed to apoptotic death display functions that are also typical of early cell cycle traverse including transitory expression of the early G_1 proteins c-Myc, c-Fos, c-Jun, and Cdc2.[18] (2) Cell death can result from a relaxation of negative control at the G_1 restriction point (R-point). The retinoblastoma gene (*rb*) product p105 (Rb protein) is a negative regulator of the R-point transition that also functions to inhibit apoptosis.[19,20] Studies of knockout mice indicate that genetic inactivation of *rb* leads to inappropriate cell proliferation *and* massive apoptosis.[21] (3) Growth factors and oncogene products that promote proliferation can also promote apoptotic death. For example, rodent fibroblasts stimulated by PDGF require a second survival signal from IGF-1 for progression through the cell cycle. In the absence of survival signaling by IGF-1, cells stimulated by PDGF undergo apoptosis.[22] Upregulated expression of certain cell cycle drivers such as c-Myc,[23,24] E2F,[21,25,26] and cyclin A[27,28] can override the growth-suppressive effect of the Rb protein, as well as other inhibitors, and activate both cell cycle transit and apoptosis. Even physiological levels of c-Myc which promote cell cycle transit in untransformed fibroblasts can induce apoptosis.[29] (4) Cells forced to proliferate die when transit through specific cell cycle checkpoints is blocked. Most cytostatic agents that increase the sensitivity of proliferating cells to apoptosis also induce cell cycle arrest as part of the cell cycle checkpoint response to DNA damage.[24] Typically, transition through these checkpoints is negatively regulated by expression of the tumor suppressor protein p53 (reviewed in Reference 30). Overexpression of p53 mimics the effect of cytostatic agents in that it arrests cell cycle transit in normal cells and induces apoptosis in cells driven by upregulated cell cycle promoters such as c-Myc.[31,32] (5) In vivo, apoptosis is detected primarily during periods of rapid cell proliferation in developing or repairing tissues (reviewed in References 33–35).

Summary

The available experimental data support the idea that cell cycle transit is a potentially lethal condition unless specific environmental signals prevent this fate. Cell death signaling apparently results when there are conflicting signals from negative and positive cell cycle regulators, and thus cells with aberrant growth control are eliminated. Growth factors play a dual role in the regulation of apoptosis. They activate cell cycle reactions that can stimulate the apoptotic pathway while somehow protecting proliferating cells against the execution of this pathway. The extracellular environment therefore must coordinately activate metabolic pathways directing both proliferation and survival in order to result in cell division cycle transit without death. While recent advances in the understanding of the cell division cycle reveal how cells integrate proliferative signals with the cell cycle machinery, the molecular mechanisms and regulatory pathways that mediate growth factor survival signaling remain uncertain.

Evidence That Translational Control May Represent a Key Nodal Point in the Regulation of Proliferation and Cell Survival

The authors' previous studies of apoptotic death under conditions of inhibited translation,[8] along with numerous other observations,[36–38] indicate that blockade of translation can result in apoptosis as well as augment the effect of extracellular signals inducing apoptosis. These observations suggest that apoptotic effectors must already be present in cells, and that de novo protein synthesis is required to escape apoptotic death. Thus, many somatic cells appear to have a dual requirement to suppress apoptosis: the presence of survival signals in the extracellular milieu, and active protein synthesis to produce intracellular inhibitors of apoptosis. In some cases, survival factors can suppress apoptosis downstream of translational control. Analysis of Myc-induced apoptosis in fibroblasts indicates that IGF-1, but not PDGF, blocks Myc-induced apoptosis in the presence of cycloheximide.[39] In contrast to PDGF, IGF-1 does not directly activate cell cycle transit in fibroblasts (reviewed in reference 40). These data can be interpreted as evidence that the antiapoptotic effect of some survival cytokines can be exerted at a post-translational level, whereas other cytokines require de novo protein synthesis to stimulate cell cycle progression and suppress apoptosis. While it is of established importance in regulating cell proliferation (reviewed in References 41, 42), little has been done to examine the role of the translational apparatus in cell survival, which may provide a link between cell cycle transit and survival signaling.

An attractive candidate for coupling cytokine-induced survival signaling with cell cycle reactions is eukaryotic translation initiation factor 4E (eIF4E). An increased rate of mRNA translation is an essential component of the proliferative response (reviewed in Reference 43). Translation of all capped eukaryotic mRNA is tightly regulated by the assembly of the initiation complex. The rate-limiting step of translation initiation is transfer of the mRNA to the 40S ribosomal subunit, an event mediated by the cap-binding protein, eIF4E.[43,44] Growth factors stimulate eIF4E production through a Myc-mediated transcriptional mechanism,[45] and also activate phosphorylation events that are essential for the translation-promoting function of eIF4E. These events include growth factor-dependent phosphorylation of both eIF4E[46-48] and its inhibitory binding protein 4E-BP1.[49-52] These modifications reduce the affinity of 4E-BP1 for eIF4E, thus enabling eIF4E to activate translation.[50] Although required for translation of all capped mRNA, increased expression of eIF4E leads to a relatively selective increase in translation of mRNA species that direct production of cell cycle-related proteins and are typically downregulated in quiescent cells.[43,53] Enforced overexpression of eIF4E results in selective enhancement of key regulators of cell cycle progression including ornithine decarboxylase,[54] Ras,[55] and cyclin D1.[45,56] As a result, overexpression of eIF4E decreases the growth factor requirement for cell cycle progression and mimics the ability of growth factors to stimulate cell proliferation[57] as well as morphogenesis.[58] In addition, enhanced expression of eIF4E in established or primary fibroblasts causes malignant transformation.[59,60] Taken together with studies that document the ability of eIF4E to interdict apoptosis in growth factor-restricted fibroblasts,[9] these findings place eIF4E at a strategic nodal point in growth factor signaling pathways, influencing both proliferation and survival.

Experimental Approaches to Examining Translational Control as the Link Between Cell Cycling and Survival

Myc-Induced Apoptosis

The authors have chosen to examine cell survival during proliferation, beginning with Myc-induced fibroblast apoptosis under growth-restricting conditions as the model system because it affords several experimental advantages. One advantage of this model is that the role of c-Myc as an essential regulator of gene transcription, cell cycle progression, differentiation, survival, and malignancy has been extensively studied. A second advantage is that more information is available about the biological effects of Myc than about any other inducer of cell cycle-dependent apoptosis (reviewed in References 39, 61, 62). A third advantage is the ready availability of different vectors conditionally or constitutively expressing either c-Myc or v-Myc.

Model Depicting The Hypothesis

Growth factors activate both Myc- and eIF4E-dependent signaling pathways. Myc has a dual function, promoting cell cycle transit under growth-promoting conditions or promoting apoptosis under growth-restricting conditions. When cell cycle arrest is signaled by the environment, normal cells downregulate Myc along with many other growth promoters. This renders the Myc-induced cell growth/death pathways inactive. As a result, normal cells become quiescent but remain viable. In contrast, cells constitutively expressing Myc (or most other strong growth-promoting signals) overcome growth arrest, cycle, and die under the same conditions. Thus, a dynamic balance between intracellular negative and positive regulators determines whether a cell divides, rests, or dies. The authors suggest that growth factors trigger an eIF4E-mediated salvage pathway to protect cells from apoptotic death in the course of normal cell cycle control. Their model predicts that there will be one or more downstream effectors of the salvage pathway whose rate of translation is *selectively* activated by eIF4E. One candidate downstream effector that is translationally activated by eIF4E is cyclin D1.[45,56] Association of cyclin D1 and cell cycle inhibitor p27 leads to sequestration of p27.[63] At least in some experimental systems, D-type cyclins are activated during suppression of apoptosis,[64] and they inhibit Myc-induced apoptosis.[65]

Data Summary

A recently published manuscript by Polunovsky et al[9] serves as the principle source of data for this chapter. This manuscript is summarized here, and supplemented with preliminary unpublished experiments. In these studies, using molecular and pharmacological tools, the authors manipulated the level and activity of eIF4E in cells forced to cycle by deregulated Myc or Ras under growth-restricted conditions. They found a direct relationship between viability and eIF4E. They also evaluated the relative abundance of cyclin D1, a candidate downstream effector, and its potentially pro-apoptotic binding partner, p27. They found that when Myc is deregulated and apoptosis is induced by subjecting cells to growth-restricted conditions, p27 is present in excess of cyclin D1, leaving it free to form pro-apoptotic complexes with other potential binding partners. Rescue of these cells by overexpression of eIF4E is accompanied by a complete change in the relationship between cyclin D1 and p27. Then the physiological pattern observed during normal G1 transit, in which all p27 is bound to cyclin D1 making it unavailable to potential pro-apoptotic binding partners, is observed. Excess cyclin D1 is free to partner with kinases that drive the G_1/S transition (ie, Cdk4 and Cdk6).

Speculation

The rate of progression through G1 is thought to be determined by an interplay between positive (cyclins) and negative (Cdk inhibitors) cell cycle regulators. The available data in fibroblasts favor a model in which adjustable levels of cyclin D1 and Cdk inhibitors determine whether that threshold level of Cdk4 activity necessary for G1 progression will be reached.[16,17,63] Data indicates that G1 blockers are the most potent inducers of apoptosis in REF/Myc cells. In addition, cyclin

A and cyclin A-dependent kinases are essential for Myc-induced apoptosis.[27,66] Based on this, the authors suggest that lovastatin and other G1 blockers, in combination with upregulated Myc, might stimulate expression of conflicting signals that trigger the apoptotic pathway: cyclin A, which leads to cell cycle progression, and Cdk inhibitors signaling G1 arrest. One candidate Cdk inhibitor is p27[KIP1] (p27), which is unique among the Cdk inhibitors in that it is activated by lovastatin and required for inhibition of both D-type and cyclin A-dependent Cdk.[17] An increase in p27 is implicated in G1 arrest caused by a wide variety of cytostatic agents.[17] The level of p27 is inversely related to the level of cyclin A/Cdk2 in the cell cycle, being high in early G1 and decreasing in late G1/early S phase when cyclin A-associated kinase activity increases.[67,68] One model for the role of p27 in cycle transit is that it acts to inhibit both G1 and S/G2 cyclin-Cdk complexes.[16,17] The accumulation of cyclin D1 and cyclin D/Cdk4 in early G1 sequesters p27,[64] facilitating the formation of active cyclin E/Cdk2 and cyclin A/Cdk2 complexes free of p27. This leads to transit of late G1 and S phase. Therefore, the authors speculate that Myc-induced apoptosis results from at least two conflicting signals that normally do not occur simultaneously during physiological cycle transit: (a) upregulation of cyclin A by Myc, and (b) an abundance of free (ie, unpartnered) p27 induced by cytostatic signals. They further speculate that eIF4E rescues such cells by activating cyclin D1 expression. Associated with its partner Cdk in G1, cyclin D1 could sequester excess p27 and eliminate the conflict.

References

1. Wyllie AH. Apoptosis (The 1992 Frank Rose Memorial Lecture). *Br J Cancer* 1993;67:205–208.
2. Bellamy COC, Malcomson RDG, Harrison DJ, Wyllie AH. Cell death in health and disease: The biology and regulation of apoptosis. *Cancer Biol* 1995;6:3–16.
3. Kerr JF, Wyllie AH, Currie AR. Apoptosis: A basic biological phenomenon with wide-ranging implications in tissue kinetics. *Br J Cancer* 1972;26: 239–257.
4. Wyllie AH. Cell death. *Int Rev Cytol* 1987;17:S755–S785.
5. Steller H. Mechanisms and genes of cellular suicide. *Science* 1995;267: 1445–1449.
6. Polunovsky VA, Bitterman PB. Regulation of cell population size. In: Crystal RG, West JB, Weibel ER, Barnes PJ (eds): *The Lung: Scientific Foundations (2nd ed)*. New York: Lippincott-Raven; 1997;133–153.
7. Polunovsky VA, Chen B, Henke C, et al. Role of mesenchymal cell death in lung remodeling following injury. *J Clin Invest* 1993;92:388–397.
8. Polunovsky VA, Wendt CH, Ingbar DH, Bitterman P. Induction of endothelial cell apoptosis by TNFa. *Exp Cell Res* 1994;214:584–594.
9. Polunovsky VA, Rosenwald IB, Tan A, et al. Translational control of pro-

grammed cell death: Factor eIF4E blocks apoptosis in growth factor re-stricted fibroblasts with physiologically regulated or deregulated Myc. *Mol Cell Biol* 1996;16:6573–6581.

10. Pardee AB. G1 events and regulation of cell proliferation. *Science* 1989;246: 603–608.

11. Hartwell LH, Weinert T. Checkpoints: Controls that ensure the order of cell cycle events. Science 1989;246:629–634.

12. Zetterberg A, Larson O, Wiman KG. What is the restriction point? *Curr Opin Cell Biol* 1995;7:835–842.

13. Hunter T, Pines J. Cyclins and cancer II: Cyclin D and CDK inhibitors come of age. *Cell* 1994;79:573–582.

14. Reed SI, Bailly E, Dulic V, Hengst L, Resnitzky D, Slingerland J. G1 con-trol in mammalian cells. *J Cell Sci* 1994;18:69–73.

15. Lees E. Cyclin dependent kinase regulation. *Curr Opin Cell Biol* 1995;7: 773–780.

16. Massague J, Polyak K. Mammalian antiproliferative signals and their tar-gets. *Curr Opin Genet Dev* 1995;5:91–96.

17. Sherr CJ, Roberts JM. Inhibitors of mammalian G1 cyclin-dependent ki-nases. *Genes Dev* 1995;9:1149–1163.

18. Pandey S, Wang E. Cells en route to apoptosis are characterized by the up-regulation of c-fos, c-Myc, c-jun, cdc2, and RB phosphorylation, resem-bling events of early cell-cycle traverse. *J Cell Biochem* 1995;58:135–150.

19. Haupt Y, Rowan S, Oren M. p53-mediated apoptosis in HeLa cells can be overcome by excess pRB. *Oncogene* 1995;10:1563–1571.

20. Slack RS, Skerjanc IS, Lach B, Craig J, Jardine K, McBurney MW. Cells dif-ferentiating into neuroectoderm undergo apoptosis in the absence of functional retinoblastoma family proteins. *J Cell Biol* 1995;129:779–788.

21. Almasan A, Yin YX, Kelly RE, et al. Deficiency of retinoblastoma protein leads to inappropriate S-phase entry, activation of E2F-responsive genes, and apoptosis. *Proc Natl Acad Sci U S A* 1995;92:5436–5440.

22. Kim HRC, Upadhyay S, Li G, Palmer KC, Deuel TF. Platelet-derived growth factor induces apoptosis in growth-arrested murine fibroblasts. *Proc Natl Acad Sci U S A* 1995;92:9500–9504.

23. Askew DS, Ashmun RA, Simmons BC, Cleveland JL. Constitutive c-myc expression in an IL-3-dependent myeloid cell line suppresses cell cycle ar-rest and accelerates apoptosis. *Oncogene* 1991;6:1915–1922.

24. Evan GI, Wyllie AH, Gilbert C, et al. Induction of apoptosis in fibroblasts by c-myc protein. *Cell* 1992;69:119–128.

25. Wu X, Levine AJ. p53 and E2F-1 cooperate to mediate apoptosis. *Proc Natl Acad Sci U S A* 1994;91:3602–3606.

26. Hiebert SW, Packham G, Strom DK, et al. E2F-1:DP-1 induces p53 and overrides survival factors to trigger apoptosis. *Mol Cell Biol* 1995;15:6864–6874.

27. Hoang AT, Cohen KJ, Barrett JF, Bergstrom DA, Dang VC. Participation of cyclin A in Myc-induced apoptosis. *Proc Natl Acad Sci U S A* 1994;91: 6875–6879.

28. Meikrantz W, Gisselbrecht S, Tam SW, Schlegel R. Activation of cyclin A-dependent protein kinases during apoptosis. *Proc Natl Acad Sci U S A* 1994;91:3754–3758.

29. Bennet MR, Evan GI, Schwartz SM. Apoptosis of rat vascular smooth muscle cells is regulated by p53-dependent and -independent pathways. *Circ Res* 1995;77:266–273.

30. Hartwell LH, Kastan MB. Cell cycle control and cancer. *Science* 1994;266: 1821–1828.
31. Canman CE, Kastan MB. Induction of apoptosis by tumor suppressor genes and oncogenes. *Cancer Biol* 1995;6:17–25.
32. Elledge RM, Lee WH. Life and death by p53. *Bioessays* 1995;17:923–930.
33. Raff MC. Social controls on cell survival and cell death. *Nature* 1992;356: 397–400.
34. Wyllie AH. Apoptosis and the regulation of cell numbers in normal and neoplastic tissues: An overview. *Cancer Metastasis Rev* 1992;11:95–103.
35. Wyllie AH. The genetic regulation of apoptosis. *Curr Opin Genet Dev* 1995;5:97–104.
36. Martin SJ, Lennon SV, Bonham AM, Cotter TG. Induction of apoptosis (programmed cell death) in human leukemic HL-60 cells by inhibition of RNA or protein synthesis. *J Immunol* 1990;1859–1867.
37. Ledda-Columbano GM, Coni P, Faa G, Manenti G, Columbano A. Rapid induction of apoptosis in rat liver by cycloheximide. *Am J Pathol* 1992;140: 545–549.
38. Gong J, Li X, Darzynkiewicz Z. Different patterns of apoptosis of HL-60 cells induced by cycloheximide and camptothecin. *J Cell Physiol* 1993;157: 263–270.
39. Harrington EA, Bennett MR, Fanidi A, Evan GI. c-Myc-induced apoptosis in fibroblasts is inhibited by specific cytokines. *EMBO J* 1994;13:3286–3295.
40. Baserga R. The insulin-like growth factor I receptor: A key to tumor growth? *Cancer Res* 1995;55:249–252.
41. Brooks RF. Continuous protein synthesis is required to maintain the probability of entry into S phase. *Cell* 1977;12:311–317.
42. Mader S, Sonenberg N. Cap binding complexes and cellular growth control. *Biochimie* 1994;77:40–44.
43. Sonenberg N. mRNA 5′ cap binding protein eLF4E and control of cell growth. In: Hershey JW, Matthews MB, Sonenberg N (eds): *Translational Control.* Cold Spring Harbor, NY: Cold Spring Harbor Laboratory Press; 1996;245–269.
44. Hernanedes G, Sierra JM. Translation initiation factor eIF4E from drosophila-cDNA sequence and expression of the gene. *Biochim Biophys Acta* 1995;1261:427–431.
45. Rosenwald IB, Rhoads DB, Callanan LD, Isselbacher KJ, Schmidt EV. Increased expression of eukaryotic translation initiation factors e1F-4E and e1F-2a in response to growth induction by c-myc. *Proc Natl Acad Sci U S A* 1993;90:6175–6178.
46. Frederickson RM, Montine KS, Sonenberg N. Phosphorylation of eukaryotic translation initiation factor 4E is increased in Src-transformed cell lines. *Mol Cell Biol* 1991;11:2896–2900.
47. Joshi B, Cai A-L, Keiper BD, et al. Phosphorylation of eukaryotic protein synthesis initiation factor 4E at Ser-209. *J Biol Chem* 1995;270:14597–14603.
48. Zhang Y, Klein HL, Schneider RJ. Role of Ser-53 phosphorylation in the activity of human translation initiation factor eIF4E in mammalian and yeast cells. *Gene* 1991;163:283–288.
49. Pause A, Belsham GJ, Gingras A-C, et al. Insulin-dependent stimulation of protein synthesis by phosphorylation of a regulator of 5′-cap function. *Nature* 1994;371:762–767.
50. Lin T-A, Kong X, Haystead TAJ, et al. PHAS-1 as a link between mitogen-

activated protein kinase and translation initiation. *Science* 1994;266: 653–656.

51. Hagstead TAJ, Haystead CMM, Hu C, Lin T-A, Lawrence JC Jr. Phosphorylation of PHAS-1 by mitogen-activated protein (MAP) kinase. *J Biol Chem* 1994;269:23185–23191.

52. Graves LE, Bornfeldt KE, Argast GM, et al. cAMP-and rapamycin-sensitive regulation of the association of eukaryotic initiation factor 4E and the translational regulator PHAS-1 in aortic smooth muscle cells. *Proc Natl Acad Sci U S A* 1995;92:7222–7226.

53. Rhoads RE. Regulation of eukaryotic protein synthesis by initiation factors. *J Biol Chem* 1993;268:3017–3020.

54. Shantz LM, Pegg AE. Overproduction of ornithine decarboxylase caused by relief of translational repression is associated with neoplastic transformation. *Cancer Res* 1994;54:2313–2316.

55. Lazaris-Karatzas A, Smith MR, Frederickson RM, et al. Ras mediates translation initiation factor 4E-induced malignant transformation. *Genes Dev* 1992;6:1631–1642.

56. Rosenwald IB, Kaspar R, Rosseau D, et al. Eukaryotic translation initiation factor 4E regulates expression of cyclin D1 at transcriptional and post-transcriptional levels. *J Bio Chem* 1995;270:21176–21180.

57. Smith MR, Jaramillo M, Liu Y, et al. Translation initiation factors induce DNA synthesis and transform NIH 3T3 cells. *New Biologist* 1990;2:648–654.

58. Klein PS, Melton DA. Induction of mesoderm in xenopus laevis embryos by translation initiation factor 4E. *Science* 1994;265:803–806.

59. Lazaris-Karatzas A, Montine KS, Sonenberg N. Malignant transformation by a eukaryotic initiation factor subunit that binds to mRNA 5' cap. *Nature* 1990;345:544–547.

60. Lazaris-Karatzas A, Sonenberg N. The mRNA 5' cap-binding protein, eIF4E, cooperates with v-myc or E1A in the transformation of primary rodent fibroblasts. *Mol Cell Biol* 1992;12:1234–1238.

61. Evan GI, Brown L, Whyte M, Harrington E. Apoptosis and the cell cycle. *Curr Opin Cell Biol* 1995;7:825–834.

62. Packham G, Cleveland JL. c-Myc and apoptotis. *Biochim Biophys Acta* 1994;1242:11–28.

63. Poon RYC, Toyoshima H, Hunter T. Redistribution of the CDK inhibitor p27 between different cyclin CDK complexes in the mouse fibroblast cell cycle and in cells arrested with lovastatin or ultraviolet irradiation. *Mol Biol Cell* 1995;6:1197–1213.

64. Kinishita T, Yokota T, Arai K, Miyajima A. Suppression of apoptotic death in hematopoietic cells by signaling through the IL-3/GM-CSF receptors. *EMBO J* 1995;14:266–275.

65. Rhee K, Bresnahan W, Hirai A, Hirai M, Thompson EA. c-Myc and cyclin D3 (CcnD3) genes are independent targets for glucocorticoid inhibition of lymphoid cell proliferation. *Cancer Res* 1995;55:4188–4195.

66. Meikrantz W, Schlegel R. Suppression of apoptosis by dominant negative mutants of cyclin-dependent protein kinases. *J Biol Chem* 1996;17:10205–10209.

67. Hengst L, Reed SI. Translational control of p27[Kip1] accumulation during the cell cycle. *Science* 1995;271:1861–1864.

68. Resnitzky D, Hengst L, Reed SI. Cyclin A-associated kinase activity is rate limiting for entrance into S phase and is negatively regulated in G1 by p27[Kip1]. *Mol Cell Biol* 1995;15:4347–4352.

Chapter 23

Is There a Genetic Susceptibility That May Predispose to the Development of the Acute Respiratory Distress Syndrome (ARDS)?

Norbert F. Voelkel, MD, Jenny Allard, BS, and Steven Abman, MD

Introduction

Acute respiratory distress associated with the development of noncardiogenic pulmonary edema and histologically diffuse alveolar damage is a catastrophic event which we call—for lack of a better term—the acute respiratory distress syndrome (ARDS). Because of the very prominent inflammatory disease component, in particular the element of intravascular inflammation, it has been suggested that ARDS be renamed "inflammatory pulmonary edema."[1,2]

Although the incidence of ARDS varies among different groups of patients, risk factor categories, and combinations of risk factors,[3,4] it is the experience of every intensivist that one cannot predict which particular patient "at risk" will or will not develop ARDS. While most clinicians agree upon the risk factors that predispose patients to the development of ARDS, it is not clear why the majority at risk do not develop the syndrome.[3,4] This point was made clear for the first time in the prospective study by Fowler et al,[3] who showed that only 88 patients out of a cohort of 993 patients with appropriate risk factors developed

Supported by an NIH Vascular Academic Award #HL02825.

From: Weir EK, Reeves JT (eds). *Pulmonary Edema*. Armonk, NY: Futura Publishing Company, Inc.; ©1998.

ARDS. Perhaps the incidence of <10% in this first prospective survey may have been low, since a more recent study by Hudson et al[4] found that 26% of 695 patients at risk went on to develop ARDS. Regardless, whether the incidence in the at-risk population is 10% or closer to 25%, the fact remains that not everyone at risk develops ARDS. If the biological response to the insult *is not* determined by a dose-response relationship (either magnitude or duration of insult), this poses the question, what important risk factors have thus far remained unidentified, or is there perhaps a genetic disposition which plays a pivotal role? When clinicians say that 75% to 90% of the at-risk patients are "doing something right" and 10% to 25% are "doing something wrong," they are probably working from the premise that there are genetic factors tipping the scale between "at risk" and ARDS. If, indeed, this is the case, where in the chain of pathogenetic events leading to ARDS could this balance be tipped? Figure 1 provides one possible scenario for ARDS development in patients with the sepsis syndrome. Considering ARDS and bacterial infection, it is clear that 100% of the patients will have bacteremia and endotoxemia. Circulating endotoxin levels, von Willebrand factor antigen, endotoxin, tumor necrosis factor, the terminal complement complex, and neutrophil elastase have all been measured and found not to discriminate between at-risk patients and ARDS patients.[5-9]

What is not known is whether the same degree of neutrophil activation and chemotaxis to the lung capillaries occurs in all infected patients. If there were clear differences in the neutrophil behavior between at-risk patients and ARDS patients, one could study the neutrophils from ARDS survivors. When Rocker et al[9] measured plasma- and bronchoalveolar lavage fluid neutrophil elastase, they found the elastase levels increased in at-risk patients, indicating that inflammation (and neutrophil activation) occurred in patients who did not develop ARDS. The authors hypothesize that the earliest "ARDS decision" is made in the lung vascular compartment as a result of cell-cell interactions.

Host Resistance to ARDS

Host resistance to ARDS is presently a postulate awaiting the definition of a host resistance phenotype, however, *host resistance to infection* has been recognized for many years. New insights into the problem of resistance to granulomatous diseases and to parasitic infections has been gained from experiments using a variety of mouse strains. In the mouse, the Bcg gene controls macrophage priming for activation and is a major gene for susceptibility to infection with mycobacteria.[10]

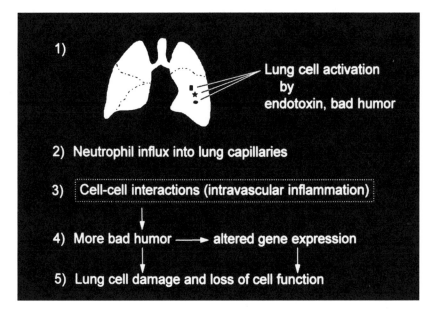

Figure 1. This schematic is built on the assumption that in order for the catastrophic event (which we call ARDS) to occur, a state of lung cell activation is required. The challenge leading to lung cell activation can be delivered via the airways or intravascularly. Chemotactic factors will have attracted neutrophils to the lung capillaries. Up to this point, the scenario may be common for at-risk patients who do not develop ARDS and for patients who do develop ARDS. The difference between at-risk and development of ARDS may depend on the intensity of the intravascular inflammation and the resulting activation of mediator cascades. Local mediator release may alter the expression of several genes in lung target cells, including alveolar macrophages, endothelial cells, and alveolar epithelial cells. Both mediator cascades and the alteration in gene expression may then lead to severe lung cell damage and loss of cell function.

A candidate gene for Bcg was identified by positional cloning and was designated "natural resistance-associated macrophage protein gene" (Nramp 1), and the human homologue NRAMP1 has recently been cloned. It is hypothesized that Nramp might function as a nitrate transporter and may play a role in the antimicrobial activity of macrophages against intracellular pathogens.

Resistance to murine cytomegalovirus is controlled by two genes: one mapping to the major histocompatibility complex (MHC), and the other mapping to the Cmv-1 locus on mouse chromosome 6.[11] Resistance to listeria infection is controlled by a single gene locus on chromosome 2, while resistance to influenza virus infection is controlled by Mx1. In humans, two Mx proteins have been identified; MXA protects cultured cells against influenza virus infection, but MXB does not.[11]

Host resistance to oxidant stress also has been recognized.[12,13] Both species and strain variations in lung oxidant enzyme are known to occur.[12,14] There are many enzyme systems that can determine resistance or susceptibility to oxidant stress and oxidant-induced lung injury. One system is the cytochrome P450 family of enzymes. The lung cytochrome P450 may produce active oxidant species and potent arachidonic acid metabolites,[15] and inhibition of lung Cyt P450 activity has been shown to reduce oxygen-induced lung injury.[16,17] It is known that there are genetic differences in response to Cyt P450 inducers. For example, Mansour et al[12] showed differences in Cyt P450 induction by β-naphthoflavone between C57BL/6J and DBA/2J mice, and the Cyt P450-inducible strain was protected against lethal hyperoxia. Whereas in this example "inducibility" correlates with protection, one might also consider the opposite—namely, that an induced (ready to go) Cyt P450 system (induced perhaps by chronic alcoholism) might greatly amplify a number of Cyt P450-dependent reactions and cause injury. This may be illustrated by the hepatic and pulmonary membrane damage observed in rats following disulfiram feeding. Disulfiram is widely used as an adjunct in the supportive treatment of patients with alcohol disease; its organ toxicity is likely caused by Cyt P450-catalyzed metabolites.[18] Oxidant stress causes alterations in gene expression. In particular, heat shock proteins and heme oxygenase-1 are upregulated by oxidants,[19] in part with the participation of transcriptional regulators like NF-KB. Heme oxygenase-1 induction during oxidant stress may play a beneficial role in lung injury due to the production of the antioxidant bilirubin, or may have detrimental effects because the oxidative cleavage of heme also yields carbon monoxide (CO), which may have similar actions as ·NO (including participation in lung vascular tone control).

Figure 2 lists a number of factors that can participate in signal amplification. Amplifiers can be proteins, like cytochromes or kinases. Membrane phospholipids, phospholipases, or increased Ca^+ levels are other candidates.

The Fischer 344 Rat Model of Acute Lung Injury

The Fischer 344 rat strain is of interest because of its susceptibility to development of spontaneous cancers due to premature aging and because of its susceptibility to oxidant stress.[20,21] Smith et al[22] were the first to recognize that Fischer rats developed liver cell necrosis after diquat treatment when other rat strains—in particular, Sprague-Dawley rats—did not. The authors wondered whether the lungs from Fischer rats were also vulnerable when exposed to oxidants. One interesting

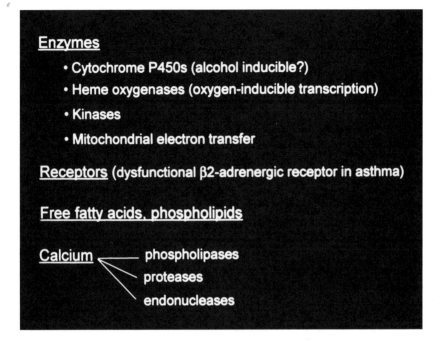

Figure 2. Examples for "Amplifiers."

difference between Fischer 344 and Sprague-Dawley lungs is their vascular reactivity; Fischer rats are hyporesponsive to vasoconstricting stimuli. Hypoxic vasoconstriction is very weak in unanesthetized Fischer rats and also in their isolated perfused lungs.[23] Isolated main pulmonary arteries from Fischer rats show a reduced contraction to KCl or angiotensin II when compared with those from age-matched Sprague-Dawley rats. Having characterized the differences in pulmonary vascular reactivity between Fischer 344 and Sprague-Dawley rats, the authors exposed the isolated lungs from each strain to 3 hours of hyperoxia (95% oxygen ventilation). The Fischer rat lungs developed edema within 3 hours of ventilation with 95% oxygen.[13] The edema formation was reduced by addition of catalase or of N^wnitro-L-arginine methyl ester (L-NAME) to the perfusate (Figure 3). When lungs from both strains were homogenized and analyzed for their levels of reduced glutathione, conjugated dienes catalase (glutathione peroxidase), and Cyt P450 activities, no differences were found. Lung tissue ATP levels were lower in Fischer rats[13] and so was the amount of nitric oxide synthase (eNOS) protein (by Western blotting) (Figure 4). The NOS inhibitor, L-NAME ($10-4$ mol/L) inhibited the hyperoxia-induced lung edema in perfused Fischer rat lungs (Figure 5), and the abundance

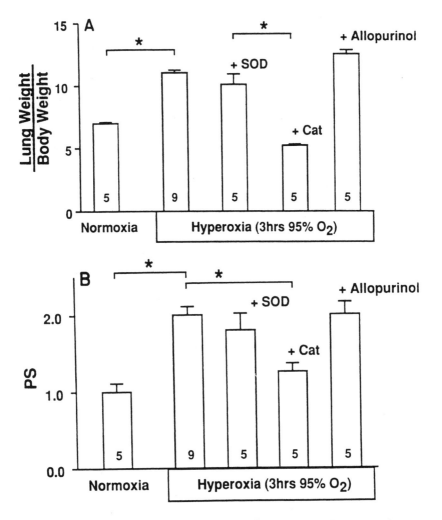

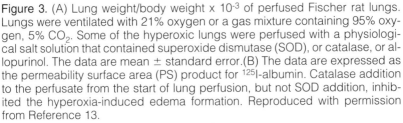

Figure 3. (A) Lung weight/body weight x 10^{-3} of perfused Fischer rat lungs. Lungs were ventilated with 21% oxygen or a gas mixture containing 95% oxygen, 5% CO_2. Some of the hyperoxic lungs were perfused with a physiological salt solution that contained superoxide dismutase (SOD), or catalase, or allopurinol. The data are mean ± standard error.(B) The data are expressed as the permeability surface area (PS) product for ^{125}I-albumin. Catalase addition to the perfusate from the start of lung perfusion, but not SOD addition, inhibited the hyperoxia-induced edema formation. Reproduced with permission from Reference 13.

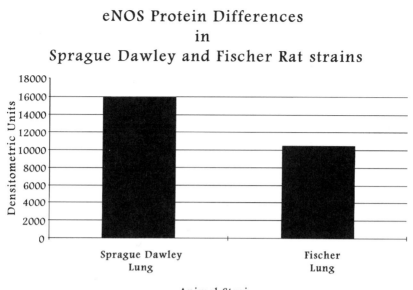

eNOS Protein Differences in Sprague Dawley and Fischer Rat strains

Figure 4. Perfused Fischer rat lungs (perfused under normoxic or hyperoxic conditions) show a significant decrease in eNOS protein (by Western blotting) as compared to perfused Sprague-Dawley lungs studied under comparable conditions.

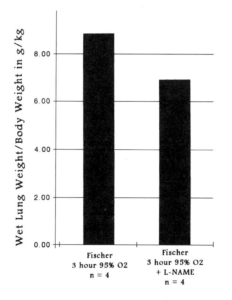

Figure 5. Lungs obtained from Fischer rats were perfused under similar conditions as described for Figure 3. The NOS inhibitor L-NAME had been added to the perfusate at the beginning of lung perfusion.

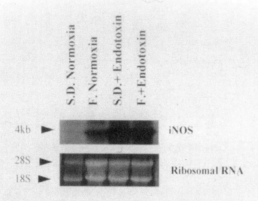

Normoxic perfused Fisher rat lungs express more RNA for iNOS than normoxic perfused Sprague Dawley rat lungs.

Figure 6. Northern blot data: perfused lungs from Fischer rats have a greater abundance for the induceable NOS than lung tissue obtained from perfused Sprague-Dawley rats. The induction of the iNOS gene within 2 hours following i.p. injection of salmonella typhimurium endotoxin appears to be comparable for both rat strains.

of iNOS mRNA in Fischer rat lungs was greater than that in Sprague-Dawley rat lungs (Figure 6). Thus, there are metabolic differences which may explain the decreased vascular reactivity and increased susceptibility to hyperoxic damage in the Fischer rat lungs as compared to the Sprague-Dawley strain. An increase in the mRNA for the inducible NOS and protection against weight gain of the hyperoxic lungs by L-NAME would be consistent with higher ˙NO production by the Fischer rat lungs. Ishizaki et al[24] have recently shown that ˙NO can promote acute lung injury. Higher ˙NO output can cause mitochondrial energy metabolism impairment[25] and account for the low lung ATP levels in the Fischer rat. It is now appreciated that ˙NO can cause surfactant dysfunction[26,27] and that nitrovasodilators can enhance tumor necrosis factor-(TNF) induced lung edema formation[28] and alter alveolar type II cell metabolism.[29]

Conclusions and Outlook

To seriously consider a genetic ARDS susceptibility, it is first necessary to define the host resistance/susceptibility phenotype, ie, we must gain some understanding—on the cellular and molecular level—of the difference between at-risk patients and ARDS patients. If there is a genetic ARDS susceptibility, then it is more likely that the predisposition will be polygenic rather than explainable by a single gene locus.[30,31] In this context, it is of interest that an increased incidence of ARDS has been reported for a rare inherited disease called lysinuric protein intolerance. This disorder is characterized by intestinal, renal, and liver transport defects for diamino acids and for arginine, ornithine, and lysine,[32] as well as by familial differences in the endothelin-triggered TNF response.[33] It would be reasonable to speculate that ethanol[34] abuse and hyperoxia,[35] as ARDS risk factors, point towards a participation of the cytochrome enzyme family in the ARDS pathogenesis.

More than 1500 different strains of mice have been developed for research and more than 500 mutant genes with adverse phenotypic consequences have been described. Based on a better understanding of the ARDS phenotype, appropriate mouse strains can be selected to test a specific hypothesis.

An alternative approach is to test a specific hypothesis by comparing test data from ARDS survivors to those from patients at risk. Differential display techniques can be used, as can pharmacological approaches similar to those which established the concept of fast and slow "drug metabolizers."

Acknowledgments The authors are indebted to Dr. Alan Jobe, who provided the information regarding the lysinuric protein intolerance.

References

1. Effros RM, Mason GR. An end to "ARDS." Chest 1986;89:162–163.
2. Voelkel NF. The adult respiratory distress syndrome. *Klin Wocheschr* 1989;67:559–567.
3. Fowler AA, Hamman RF, Good JT, et al. Adult respiratory distress syndrome: Risk with common predispositions. *Ann Intern Med* 1983;98: 593–597.
4. Hudson LD, Milberg JA, Anardi D, et al. Clinical risks for development of the acute respiratory distress syndrome. *Am J Respir Crit Care Med* 1995; 151:293–301.
5. Moss M, Ackerson L, Gillespie MK, et al. Von Willebrand factor antigen levels are not predictive for the adult respiratory distress syndrome. *Am J Respir Crit Care Med* 1995;151:15–20.
6. Parsons PE, Giclas PC. The terminal complement complex (sCb-9) is not specifically associated with the development of the adult respiratory distress syndrome. *Am Rev Respir Dis* 1990;141:98–103.
7. Parsons PE, Moore FA, Moore EE, et al. Studies on the role of tumor necrosis factor in adult respiratory distress syndrome. *Am Rev Respir Dis* 1992; 146:694–700.
8. Parsons PE, Worthen GS, Moore EE, et al. The association of circulating

endotoxin with the development of the adult respiratory distress syndrome. *Am Rev Respir Dis* 1989;140:294–301.

9. Rocker GM, Pearson D, Wiseman SM, et al. Diagnostic criteria for adult respiratory distress syndrome: Time for reappraisal. *Lancet* 1989;1(8630): 120–123.

10. Liu J, Fujiwara TM, Buu NT, et al. Identification of polymorphisms and sequence variants in the human homologue of the mouse natural resistance-associated macrophage protein gene. *Am J Hum Genet* 1995; 56:845–853.

11. Malo D, Skamene E. Genetic control of host resistance to infection. *Trends Genet* 1994;10(10):365–371.

12. Mansour H, Levacher M, Azoulay-Dupuis E, et al. Genetic differences in response to pulmonary cytochrome P-450 inducers and oxygen toxicity. *J Appl Physiol* 1988;64(4):1376–1381.

13. He L, Chang S-W, Montellano O, et al. Lung injury in Fischer but not Sprague-Dawley rats after short-term hyperoxia. *Am J Physiol* 1990; 259(3):L451–L458.

14. Bryan DL, Jenkinson SG. Species variation in lung oxidant enzyme activities. *J Appl Physiol* 1987;63:597–602.

15. Capdevila JH, Falck JR, Estabrook RW. Cytochrome P450 and the arachidonate cascade. *FASEB J* 1992;6:731–736.

16. Hazinski TA, France M, Kennedy KA, Hansen TN. Cimetidine reduces hyperoxic lung injury in lambs. *J Appl Physiol* 1989;67:2486–2492.

17. Hazinski TA, France M, Kennedy KA, Hansen TN. Pulmonary oxygen toxicity in young lambs: Physiological and biochemical effects of endotoxin infusion. *J Appl Physiol* 1988;65:1579–1585.

18. Berlin RG. Disulfiram hepatotoxicity: A consideration of its mechanism and clinical spectrum. *Alcohol Alcohol* 1989;24(3):241–246.

19. Choi AMK, Alam J. Heme oxygenase-1: Function, regulation, and implication of a novel stress-inducible protein in oxidant-induced lung injury. *Am J Respir Cell Mol Biol* 1996;15:9–19.

20. Cox RH, Tulenko TN. Effects of aging on agonist-activated ^{86}Rb efflux in arteries of Fischer 344 rats. *Am J Physiol* 1989;257(26):H494–H501.

21. Davey FR, Moloney WC. Postmortem observations on Fischer rats with leukemia and other disorders. *Lab Invest* 1970;23:327–334.

22. Smith CV, Hughes H, Lauterburg BH, Mitchell JR. Oxidant stress and hepatic necrosis in rats treated with diquat. *J Pharmacol Exp Ther* 1985;235: 172–177.

23. He L, Chang S-W, Voelkel NF. Pulmonary vascular reactivity in Fischer rats. *J Appl Physiol* 1991;70(4):1861–1866.

24. Ishizaki T, Shigemori K, Nakai T, et al. Leukotoxin, 9, 10-epoxy-12-octadecenoate causes edematous lung injury via activation of vascular nitric oxide synthase. *Am J Physiol* 1995;269(13)L65–L70.

25. Drapier JC, Hibbs JB. Differentiation of murine macrophages to expression-specific cytotoxicity for tumor cells results in L-arginine-dependent inhibition of mitochondrial iron- sulfur enzymes in the macrophage effector cells. *J Immunol* 1988;140:2829–2838.

26. Hallman M, Bry K, Lappalainen U. A mechanism of nitric oxide-induced surfactant dysfunction. *J Appl Physiol* 1996;80(6):2035–2043.

27. Hallman M, Waffarn F, Bry K, et al. Surfactant dysfunction after inhalation of nitric oxide. *J Appl Physiol* 1996;80(6):2026–2034.

28. Johnson A, Ferro TJ. Nitrovasodilator repletion increases TNF-α-induced pulmonary edema. *J Appl Physiol* 1996;80(6):2151–2155.

29. Miles PR, Bowman L, Huffman L. Nitric oxide alters metabolism in isolated alveolar type II cells. *Am J Physiol* 1996;271(15):L23–L30.
30. Dragani TA, Canzian F, Pierotti MA. A polygenic model of inherited predisposition to cancer. *FASEB J* 1996;10:865–870.
31. Green AS, Turki J, Halls IP, Liggett SB. Implications of genetic variability of human β_2-adrenergic receptor structure. *Pulm Pharmacol* 1995;8:1–10.
32. Hallman M, Maasilta P, Sipila I, Tahvanainen J. Composition and function of pulmonary surfactant in adult respiratory distress syndrome. *Eur Respir J Suppl* 1989;3:104s–108s.
33. Derkx HHF, Bruin KF, Jongeneel CV, et al. Familial differences in endotoxin-induced TNF release in whole blood and peripheral blood mononuclear cells in vitro: Relationship to TNF gene polymorphism. *J Eur Res* 1995;2:19–25.
34. Moss M, Moore FA, Moore EE, et al. Patients who abuse alcohol have an increased incidence of the adult respiratory distress syndrome (ARDS). *Am J Respir Crit Care Med* 1995;A71.
35. Hazinski TA, Noisin E, Hamon I, et al. Sheep lung cytochrome P4501A1 (CYP1A1): cDNA cloning and transcriptional regulation by oxygen tension. *J Clin Invest* 1995;96:2083–2089.

Treatment of Pulmonary Edema

Chapter 24

Treatment of the Adult Respiratory Distress Syndrome:
A Pathophysiological Approach

Robert J. Mangialardi, MD
and Gordon R. Bernard, MD

Introduction

The adult respiratory distress syndrome (ARDS) was first described by Ashbaugh[1] in 1967. ARDS is a true clinical syndrome defined as bilateral pulmonary infiltrates with poor oxygenation in the absence of elevated hydrostatic pressures. In reality, ARDS is a heterogeneous disease that occurs in association with a wide variety of disorders including sepsis, diffuse pneumonia, aspiration, multiple trauma, hemorrhagic shock, multiple blood transfusions, acute pancreatitis, and in a variety of inhalational lung injuries.[2] The incidence of ARDS is debatable, at least it was in the past, because of variability in how it is defined, but the incidence has been estimated to be as high as 150,000 cases per year in the United States, with an estimated mortality exceeding 50%.[3] The health care economic impact may be measured in billions of dollars. Despite the advent of many new and promising drugs, no therapy to date has proven beneficial when evaluated via placebo-controlled, randomized clinical trials.[4] Treatment remains largely supportive with attention to adequate oxygenation, mechanical ventilation, maintenance of appropriate volume status, suppression of concurrent infection, and adequate nutrition. The pulmonary dysfunction is characterized by inadequate oxygenation secondary to increased

Supported by NIH HL 19153, SCOR in Acute Lung Injury.

From: Weir EK, Reeves JT (eds). *Pulmonary Edema.* Armonk, NY: Futura Publishing Company, Inc.; ©1998.

right-to-left shunting, poor lung compliance, increased dead space fraction, and increased pulmonary vascular resistance. Histologically, there is a neutrophil alveolitis early in the course, with or without alveolar fibrosis later in the course.

This chapter describes the inflammation model of ARDS as well as a model based on pulmonary edema due to low oncotic pressures. Therapeutic modalities that have been carefully studied, as well as those currently under investigation, are described. Therapies are divided into categories based on therapeutic goals: reducing lung inflammation, vasodilation, surfactant repletion, reducing ventilator-induced lung injury, and reducing lung water via improving oncotic pressures.

Pathophysiology

Nearly 100 years ago, Frank Starling defined the relationship between hydrostatic and colloid oncotic pressures that governs the flux of fluid from the capillary to the interstitium.[5] The Starling relationship provides four mechanisms for edema formation: (1) increase in the capillary hydrostatic pressure to interstitial hydrostatic pressure gradient, (2) decrease in the capillary oncotic pressure to interstitial oncotic pressure gradient, (3) increase in capillary permeability to water and small molecules, and (4) decrease in the lymphatic drainage of the interstitium to the systemic circulation. When pulmonary edema develops because of the first mechanism, increased hydrostatic pressure gradient, it is generally referred to as hydrostatic or cardiogenic pulmonary edema. When pulmonary edema develops in the absence of an increased hydrostatic pressure gradient, it is termed nonhydrostatic pulmonary edema, and if oxygenation is sufficiently poor (usually PaO_2/FiO_2 ratio <200), clinicians apply the term ARDS. Based on the pathophysiological mechanism of lung inflammation, it is frequently implied that this type of pulmonary edema is caused by increased permeability (mechanism 3).[2] However, bedside confirmation of inflammatory lung injury is very difficult, and is subject to interpretation. No clinical trial thus far in ARDS has required proof of inflammation. The inclusion criteria in these trials have typically been bilateral pulmonary infiltrates, poor oxygenation, and no evidence of elevated hydrostatic pressures.

There is a large amount of circumstantial evidence that pulmonary edema in ARDS patients is caused by acute lung inflammation. Several investigators have shown that both patients with sepsis and patients with ARDS typically have marked elevations in pro-inflammatory cytokines, principally tumor necrosis factor-α (TNFα), interleukin-1 (IL-1), and interleukin-6 (IL-6).[6,7] These cytokines are released by monocytes and other cells in response to a variety of stimuli, most notably lipopolysaccharide (LPS or endotoxin).[2] These pro-inflammatory cytokines induce lung endothelial cells to produce chemotaxins such as interleukin-8 (IL-8) and neutrophil adhesion molecules such as intercellular adhesion molecule-1 (ICAM-1) and IL-8. Under the influence of these pro-inflammatory cytokines, neutrophils migrate to the lung, bind to the endothelium, and cross the basement membrane into the interstitium and alveolus. There, they release oxidant products such as superoxide (O2−), which is enzymatically converted to other oxidants such as the hydroxyl radical (·OH−).[8] These oxidants have been shown in experimental models to damage endothelial cell membranes by lipid peroxidation, which may lead to cell rupture and death. Peroxylipid products have been described in bronchoalveolar lavage (BAL) samples in both animal models of ARDS and in humans. Other investigators have found elevated quantities of cyclooxygenase products, typically thromboxane A_2 (TXA$_2$) and prostacycline (PGI$_2$).[9] Thromboxane is a potent vasoconstrictor while prostacylcin is a potent vasodilator and, together, these may mediate derangements in pulmonary vascular autoregulation in ARDS that are responsible for increased right-to-left shunting and hypoxemia. Furthermore, thromboxane may serve as a pro-inflammatory product, leading to further neutrophil recruitment and activation. Patients with sepsis or ARDS tend to have marked elevations in both plasma and BAL levels of TNF, IL-1, IL-6, and IL-8, and these levels remain elevated while the patient has ARDS, but slowly resolve in patients who recover.

The inflammatory model of ARDS provides numerous points for iatrogenic intervention to interrupt the autoinflammation process, and it has led to numerous clinical trials of such interventions. These interventions have universally looked promising in animal models and in uncontrolled human studies, but no intervention that has been subjected to the scrutiny of large-scale randomized clinical trials has proven to be better than placebo. Many of these studies have focused on patients with sepsis, in the hopes of preventing the inflammatory cascade from causing ARDS, because sepsis is the most common clinical event associated with ARDS. These interventions have included corticosteroids, anti-endotoxin antibodies, anti-TNF antibodies, IL-1 receptor antagonists, nonsteroidal anti-inflammatory drugs, N-acetylcysteine, and prostaglandin E1.

Corticosteroids

Corticosteroids were among the first anti-inflammatory agents studied in patients with either sepsis or ARDS. Based on a suggestion of improved survival in sepsis patients treated with corticosteroids, several large-scale randomized trials have been completed, but none has shown benefit over placebo. These studies are listed and compared in Table 1. There have been a few uncontrolled studies of cortico-steroids late in the course of ARDS that purport to show some benefit in lung function, but this finding has yet to be verified by randomized placebo-controlled trials.[6]

Anti-Endotoxin Antibodies

There are a variety of antibody preparations available against various moieties of the endotoxin molecule and at least three of these have been studied in large, randomized, clinical trials of patients with sepsis. These are summarized in Table 2. None of the studies reported on development or resolution of ARDS as a clinical endpoint.

Anti-TNF Antibodies and IL-1 Receptor Antagonists

Because clinical studies of anti-endotoxin modalities have only shown benefit in patients with demonstrated gram-negative bacterial infection, and because such infection can only be demonstrated in a fraction of all patients with sepsis syndrome who progress to ARDS, other investigators have studied interventions to block the inflammatory cascade at the level of cytokine production, theorizing that such intervention may be more clinically applicable. Both anti-TNF antibody and IL-1 receptor antagonist (a naturally occurring biological product) have proven beneficial in protecting animals from otherwise lethal doses of bacteria or endotoxin. Fisher et al[18] compared IL-1ra to placebo in 893 patients with sepsis syndrome and found no overall survival advantage, although retrospective analysis suggested some increase in survival time among patients with greater than one organ failure or among patients with high initial prediction of mortality. A phase II trial[19] evaluating murine anti-TNF antibody in patients with sepsis also failed to demonstrate improved survival in the overall population, but there was some suggestion of better outcome in patients with higher initial TNF levels.

Antioxidant Therapies

The terminal end of the inflammatory cascade involves direct tissue injury by oxidants released from activated inflammatory cells. This raises the possibility that antioxidant therapies may be beneficial for patients with ARDS. These interventions include repletion of glu-

Table 1

Major Randomized Clinical Trials of Corticosteroids in Sepsis or ARDS

Patients/ Study	Disease	Time of Dose	Dosing	Findings
Sprung[10]	59/sepsis	mean 17.5 hours after onset of shock	High dose methylpred-nisilone or dexametha-sone; 1 to 2 doses only	Patients dosed within 4 hours of shock onset had faster reversal of shock; treated patients had lower mortality at 133 hours but no mortality difference in overall hospital mortality.
Bernard[11]	99/ARDS	mean approx. 30 hours after onset of ARDS	30 mg/kg methylpred-nisolone q 6h × 4 doses	No difference between drug and placebo in 45-day mortality or rate of ARDS reversal.
Bone[12]	382/ sepsis	within 2 hours of meeting entry criteria	30 mg/kg methylpred-nisolone q 6 h × 4 doses	No difference in prevention of shock, reversal of shock, overall mortality. Increased 14-day mortality in treated patients (vs placebo) who had serum creatinine > 2 mg/dL at entry.
VA[13] Cooper-ative Study	223/ sepsis	mean 2.8 hours from diagnosis of sepsis	30 mg/kg methylpred-nisolone bolus then 5 mg/kg/h × 9 h infusion	No difference in 14-day mortality. Placebo-treated patients had a higher incidence or resolution of secondary infection by 14 days.
Luce[14]	87/sepsis	mean 1.1 hours after onset of septic shock	30 mg/kg methylpred-nisolone q 6 h × 4 doses	No difference in incidence of ARDS or in hospital mortality between treatment and placebo.

Table 2

Studies of Anti-Endotoxin Antibodies in Patients with Sepsis

Study	Patients	Antibody	Findings
Calandra[15]	100 (71 w/documented gram-negative infection)	human IgG against E. coli J5 strain	No difference in systemic complications, reversal of shock or overall mortality
Greenman[16]	486 (316 w/documented gram-negative sepsis)	murine monoclonal Ab against gram-neg endotoxin E5	No difference in mortality for all patients. Greater survival in nonshock patients with documented gram-negative infection
Ziegler[17]	543 (200 w/positive blood cultures for gram-negative organisms)	HA-1A human monoclonal IgM (binds to lipid A domain of endotoxin)	No benefit among 343 patients without documented bacteremia; reduced mortality among 200 patients w/bacteremia vs placebo (both with and without shock)

tathione stores with N-acetylcysteine (NAC) administration and antioxidant vitamins such as selenium, vitamin E, and vitamin C. Of these, NAC has been most extensively studied, and the results have been mixed. Jepsen et al[20] evaluated high-dose NAC in 66 ARDS patients and found no benefit in respiratory endpoints or mortality in NAC-treated patients. In fact, there was a trend toward more pulmonary complications in the treated group. Suter et al[21] evaluated NAC therapy in 61 patients with mild lung injury (not ARDS) and with predisposing factors to ARDS. They also failed to demonstrate any differences in mortality or ARDS development between NAC and placebo groups, but they did find some improvement in oxygenation and reduced need for ventilatory support in the NAC-treated group. Antioxidant vitamins have shown some potential in animal models of ARDS but have yet to be validated in human trials.[22]

Interleukin-10

The authors are currently planning a randomized clinical trial of interleukin-10 (IL-10) versus placebo in ARDS patients. IL-10 is a naturally occurring cytokine that has potent anti-inflammatory properties.[23] Specifically, it inhibits monocyte production of IL-1, IL-6, and TNF in response to endotoxin and downregulates production of antigen presenting proteins by monocytes, but it does not decrease production of IL-1ra or soluble TNF receptors. Elevated IL-10 levels have been demonstrated in patients with sepsis in one study.[24] Another study reported low IL-10 levels in the BAL of patients with ARDS who died, compared to higher IL-10 levels in ARDS patients who survived, raising the possibility of an imbalance between naturally occurring proinflammatory and anti-inflammatory cytokines in this disease.[25] Thus, IL-10 specifically interferes with several steps in the current pathophysiological model of ARDS and it may be of benefit, but it must be investigated in prospective clinical trials.

Cyclooxygenase Inhibitors

Cyclooxygenase products are elevated in patients with ARDS, and these products are known to cause both increased inflammation and derangements in vascular autoregulation.[9] There has been clinical interest in the use of ibuprofen in sepsis and ARDS because nonsteroidal anti-inflammatory drugs (NSAIDs) inhibit thromboxane and prostacyclin production. NSAIDs have been shown to attenuate lung injury in animal models of sepsis, and in a 30-patient placebo-controlled study, ibuprofen treatment reduced fever, tachycardia, and peak airway pressures relative to placebo.[26] A recently completed large, multicenter, randomized, blinded clinical trial confirmed several beneficial physiological effects of ibuprofen but failed to show a mortality benefit in septic patients.

Vasodilators: Nitric Oxide and Prostaglandin E_1

Nitric oxide and prostaglandin E_1 (PGE_1) have been evaluated for their vasodilatory properties in ARDS patients, especially in light of the finding that mortality correlates with lower cardiac output. Bone et al[27] conducted a 100-patient, blinded, randomized study of PGE_1 in ARDS patients and found no mortality benefit versus placebo. Treated patients did have significant reductions in systemic and pulmonary vascular resistance and reduced blood pressures, with concomitant increases in cardiac output, stroke volume, and heart rate. Others have shown that this hemodynamic benefit is also associated with worsening oxygenation, presumably because PGE_1 may vasodilate lung units that are poorly ventilated, thus increasing right-to-left shunt. Inhaled nitric oxide may offer many of the vasodilatory and hemodynamic benefits of PGE_1 without worsening oxygenation because the drug is only delivered to ventilated lung units. An uncontrolled study of NO in

ARDS patients showed that inhaled NO can allow a reduction of FiO_2 by approximately 15%, though many questions remain regarding the overall benefit of such therapy.[28]

Surfactant

Surfactant has been shown to be quantitatively deficient as well as qualitatively abnormal in patients with ARDS, raising the possibility that ARDS is primarily a disease of surfactant deficiency.[29] This is certainly true in the neonatal respiratory distress syndrome, and exogenously administered surfactant in neonates improves outcome. Early clinical trials of artificial surfactants suggested some benefit in ARDS patients. However, a recent large, multicenter, randomized, blinded clinical trial failed to demonstrate any survival or respiratory mechanics benefit for continuously aerosolized surfactant for up to 5 days in patients with ARDS.[30]

Improvements in Supportive Care

Mechanical ventilation, especially at the high airway pressures frequently encountered in ARDS patients, can induce lung injury in animals that is indistinguishable from ARDS.[31] Furthermore, lung disease in ARDS patients is heterogeneous with the greater amounts of diseased alveoli in dependent lung regions. Some alveoli are functionally normal. These observations raise the possibility that the ventilator itself may perpetuate lung injury in ARDS patients, and they have led to the development of ventilator strategies to minimize airway pressures. Hickling et al[32] demonstrated improved mortality versus historical controls in 50 ARDS patients, where mechanical ventilation was limited to peak airway pressures of 35 cm H_2O, even if this resulted in hypoventilation and severe hypercapnic respiratory acidosis. Based on this observation, a large, randomized, multicenter clinical trial is currently underway to compare a low-pressure ($+/-$ hypercapnic) ventilator strategy to conventional higher-pressure (normocapnic) ventilation. Other ancillary strategies such as extracorporeal oxygenation and carbon dioxide removal, intravenacaval oxygenators (IVOX), pressure-controlled inverse-ratio ventilation, and prone positioning have been developed to facilitate gas exchange, but thus far these techniques have not survived the scrutiny of randomized trials.[33,34] A new potentially beneficial therapy that is not yet clinically available is liquid ventilation.[35] This therapy involves filling the patient's lungs with a low-surface-tension perfluourocarbon liquid that has surfactant and oxygen transport properties but that is otherwise inert. The patient is then ventilated with conventional gas ventilation. This approach has been tested in animals and in a small number of humans and it seems to produce dramatic improvements in oxygenation and lung compliance, and a histologic reduction in inflammatory alveolitis.

Diuretics and Oncotic Pressure

Despite the fact that ARDS is widely recognized as a disease of pulmonary edema, there has never been a large-scale clinical trial comparing diuretics to placebo.[4] In fact, there is considerable controversy over the role of diuretics in this process. Proponents of diuretic therapy cite animal models of permeability pulmonary edema that show that the degree of lung water correlates with hydrostatic filling pressures even when the pulmonary capillary wedge pressure is in the normal range. Thus, they argue for the use of diuretics to keep the filling pressures as low as possible, consistent with reasonable blood pressure and cardiac output. Critics of diuretic therapy note that diuretics may reduce cardiac output, and that survival in ARDS has been correlated with tissue oxygen delivery and not with the amount of lung water. Furthermore, the critics note that aggressive use of diuretics may ultimately impair renal function, and impaired renal function is an independent predictor of poor outcome.

Mitchell et al[36] compared an aggressive diuretic strategy based on extravascular lung water measurements to a more standard diuretic approach based on elevated pulmonary capillary wedge pressure (PCWP) in 100 patients with pulmonary edema (mixed CHF and ARDS). Overall, they found a statistically significant reduction in number of ventilator days and number of ICU days in the more aggressive diuretic group. Among patients with ARDS only, they noted the same trend but the results did not reach statistical significance. In a retrospective study, Simmons et al[37] examined the influence of weight change on outcome in ARDS. They retrospectively reviewed the records of 213 patients who were prospectively enrolled in an ARDS data base. They compared baseline weight to weight on day 14 after study entry, and found that patients who lost 3 or more kilograms had significantly better survival than those who gained 3 or more kilograms (67% versus 0%, $P<0.0001$). Humphrey et al[38] retrospectively compared survival in ARDS patients based on change in pulmonary artery occlusion pressure. Patients with a 25% reduction in PCWP over the course of their ICU stay had a 75% survival compared to a 30% survival in patients who did not experience such a reduction. The difference remained statistically significant after adjustments werre made for differences in age and initial Apache II scores.

The authors recently reviewed their data from 455 sepsis patients entered into the ibuprofen-in-sepsis trial. One hundred seventy-eight of these patients (39%) developed ARDS, and of these, 92% had measured serum protein levels at study entry <6.0 g/dL. Patients with low serum protein levels were twice as likely to develop ARDS as patients with normal protein levels. Furthermore, ARDS patients with normal protein levels lost significantly more weight over the first 5 days of the study than did patients with low protein (who gained significant weight). ARDS patients with low protein levels were three times as likely to die as patients with normal protein levels. Logistic regression analysis was performed to control for other variables such as Apache scores. This analysis revealed that the strongest predictor of mortality in ARDS patients was the direction of protein change over the first 5 days (rising protein correlated with improved survival), and after controlling for direction of protein change, the Apache II score, which was designed to predict mortality, became an insignificant predictor of mortality in this patient population. This was not true in sepsis patients without ARDS.

These findings raise the possibility that serum protein levels, the principal determinant of serum oncotic pressure, may be the missing link explaining the association between weight gain and poor outcome. Based on these findings, the authors have begun the process of implementing a randomized clinical trial comparing combination therapy with intravenous albumin and diuretics to diuretics alone and to placebo in hypoproteinemic ARDS patients.

Summary

Despite extensive research over the last 30 years, effective pharmacotherapy for ARDS remains elusive. By current definition of ARDS, there are a variety of underlying diseases and perhaps a variety of underlying pathophysiological mechanisms. There are many interesting new modalities currently being tested. The ultimate effective clinical approach to patients with ARDS may be a multifaceted effort involving minimization of inflammatory injury, minimization of ventilator-induced lung injury, enhancement of surfactant action, and minimization of lung water by use of diuretics with or without colloid.

References

1. Ashbaugh DG, Bigelow DB, Petty TL. Acute respiratory distress in adults. *Lancet* 1967;2:319.
2. Demling RH. The modern version of the adult respiratory distress syndrome. *Annu Rev Med* 1995;46:193–202.

3. Bernard GR, Artigas A, Brigham KL, et al. The American-European consensus conference on ARDS. Definitions, mechanisms, relevant outcomes, and clinical trial cooridination. *Am J Respir Crit Care Med* 1994;149: 818–824.
4. Shuster DP. Fluid management in ARDS: "Keep them dry" or does it matter. *Intensive Care Med* 1995;21:101–103.
5. Kaminski MV Jr, Haase TJ. Albumin and colloid osmotic pressure implications for fluid resuscitation. *Crit Care Clin* 1992;8:311–321.
6. Meduri GU, Headley S, Tolley E, et al. Plasma and BAL cytokine response to corticosteroid rescue treatment in late ARDS. *Chest* 1995;108:1315–1325.
7. Meduri GU, Kohler G, Headley S, et al. Inflammatory cytokines in the BAL of patients with ARDS. *Chest* 1995;108:1303–1314.
8. Brigham KL. Oxidant stress and adult respiratory distress syndrome. *Eur Respir J* 1990;3(suppl 11):482S–484S.
9. Wheeler AP, Hardie WD, Bernard GR. The role of cyclooxygenase products in lung injury induced by tumor necrosis factor in sheep. *Am Rev Respir Dis* 1992;145:632–639.
10. Sprung CL, Caralis PV, Marcial EH, et al. The effects of high dose corticosteroids in patients with septic shock. *New Engl J Med* 1984;311:1137–1143.
11. Bernard GR, Luce JM, Sprung CL, et al. High dose corticosteroids in patients with the adult respiratory distress syndrome. *New Engl J Med* 1987;317:1565–1570.
12. Bone RC, Fisher CJ, Clemmer TP, et al. Early methylprednisolone treatment for septic syndrome and the adult respiratory distress syndrome. *Chest* 1987;92:1032–1046.
13. VA Cooperative Study Group. Effect of high dose glucocorticoid therapy on mortality in patients with clinical signs of systemic sepsis. *New Engl J Med* 1987;317:659–665.
14. Luce JM, Montgomery AB, Marks JD, et al. Ineffectiveness of methylprednisolone in preventing parenchymal lung injury and improving mortality in patients with septic shock. *Am Rev Respir Dis* 1988;138:62–68.
15. Calandra T, Glauser MP, Schellekens J, et al. Treatment of gram negative septic shock with human IgG antibody to Escherichia coli J5: A prospective, double-blind, randomized trial. *J Infect Dis* 1988;158:312–319.
16. Greenman RL, Schein RMH, Martin MA, et al. A controlled clinical trial of E5 murine monoclonal IgM antibody to endotoxin in the treatment of gram negative sepsis. *JAMA* 1991;266:1097–1102.
17. Ziegler EJ, Fisher CJ, Sprung CL, et al. Treatment of gram negative bacteremia and septic shock with HA-1A human monoclonal antibody against endotoxin. *New Engl J Med* 1991;324:429–436.
18. Fisher CJ, Dhainaut JFA, Opal SM, et al. Recombinant human interleukin 1 receptor antagonist in the treatment of patients with sepsis syndrome. Results from a randomized, double-blind, placebo controlled trial. *JAMA* 1994;271:1836–1843.
19. Fisher CJ, Opan SM, Dhainaut JF, et al. Influence of an anti-tumor necrosis factor monoclonal antibody on cytokine levels in patients with sepsis. *Crit Care Med* 1993;21:318–327.
20. Jepsen S, Herlevsen P, Knudsen P, et al. Antioxidant treatment with N-acetylcysteine during adult respiratory distress syndrome. A prospective, randomized, placebo-controlled study. *Crit Care Med* 1992;20:918–923.
21. Suter PM, Domenighetti G, Schaller MD, et al. N-acetylcysteine enhances recovery from acute lung injury in man. *Chest* 1994;105:190–194.

22. Sawyer MAJ, Mike JJ, Chavin K, et al. Antioxidant therapy and survival in ARDS (Abstr) *Crit Care Med* 1989;17:S153
23. Moore KW, O'Garra A, de Waal Malefyt R, et al. Interleukin-10. *Annu Rev Immunol* 1993;11:165–190.
24. Marchant A, Deviere J, Byl B, et al. Interleukin 10 production during septicaemia. *Lancet* 1994;343:707–708.
25. Donnelly SC, Strieter RM, Reid PT, et al. The association between mortality rates and decreased concentrations of interleukin-10 and interleukin-1 receptor antagonist in the lung fluids of patients with the adult respiratory distress syndrome. *Ann Intern Med* 1996;125:191–196.
26. Bernard GR, Reines HD, Halushka PV, et al. Prostacyclin and thromboxane A2 formation is increased in human sepsis syndrome. Effects of cyclooxygenase inhibition. *Am Rev Respir Dis* 1991;144:1095–1101.
27. Bone RC, Slotman G, Maunder R, et al. Randomized double-blind, multicenter study of prostaglandin E1 in patients with the adult respiratory distress syndrome. *Chest* 1989;96:114–119.
28. Rossaint R, Falke KJ, Lopez F, et al. Inhaled nitric oxide for the adult respiratory distress syndrome. *New Engl J Med* 1993;328:399–405.
29. Gunther A, Siebert C, Schmidt R, et al. Surfactant alterations in severe pneumonia, acute respiratory distress syndrome, and cardiogenic lung edema. *Am J Respir Crit Care Med* 1996;153:176–184.
30. Anzueto A, Baughman RP, Guntupalli KK, et al. Aerosolized surfactant in adults with sepsis induced acute respiratory distress syndrome. *New Engl J Med* 1996;334:1417–1421.
31. Dreyfuss D, Soler P, Basset G, et al. High inflation pressure pulmonary edema. Respective effects of high airway pressure, high tidal volume, and positive end expiratory pressure. *Am Rev Respir Dis* 1988;137:1159–1164.
32. Hickling KG, Henderson SJ, Jackson R. Low mortality associated with low volume pressure limited ventilation with permissive hypercapnia in severe adult respiratory distress syndrome. *Intensive Care Med* 1990;16:372–377.
33. Stoller JK, Kacmarek RM. Ventilatory strategies in the management of the adult respiratory distress syndrome. *Clin Chest Med* 1990;11:755–772.
34. Zwischenberger JB, Nguyen TT, Tao W, et al. IVOX with gradual permissive hypercapnia: A new management technique for respiratory failure. *J Surg Res* 1994;57:99–105.
35. Tutuncu AS, Faithfull S, Lachmann B. Intratracheal perfluorocarbon administration combined with mechanical ventilation in experimental respiratory distress syndrome: Dose dependent improvement of gas exchange. *Crit Care Med* 1993;21:962–969.
36. Mitchell JP, Schuller D, Calandrino FS, et al. Improved outcome based on fluid management in critically ill patients requiring pulmonary artery catheterization. *Am Rev Respir Dis* 1992;145:990–998.
37. Simmons RS, Berdine GG, Seidenfeld JJ, et al. Fluid balance and the adult respiratory distress syndrome. *Am Rev Respir Dis* 1987;135:924–929.
38. Humphrey H, Hall J, Sznajder I, et al. Improved survival in ARDS patients associated with a reduction in pulmonary capillary wedge pressure. *Chest* 1990;97:1176–1180.

Chapter 25

Acute and Chronic Efficacy of Nitric Oxide in the Adult Respiratory Distress Syndrome (ARDS)

R. Rossaint, MD and K. Falke, MD

Introduction

The adult respiratory distress syndrome (ARDS) is an acute and severe alteration in lung structure and function characterized by hypoxemia, reduced respiratory compliance, and diffuse radiographic infiltrates.[1] Since its first description by Ashbaugh et al[1] in 1967, the overall mortality rate of this syndrome remained slightly above 50% despite extensive clinical and laboratory research efforts.[2] Among other unknown factors, this high mortality may be influenced by the disease itself, as well as by iatrogenic factors such as ventilator settings with high airway pressures and high inspiratory oxygen concentrations (FiO_2). In the progression of ARDS, high mean airway pressures, as well as high FiO_2 may be required to ensure adequate arterial oxygen partial pressures (PaO_2). Both factors are considered harmful to the lung.[3,4] Therefore, today's therapeutic approaches aim for a reduction in peak airway pressure and application of less enriched oxygen mixtures. Conventional concepts used are pressure- and/or volume-limited ventilation with positive end-expiratory pressure (PEEP) and acceptance of an increased partial pressure of carbon dioxide, positioning, including prone position, differential lung ventilation, and avoidance of fluid overload.[5] At the beginning of this decade, the inhalation of low concentrations of nitric oxide (NO) was introduced as an experimental method in the therapy of ARDS.

Until a few years before 1990, the purpose of NO in biological tis-

From: Weir EK, Reeves JT (eds). *Pulmonary Edema*. Armonk, NY: Futura Publishing Company, Inc.; ©1998.

sue was unknown. In 1980, Furchgott and Zawadski[6] reported that the relaxing effect of acetylcholine on isolated arteries is dependent on the vascular endothelium. The authors postulated that the relaxing effect must be mediated by an unstable humoral factor, later known as the endothelium-derived relaxing factor (EDRF). In 1987, two independent research groups published results which implied that NO accounts for the action of EDRF.[7,8] This description of the essential role of the endothelium-derived NO in mediating vascular relaxation, its gaseous state, as well as its rapid inactivation by hemoglobin as soon as it enters the bloodstream, may have stimulated Higenbottam et al,[9] in 1988, to test the vasodilatory effects of 40 parts per million (ppm) NO in air in patients with primary pulmonary hypertension. They observed dilatory effects of inhaled NO on the pulmonary vasculature, however, in contrast to the infusion of prostacyclin (PGI_2), they did not find any systemic vasodilation during NO inhalation. Inhaled NO was also shown to selectively dilate, in a dose-dependent manner, the pulmonary circulation in awake, spontaneously breathing lambs that were acutely vasoconstricted, either by infusion of the stable thromboxane endoperoxide analogue, U46619, or by breathing a hypoxic gas mixture.[10] Moreover, hypoxic pulmonary vasoconstriction in mechanically ventilated sheep was completely abolished by breathing 20 ppm NO, without impairing gas exchange.[11] These studies and little evidence of toxicity of low concentrations of inhaled NO were the basis for the first clinical trials of inhaled NO to selectively reduce the pulmonary hypertension in ARDS.

Acute Effects of Inhaled NO in ARDS

In patients suffering from ARDS, a reduction of the increased pulmonary artery pressure (PAP) might be of special interest; first, in order to decrease right ventricular afterload, and second, to facilitate the resolution of alveolar and interstitial pulmonary edema. Systemically infused vasodilators lower PAP, but because of the global effect on the vasculature within the pulmonary and systemic circulation, their use is limited. The concomitant dilation of the systemic circulation causes arterial hypotension, possibly affecting the blood flow to various organs. Moreover, the vasodilation in the pulmonary vasculature increases the blood flow to areas of intrapulmonary shunt, thereby compromising oxygenation even further. In 1990, inhaled NO was first used for selective pulmonary vasodilation in an ARDS patient.[12] In this patient with pronounced pulmonary hypertension approaching systemic pressure levels, inhaled NO induced a selective reduction in PAP, improved right ventricular function, and, surprisingly, increased the PaO_2 (Figure 1).[12] The subsequent study in ten patients confirmed that NO inhalation

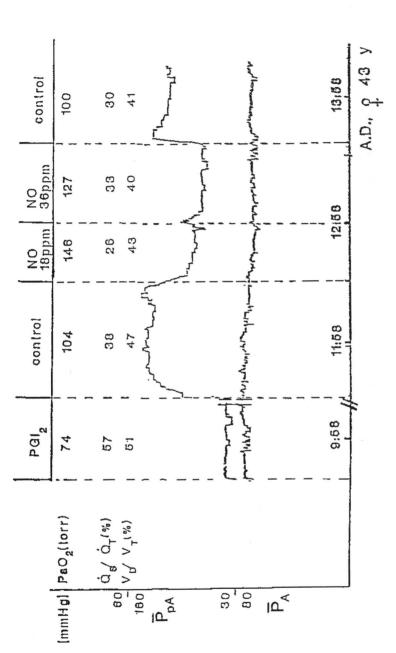

Figure 1. Effect of the first administration of nitric oxide (NO) in a patient with severe ARDS undergoing veno-venous extracorporeal gas exchange. Mean systemic arterial pressure and mean pulmonary artery pressure were continuously measured. Before inhalation of two concentrations of NO (18 and 36 parts per million) the patient received 4 ng/kg bw/min prostacyclin (PGI$_2$). The PaO$_2$, true intrapulmonary right-to-left shunt (Q_S/Q_T) and dead space (V_D/V_T) were assessed intermittently.

in patients with severe ARDS selectively reduced pulmonary hypertension and improved arterial oxygenation.[13] In this study, the investigators compared the effects of short-term low-dose NO inhalation with intravenous PGI_2. Eighteen ppm NO lowered PAP by an average of 7 mm Hg and to the same extent as the intravenous infusion of 4 ng/kg bw/min PGI_2. Whereas PGI_2 caused mean arterial pressure to fall and cardiac output to rise, these parameters remained unchanged during NO inhalation. Concomitant with the selective decrease in PAP, NO inhalation brought about a clear improvement in pulmonary oxygenation. These results were confirmed later by further studies which all demonstrated the selective effect on the pulmonary vasculature, presumably restricted to ventilated lung areas, leading to a decrease in PAP and an improvement in pulmonary gas exchange.[14-21]

Influence of NO on Ventilation/Perfusion Distributions

In order to find out the mechanisms by which inhaled NO causes the increase in PaO_2, Rossaint and colleagues analyzed the ventilation/perfusion distribution using the multiple inert gas elimination technique in nine patients with ARDS.[13] It was shown that the improved oxygenation during NO inhalation is due to redistribution of pulmonary blood flow in favor of well-ventilated lung regions, away from regions of intrapulmonary shunt (Figure 2). There is evidence that NO also participates in the regular ventilation/perfusion distributions within the healthy lungs of numerous species, including humans. NO is produced endogenously in the airways, as well as in the lung itself. Most of the endogenously produced NO is formed in the upper airways, especially in the nose and the paranasal sinuses,[22-24] whereas less than 10% is excreted in the lower airway and lungs. During normal spontaneous breathing certain amounts of NO are autoinhaled, affecting the regulation of the ventilation/perfusion ratios in the lungs.[22] This presumption is supported by observed beneficial effects of a replacement therapy with physiological concentrations of NO in intubated patients with and without ARDS. In these patients who do not autoinhale the NO synthesized in the upper airways, NO concentrations of 10 to 100 parts per billion (ppb), which are similar to the concentration continuously released in the adult human nasopharynx, improve arterial oxygenation.[25,26] In healthy adults the significance of autoinhaled NO may be minor. However, in lung diseases associated with regional alveolar hypoxia, the contribution of autoinhaled NO may act synergistically with an inhibition of the expression of endothelial constitutive NO synthase in hypoxic lung areas.[27] Both mechanisms, autoinhaled NO for vasodilating well-ventilated lung regions

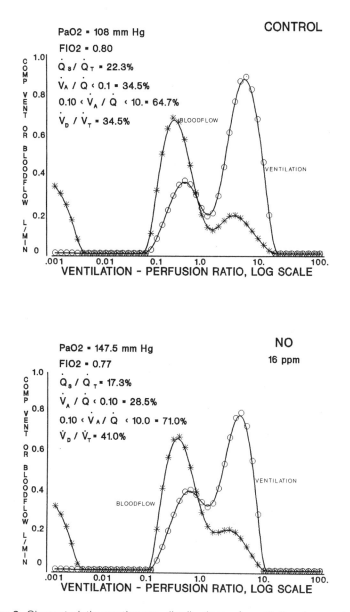

Figure 2. Characteristic continuous distributions of ventilation (open circles) and perfusion (stars) during baseline and during inhalation of 16 parts per million (ppm) nitric oxide (NO) in a patient with severe ARDS. **Baseline graph:** Ventilation-perfusion mismatching, a high fractional blood flow to Q_S/Q_T (blood flow to areas of the lung with VA/Q ratios <0.0005) and to areas with low V_A/Q ratios (blood flow to areas of the lungs with V_A/Q ratios between 0.0005 and 0.10) contribute strongly to the disturbed pulmonary gas exchange of this patient. **NO graph:** A decreased Q_S/Q_T fraction and no change in the blood flow to areas of low V_A/Q ratios has resulted in an increase in the blood flow to areas of normal V_A/Q ratios (blood flow to areas of the lungs with V_A/Q ratios between 0.10 and 10.0). Although there is a persistent mismatching of the ventilation-perfusion distributions, the change of blood flow from areas of Q_S/Q_T to areas with normal V_A/Q ratios has resulted in an improved PaO_2.

and reduced production of NO in shunt areas, may maintain pulmonary gas exchange in acute lung injury. In intubated, anesthesized, and mechanically ventilated patients, NO autoinhalation is interrupted and, in addition, ventilation/perfusion mismatch may occur due to development of compression atelectasis. Therefore, replacement of even physiological levels of NO may contribute to the redistribution of blood flow to well-ventilated lung regions, which will cause an improvement of arterial oxygenation.

NO and Pulmonary Edema

Inhaled NO has the capability to reduce pulmonary hypertension in ARDS, however, inhaling NO does not reduce the PAP to a normal level, probably because pulmonary vascular occlusion or compression is present. Studies by Benzing and Geiger[14,28] demonstrated that the decrease in PAP, with the associated change of the hydrostatic pressure in the pulmonary capillary bed, is of sufficient magnitude to enhance the resolution of interstitial pulmonary edema. In a first study, these authors reported that, in patients with acute lung injury, inhalation of 40 ppm NO causes predominantly vasodilation of the pulmonary venous vasculture, thereby decreasing the pulmonary capillary pressure.[14] It was assumed that NO will decrease fluid filtration because the hydrostatic pressure in the capillaries (and not the PAP by itself) becomes the decisive factor of net fluid filtration into the interstitial space when microvascular permeability is enhanced. In order to prove this hypothesis, Benzing et al performed a further investigation in nine patients with acute lung injury to analyze the effect of the same concentration of inhaled NO on transvascular albumin flux measured by a double radioisotope method, with use of ^{99m}Tc-labeled albumin and ^{51}Cr-labeled autologous red blood cells.[28] With this short-term study, the authors could show that the decrease in pulmonary capillary pressure during NO inhalation is associated with reduced transvascular albumin flux. Although there is now evidence that inhaled NO can reduce pulmonary edema, the long-term effect on transcapillary fluid filtration and dose response of NO have yet to be established.

NO and Right Ventricular Function

In patients with ARDS, pulmonary hypertension may result from the combined effects of hypoxic pulmonary vasoconstriction, release of mediators, and microthrombosis in the pulmonary circulation. This pulmonary hypertension represents an increase in the outflow pressure load on the right ventricle, which may cause a decrease in right ventricular ejection fraction (RVEF) and increases in right ventricular volumes. When inhaled NO was given for the first time to a patient with severe ARDS, the selective pulmonary vasodilation resulted in an increased RVEF.[12] Recently, this observation was confirmed by Fierobe and coworkers.[17] In 13 patients with severe ARDS, they examined whether inhaled NO improved right ventricular function and whether the changes in pulmonary hemodynamics and right ventricular function were related to changes in arterial oxygenation. Inhalation of 5 ppm NO was followed by a decrease in PAP from 36 ± 5 mm Hg to 31 ± 6 mm Hg ($P<0.01$) and in pulmonary vascular resistance from 211 ± 43 dyne·s·cm^{-5} to 180 ± 59 dyne·s·cm^{-5} ($P<0.05$), which was associated with an increase in RVEF from $32\pm5\%$ to $36\pm6\%$ ($P<0.05$) and a trend toward decreased right ventricular volumes. The increase in PaO_2/FiO_2 (103 ± 47 mm Hg versus 142 ± 63 mm Hg) was not related to hemodynamic changes. Similar findings were described in a study by Rossaint and coworkers.[21] They compared the effects of inhaled NO and infused PGI_2 on right ventricular function parameters assessed by the thermodilution technique in patients with ARDS. Ten patients inhaled 18 ppm NO and 36 ppm NO, randomized to be preceded or followed by an intravenous infusion of PGI_2 (4 ng·kg^{-1}·min^{-1}). Inhaling 18 ppm NO reduced the PAP from 33 ± 2 mm Hg to 28 ± 1 mm Hg ($P=0.008$), increased RVEF, as assessed by thermodilution technique, from $28\pm2\%$ to $32\pm2\%$ ($P=0.005$), decreased right ventricular end-diastolic volume index from 114 ± 6 mL·m^{-2} to 103 ± 8 mL·m^{-2} ($P=0.005$), and decreased right ventricular end-systolic volume index from 82 ± 4 mL·m^{-2} to 70 ± 5 mL·m^{-2} ($P=0.009$). Mean arterial pressure and cardiac index did not change significantly. The effects of 36 ppm NO were not different from the effects of 18 ppm NO. Infusion of PGI_2 also reduced PAP from 34 ± 2 mm Hg to 30 ± 2 mm Hg ($P=0.02$) and increased RVEF from $29\pm2\%$ to $32\pm2\%$ ($P=0.02$), but in contrast to inhaled NO, right ventricular end-diastolic and end-systolic volume indices did not change significantly, mean arterial pressure decreased from 80 ± 4 mm Hg to 70 ± 5 mm Hg ($P=0.03$), and cardiac index increased from 4.0 ± 0.5 L·min^{-1}·m^{-2} to 4.5 ± 0.5 L·min^{-1}·m^{-2} ($P=0.02$).

Both studies demonstrate that, in a group of hemodynamically stable ARDS patients, inhaled NO slightly improved RVEF, which was not associated with an increase in cardiac index. These changes indicate that the right ventricle is working on another part of its pressure-volume relationship, since during NO inhalation, the increase of RVEF was accompanied by decreased right ventricular volumes at a constant cardiac index; that is a normal physiological response of the right ventricle in the presence of different loading conditions. However, these data also show that cardiac index could not be influenced by the alterations in right ventricular parameters obtained in this group of hemodynamic stable ARDS patients. The increase in cardiac index observed during the infusion of i.v. vasodilators such as PGI_2 is probably due to reduction in systemic vascular resistance, since in the study of Rossaint et al,[21] the decrease of PAP and the corresponding increase of RVEF were similar during the administration of either vasodilator. The right ventricular end-diastolic volume did not decrease during the infusion of PGI_2, probably due to augmented venous return. However, even if in these studies the increased RVEF during NO inhalation did not result in an augmented cardiac index, one should be well aware that in patients with right ventricular failure, inhaled NO may cause in improvement in right ventricular function presumably leading to a rise in cardiac index, as demonstrated in four patients by Wysocki et al.[29]

Dose-Response Relationships of Inhaled NO

In 1991, Frostell et al[10] demonstrated that, in awake lambs, increasing concentrations of inhaled NO resulted in a dose-dependent reduction of hypoxia-induced pulmonary hypertension. Dyar and coworkers examined the effect of inhaled NO using concentrations between 4 ppm and 512 ppm in six sheep with pulmonary hypertension induced with hypoxia and endotoxin.[30] They found that the maximum decrease in PAP occurred with 64 ppm and that increasing the dose to 512 ppm had no further effect. Gerlach et al evaluated the optimal concentration of inhaled NO for reducing pulmonary hypertension and improving arterial oxygenation in 12 patients with ARDS.[25] They studied the dose-response and time course of the pulmonary effects of five concentrations of NO (0.01 ppm, 0.1 ppm, 1 ppm, 10 ppm, and 100 ppm). Arterial oxygenation improved at much lower concentrations of NO than those needed to reduce PAP; analysis of the dose responses demonstrated that the effect of NO on PaO_2 was significant at 0.1 ppm, whereas the effect of NO on PAP was only significant with concentrations of 1 ppm and more. The idealized dose-response curves for PaO_2 and PAP showed different patterns: the improvement in oxygenation, with 50% maximal response (ED_{50}) at approximately 0.1 ppm, had a maximum at 10 ppm NO and, at the highest tested concentration (100 ppm), drifted back towards the baseline data, whereas PAP presented a continuous, dose-dependent downwards tendency, with an ED_{50} of approximately 2 ppm NO to 3 ppm NO. In two patients, the authors found that 40% of the maximal achieved increase in PaO_2, which was registered at 1 ppm, occurred at 0.01 ppm. Furthermore, using 100 ppm NO or more, the PaO_2 decreased back towards the baseline. This observation may be based on a diffusion of NO at high concentrations through the lung tissue, from ventilated to nonventilated lung segments, potentially dilating blood vessels in shunt and low ventilations/perfusions areas. Thereby, the intrapulmonary shunt increases and the arterial oxygenation deteriorates. This presumption is supported by the fact that PAP decreased further as NO concentration was increased.

Slightly different results were obtained by Puybasset et al.[20] They determined the dose-response curve of eight concentrations of inhaled NO (between 0.1 ppm and 5 ppm), in terms of pulmonary vasodilation and improvement in PaO_2 in six patients with ARDS. In accordance with the study by Gerlach et al,[25] they found that the inhalation of 0.1 ppm NO to 2 ppm NO induced a dose-dependent decrease of PAP and a dose-dependent increase in PaO_2. However, in contrast, they could not confirm that the PAP decreased further when the NO concentration increased to 5 ppm. In two patients, 91% and 74% of the pulmonary vasodilating effect was observed at a concentration of 0.1 ppm, suggesting that lower concentrations would also have been effective. Since these authors did not test concentrations higher than 5 ppm, it remains speculative whether a further decrease in PAP might have occurred if they had increased the NO concentration to higher levels. However, the available data demonstrate that individual dose-response studies should be performed before starting NO inhalation therapy. Since significant improvements of PaO_2 in patients with ARDS are already induced by doses of NO, which are much lower than those used in the first clinical NO studies and which are similar to those inhaled in normal breathing humans due to atmospheric concentrations and due to NO produced in the nasopharynx,[22] the risk of toxicity related to NO inhalation can be reduced if an improvement of PaO_2 is the primarily goal of NO inhalational therapy. Therefore, clinicians must decide individually whether they predominantly want to reduce the patient's PAP or to increase the PaO_2. Moreover, since from the authors' experience, both parameters in severe ARDS are differently influenced by NO over a range from 0.01 ppb to at least 100 ppm, it is difficult to determine an "optimal" concentration for the individual patient, especially as the dose-response relationship may differ from day to day.

Ratio of Responders to Nonresponders

For unknown reasons, some patients with severe ARDS did not show any improvement in oxygenation or any reduction in PAP. Rossaint and coworkers[31] analyzed systemic and pulmonary hemodynamics and gas exchange variables immediately before inhalation and after 30 minutes of first inhalation of 10 ppm NO to 20 ppm NO in 30 patients. In only 83% of these patients, NO increased PaO_2/FiO_2 by ≥ 10 mm Hg; in 87%, NO reduced venous admixture by $\geq 10\%$; and in 63%,

NO decreased PAP by $\geq$3 mm Hg. In 5 of these 30 patients, NO inhalation failed to improve arterial oxygenation. Rossaint and colleagues also could not identify any cause for the failure of inhaled NO to improve pulmonary gas exchange and reduce pulmonary hypertension, and they could only speculate on the cause for the nonresponsiveness to inhaled NO in their patients. Inhalation of NO dose-response studies were not performed. Therefore, it cannot be ruled out that other concentrations of NO would have been more effective. Interestingly, in these first 30 patients treated with NO inhalation, it was observed that some of the initial nonresponders demonstrated significant increases in PaO_2 or a reduction of pulmonary hypertension during inhalation of NO a few days later.

In an attempt to find factors that influence the effect of inhaled NO, Rossaint and colleagues[31] analyzed the correlation between several parameters. However, the increase in PaO_2/FiO_2 due to NO inhalation did not correlate with the pulmonary vascular resistance index, and the decrease in PAP following NO inhalation was not dependent on venous admixture before NO inhalation. In contrast to a report by Bigatello et al,[15] who demonstrated in seven patients with ARDS that the magnitude of the vasodilator response during NO inhalation correlated with the pulmonary vascular resistance when stopping NO inhalation, Rossaint and coworkers found no correlation between the effect of NO inhalation on PAP and PAP before NO inhalation. Furthermore, also in contrast to results found by Bigatello et al,[15] they could not demonstrate that the decrease in venous admixture due to NO inhalation correlated with venous admixture before NO inhalation or that the effect of NO inhalation correlated with cardiac output. In addition, they observed responders and nonresponders independent of the necessity for extracorporeal membrane oxygenation (ECMO) or intravenous catecholamine infusions. In agreement with the observations of Rossaint and coworkers, Krafft et al[18] could not identify any factor predicting the response to inhaled NO in patients with septic ARDS. However, they found that inhaled NO induced marked improvement in hemodynamics and oxygenation in only 40% of patients with ARDS. If the patients were NO responders, they presented higher RVEF, higher cardiac indices, and higher oxygen delivery values than NO nonresponders. In addition, Puybasset et al[32] reported a NO response rate of 100% for 11 patients without septic shock, while only 3 of 6 patients with septic shock were responders. Therefore, these authors concluded that inhaled NO is less effective in patients with septic shock. Furthermore, this group found that factors determining NO-induced improvement in arterial oxygenation and pulmonary vascular effects are the possibility of PEEP-induced alveolar recruitment and the baseline level of pulmonary vascular resistance.[19]

Long-Term Effects of NO Inhalation in ARDS

To the authors' knowledge, only a few studies exist that investigate the effects of long-term NO inhalation in ARDS patients.[13,15,27,31,33] These studies include more than 65 patients who inhaled 0.1 ppm NO to 40 ppm NO for a duration between 2 days and 53 days. The effect of NO inhalation on PAP and on PaO_2 persisted throughout the entire exposure period (Figure 3 and Figure 4). No tachyphylaxis or severe toxic side effects were described in these studies. Whereas NO treatment with concentrations below 20 ppm NO were not associated with any clinically important formation of methemoglobin, maximum methemoglobin in patients treated with 40 ppm NO was reported to be $3.0 \pm 0.3\%$.[16] However, it has been observed that in some patients after long-term NO inhalation, a rebound phenomenon occurred.[34,35] Discontinuation of NO led, for various time periods, to extremely high PAP and low PaO_2. After this period, without any interventions, the PAP decreased and PaO_2 increased again, even if not to the same values as during NO inhalation. The authors suspect that in these patients a negative feedback mecha-

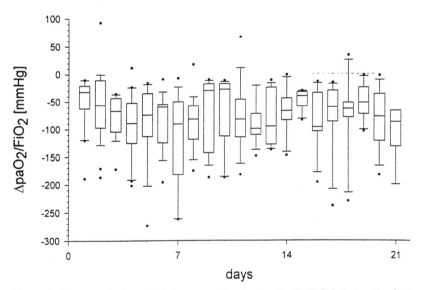

Figure 3. Changes in the arterial oxygenation index (PaO_2/FiO_2) during the first 3 weeks when briefly stopping continuous NO inhalation. 11.5 ± 1.4 ppm NO was inhaled in 30 patients for 17 ± 2.4 days. Box-and-whisker plot: The five horizontal lines on the box show the 10th, 25th, 50th (median), 75th, and 90th percentiles. The values above and below the 10th and 90th percentile are represented as data points.

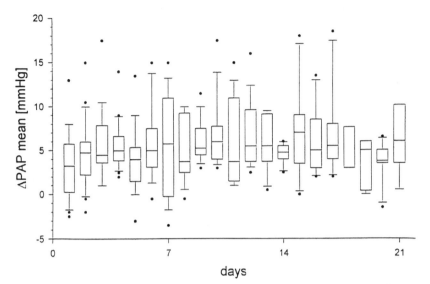

Figure 4. Changes in mean pulmonary artery pressure (PAP) during the first 3 weeks when briefly stopping continuous NO inhalation. 11.5±1.4 ppm NO was inhaled in 30 patients for 17±2.4 days. Box-and whisker plot: The five horizontal lines on the box show the 10th, 25th, 50th (median), 75th, and 90th percentiles. The values above and below the 10th and 90th percentile are represented as data points.

nism is present; inhaled NO suppresses the endogenous NO production, especially in ventilated lung areas. Therefore, stopping the exogenous NO administration causes in the normally vasodilated lung areas vasoconstriction resulting in the observed increase in PAP and, furthermore, in shift of pulmonary blood flow toward intrapulmonary shunt areas. In some of these patients the sometimes extensive increase in PAP may lead to right ventricular failure and death.[35] The hypothesis of the rebound phenomenon is supported by the observation that in vitro studies demonstrated an inhibition of the constitutive as well as the inducible NO synthase by high NO concentrations.[36,37]

Although there is ample evidence that low-dose NO induces a selective vasodilation in ventilated lung areas resulting in a significant rise in PaO_2, so far it has not been shown that NO inhalation influences the course and mortality of ARDS. In 1995, the first study was published that evaluated retrospectively the efficacy of NO inhalation regarding mortality in patients suffering from severe ARDS.[31] The authors formed matched pairs consisting of patients comparable regarding etiology and severity of their ARDS and number of other failed organs, who were or were not treated with NO. The survival rate in both groups (26 pairs) was 69%. In 1996, the preliminary results of a first prospective controlled study were reported: the mortality rate for both NO-treated patients and placebo patients was 30%.[38] Thus, presently there is no proof that inhalation of NO reduces mortality of ARDS in general or dependent on certain causes of ARDS.

Side Effects of Inhaled NO

Beside the aforementioned rebound phenomenon after discontinuation of long-term NO inhalation, one must be aware that NO inhalation may influence coagulation. Endogenously formed NO, acting synergistically with PGI_2, is known to have potent platelet antiaggregating and disaggregating properties by increasing the concentrations of cyclic guanosine monophosphate intracellularly.[39,40] Högman and coworkers observed that inhalation of low concentrations of NO prolonged bleeding time in anesthetized rabbits inhaling 30 ppm NO for 15 minutes, from 51 ± 5 seconds during baseline to 72 ± 7 seconds during NO inhalation.[41] In contrast, Samama et al[42] demonstrated that the beneficial effects of NO inhalation on pulmonary circulation and gas exchange in patients with ARDS are associated with a reduced in vitro aggregation of platelets to collagen, adenosine diphosphate, and ristocetin, but that this antithrombotic effect did not cause a significant prolongation of the bleeding time. Nevertheless, certain anticoagulatory effects should be taken into account when NO inhalation is used in patients who carry a high risk of bleeding complications, ie, premature newborns or postsurgical patients. On the other hand, this anticoagulatory effect of NO inhalation may be beneficial in severe ARDS, since ARDS lungs often show extensive formation of thrombi throughout the lung vasculature. This view may be supported by a prospective randomized animal study showing that NO inhalation is able to attenuate the accumulation of platelets as well as neutrophils in the lungs, when a sham hemodialysis model is used.[43]

In addition, the possibility must be considered that increased production of endogenous NO plays an important role in the development of acute lung injury. At least the involvement of endogenous NO production has been demonstrated in models of acute lung injury, which are oxygen radical-dependent.[44] In tissues, NO may react with O_2, yielding the nitrosodioxyl radical ($ONOO^-$). Under normal physiological conditions, little $ONOO^-$ is formed. Pathological conditions such as acute lung injury involve simultaneous increases in endogenous NO and O_2^-, resulting in increased formation of $ONOO^-$, which then, in turn, may facilitate lipid peroxidation.[45] However, on the other hand, this reaction may scavenge O_2^- from further reactions, leading to more potent oxidants such as hydroxyl radical. Since both reactions may result in potentially harmful molecules, it remains speculative whether the net effect of exogenous NO is protective against oxidant-mediated lung injury or whether it enhances ARDS.

Furthermore, NO and its oxidized version NO_2 may exert a direct toxic effect. In animal experiments and in humans, NO concentrations above 5000 ppm seem to rapidly lead to methemoglobinemia and a toxic pulmonary edema.[46,47] However, if NO is inhaled in concentrations of <50 ppm, it appears to have no acute toxic effects. In 1975, Oda et al[48] reported that there are only very low NO-Hb concentrations in the blood (0.13% of the total Hb) and low methemoglobin levels (0.2% of the total Hb) when 10 ppm NO are inhaled. Mice have been exposed to 10 ppm NO for 6 months without a rise in methemoglobin but with a slight enlargement of the spleen and a small rise in bilirubin.[49] In general, the clinical reports on methemoglobin during NO inhalation confirm that methemoglobin levels remain in a safe range. However, the authors observed in one newborn who received 50 ppm NO for treatment of severe pulmonary hypertension after cardiac surgery, a methemoglobin level of 15% which might be explained by an insufficiency of methemoglobin reductase. Therefore, they believe that the intermittent measurement of the methemoglobin level is obligatory when using NO inhalation. Nevertheless, techniques of NO administration must take into consideration the conversion of NO to NO_2, which occurs in proportion to the concentration of NO and the environmental FiO_2. NO_2, which is a strong oxidizing gas, initiates lipid peroxidation, resulting in cell injury or cell death.[50] Acute effects inducing pulmonary edema could be observed during controlled exposure to NO_2 in concentrations above 50 ppm.[46,47] However, even the prolonged exposure to such low concentrations as 2.3 ppm NO_2 may cause delayed effects, as it reduces the glutathione peroxidase activity, which offers antioxidative defense, by 14%.[51] The same concentration also decreases alveolar permeability, measured as the [99m]Technitium-Diethylenetriamine pentaacetic acid clearance rate, which is considered to be a noninvasive assessment of the integrity of the alveolar epithelium, by 22%.[51] These findings stress the importance of avoiding, or at least minimizing, NO_2 exposure. Therefore, the concentrations of NO should be as low as possible and furthermore, with use of adequate techniques of NO administration, the contact time between oxygen and NO should be as short as possible.

Conclusion

In patients with severe ARDS, inhalation of NO decreased pulmonary hypertension and improved arterial oxygenation to a clinically relevant extent by diverting blood flow away from areas of intrapulmonary shunt to areas of normal ventilation/perfusion ratio. Adding NO to the inhaled gas allowed for reduction of the FiO_2 by approximately 15%, which minimizes exposure to high concentrations of inhaled oxygen and may reduce its pulmonary toxicity. Since high inspiratory oxygen concentrations as well as high airway pressures must been seen as factors which, in themselves, contribute to the progression of the disease, NO inhalation represents a further strategy to reduce aggressive ventilator settings. Therefore, NO therapy compliments—and does not replace—other means to treat ARDS, such as pressure-limited mechanical ventilation with PEEP and permissive hypercapnea, selective ventilation of the lungs, positioning, dehydration, and, finally, if all other means fail to improve arterial oxygenation, extracorporeal gas exchange. Especially in Europe, in most referral centers for treatment of ARDS, all these therapeutic options are used in combination, each part possibly improving pulmonary gas exchange to a certain extent. It is not believed that NO inhalation is superior to other treatments of ARDS, however, the parallel use of all the above-mentioned strategies might finally result in survival. No single life saving treatment exists. Neither mechanical ventilation in the prone position, adequate dehydration, nor extracorporeal lung support have been proven to increase survival in ARDS. Therefore, today, therapy of ARDS consists of a bundle of complementary therapeutic means. NO inhalation may become part of it.

References

1 Ashbaugh DG, Bigelow DB, Petty TL, Levine BE. Acute respiratory distress in adults. *Lancet* 1967;2:319–323.

2. Krafft P, Fridrich P, Pernerstorfer T, et al. The acute respiratory distress syndrome: Definitions, severity and clinical outcome. An analysis of 101 clinical investigations. *Intensive Care Med* 1996;22:519–529.

3. Barber RE, Lee J, Hamilton WK. Oxygen toxicity in man. A prospective study in patients with irreversible brain damage. *N Engl J Med* 1970;283;1478–1484.

4. Kolobow T, Moretti MP, Fumagalli R, et al. Severe impairment in lung function induced by high peak airway pressure during mechanical ventilation. An experimental study. *Am Rev Respir Dis* 1987;135:312–315.

5. Rossaint R, Slama K, Falke KJ. Therapy of acute pulmonary failure. *Dtsch Med Wochnschr* 1991;116:1635–1639.

6. Furchgott RF, Zawadzki JV. The obligatory role of endothelial cells in the relaxation of arterial smooth muscle by acetylcholine. *Nature* 1980;288:373–376.

7. Ignarro LJ, Buga GM, Wood KS, Byrns RE, Chaudhuri G. Endothelium-derived relaxing factor produced and released from artery and vein is nitric oxide. *Proc Natl Acad Sci U S A* 1987;84:9265–9269.

8. Palmer RM, Ferrige AG, Moncada S. Nitric oxide release accounts for the biological activity of endothelium-derived relaxing factor. *Nature* 1987;327:524–526.

9. Higenbottam T, Pepke-Zaba J, Scott J, Woolman P, Coutts C, Wallwork J. Inhaled "endothelium derived-relaxing factor" (EDRF) in primary hypertension. *Am Rev Respir Dis* 1988;137:107.

10. Frostell C, Fratacci MD, Wain JC, Jones R, Zapol WM. Inhaled nitric oxide. A selective pulmonary vasodilator reversing hypoxic pulmonary vasoconstriction. *Circulation* 1991;83:2038–2047.

11. Pison U, Lopez FA, Heidelmeyer CF, Rossaint R, Falke K. Inhaled nitric oxide selectively reverses hypoxic pulmonary vasoconstriction without impairing pulmonary gas exchange. *J Appl Physiol* 1993;74:1287–1292.

12. Falke K, Rossaint R, Pison U, et al. Inhaled nitric oxide selectively reduces pulmonary hypertension in severe ARDS and improves gas exchange as well as right heart ejection fraction: A case report. *Am Rev Respir Dis* 1991;143(suppl A):248.

13. Rossaint R, Falke KJ, Lopez F, Slama K, Pison U, Zapol WM. Inhaled nitric oxide in adult respiratory distress syndrome. *N Engl J Med* 1993;328: 399–405.

14. Benzing A, Geiger K. Inhaled nitric oxide lowers pulmonary capillary pressure and changes longitudinal distribution of pulmonary vascular resistance in patients with acute lung injury. *Acta Anaesthesiol Scand* 1994; 38:640–645.

15. Bigatello LM, Hurtord WE, Kacmarek RM, Roberts JD Jr, Zapol WM. Prolonged inhalation of low concentrations of nitric oxide in patients with severe adult respiratory distress syndrome. Effects on pulmonary hemodynamics and oxygenation. *Anesthesiology* 1994;80:761–770.

16. Day RW, Guarin M, Lynch JM, Vernon DD, Dean JM. Inhaled nitric oxide in children with severe lung disease: Results of acute and prolonged therapy with two concentrations. *Crit Care Med* 1996;24:215–221.

17. Fierobe L, Brunet F, Dhainaut JF, et al. Effect of inhaled nitric oxide on right ventricular function in adult respiratory distress syndrome. *Am J Respir Crit Care Med* 1995;151:1414–1419.

18. Krafft P, Fridrich P, Fitzgerald D, Koc D, Steltzer H. Effectiveness of nitric oxide inhalation in septic ARDS. *Chest* 1996;109:486–493.

19. Puybasset L, Rouby JJ, Mourgeon E, et al. Factors influencing cardiopulmonary effects of inhaled nitric oxide in acute respiratory failure. *Am J Respir Crit Care Med* 1995;152:318–328.

20. Puybasset L, Rouby JJ, Mourgeon E, et al. Inhaled nitric oxide in acute respiratory failure: Dose-response curves. *Intensive Care Med* 1994;20: 319–327.

21. Rossaint R, Slama K, Steudel W, et al. Effects of inhaled nitric oxide on right ventricular function in severe acute respiratory distress syndrome. *Intensive Care Med* 1995;21:197–203.

22. Gerlach H, Rossaint R, Pappert D, Knorr M, Falke KJ. Autoinhalation of nitric oxide after endogenous synthesis in nasopharynx. *Lancet* 1994;343: 518–519.

23. Lundberg JON, Farkas-Szallasi T, Weitzberg E, et al. High nitric oxide production in human paranasal sinuses. *Nature Medicine* 1995;1:370–373.

24. Schedin U, Frostell C, Persson MG, Jakobsson J, Anderson G, Gustafsson LE. Contribution from upper and lower airways to exhaled endogenous nitric oxide in humans. *Acta Anaesthesiol Scand* 1995;39:327–332.

25. Gerlach H, Rossaint R, Pappert D, Falke KJ. Time-course and dose-response of nitric oxide inhalation for systemic oxygenation and pulmonary hypertension in patients with adult respiratory distress syndrome. *Eur J Clin Invest* 1993;23:499–502.

26. Kelly KP, Busch T, Gerlach H, Rossaint R: Arterial oxygenation during replacement of a physiological concentration of nitric oxide in intubated patients. *Intensive Care Med* 1996;22:S137.

27. McQuillan LP, Leung GK, Marsden PA, Kostyk SK, Kourembanas S. Hypoxia inhibits expression of eNOS via transcriptional and posttranscriptional mechanisms. *Am J Physiol* 1994;267:H1921–H1927.

28. Benzing A, Brautigam P, Geiger K, Loop T, Beyer U, Moser E. Inhaled nitric oxide reduces pulmonary transvascular albumin flux in patients with acute lung injury. *Anesthesiology* 1995;83:1153–1161.

29. Wysocki M, Vignon P, Roupie E, et al. Improvement in right ventricular function with inhaled nitric oxide in patients with the adult respiratory distress syndrome (ARDS) and permissive hypercapnia. *Am Rev Respir Dis* 1993;147:A350.

30. Dyar O, Young JD, Xiong L, Howell S, Johns E. Dose-response relationship for inhaled nitric oxide in experimental pulmonary hypertension in sheep. *Br J Anaesth* 1993;71:702–708.

31. Rossaint R, Gerlach H, Schmidt-Runke H, et al. Efficacy of nitric oxide inhalation in severe ARDS. *Chest* 1995;107:1107–1115.

32. Puybasset L, Stewart T, Rouby JJ, et al. Inhaled nitric oxide reverses the increase in pulmonary vascular resistance induced by permissive hypercapnia in patients with acute respiratory distress syndrome. *Anesthesiology* 1994;80:1254–1267.

33. Kouyoumdjian C, Adnot S, Levame M, Eddahibi S, Bousbaa H, Raffestin B. Continuous inhalation of nitric oxide protects against development of pulmonary hypertension in chronically hypoxic rats. *J Clin Invest* 1994; 94:578–584.

34. Gerlach H, Pappert D, Lewandowski K, Rossaint R, Falke KJ. Long-term inhalation with evaluated low doses of nitric oxide for selective improvement of oxygenation in patients with adult respiratory distress syndrome. *Intensive Care Med* 1993;19:443–449.

35. Chiche JD, Canivet JL, Damas P, Joris J, Lamy M. Inhaled nitric oxide for hemodynamic support after postpneumonectomy ARDS. *Intensive Care Med* 1995;21:675–678.

36. Assreuy J, Cunha FQ, Liew FY, Moncada S. Feedback inhibition of nitric oxide synthase activity by nitric oxide. *Br J Pharmacol* 1993;108:833–837.

37. Rogers NE, Ignarro LJ. Constitutive nitric oxide synthase from cerebellum is reversibly inhibited by nitric oxide formed from L-arginine. *Biochem Biophys Res Commun* 1992;189:242–249.

38. Dellinger RP, Zimmerman JL, Hyers TM, et al. Inhaled nitric oxide in ARDS: Preliminary results of a multicenter clinical trial. *Crit Care Med* 1996;24(suppl 1):A29.

39. Radomski MW, Moncada S. Regulation of vascular homeostasis by nitric oxide. *Thromb Haemost* 1993;70:36–41.

40. Radomski MW, Palmer RM, Moncada S. Endogenous nitric oxide inhibits human platelet adhesion to vascular endothelium. *Lancet* 1987;2:1057–1058.

41. Högman M, Frostell C, Arnberg H, Sandhagen B, Hedenstierna G. Prolonged bleeding time during nitric oxide inhalation in the rabbit. *Acta Physiol Scand* 1994;151:125–129.

42. Samama CM, Diaby M, Fellahi JL, et al. Inhibition of platelet aggregation by inhaled nitric oxide in patients with acute respiratory distress syndrome. *Anesthesiology* 1995;83:56–65.

43. Malmros C, Blomquist S, Dahm P, Martensson L, Thorne J. Nitric oxide

inhalation decreases pulmonary platelet and neutrophil sequestration during extracorporeal circulation in the pig. *Crit Care Med* 1996;24: 845–849.

44. Berisha HI, Pakbaz H, Absood A, Said SI. Nitric oxide as a mediator of ox-idant lung injury due to paraquat. *Proc Natl Acad Sci U S A* 1994;91: 7445–7449.

45. Radi R, Beckman JS, Bush KM, Freeman BA. Peroxynitrite-induced mem-brane lipid peroxidation: The cytotoxic potential of superoxide and nitric oxide. *Arch Biochem Biophys* 1991;288:481–487.

46. Clutton-Brock J. Two cases of poisoning by contamination of nitrous ox-ide with higher oxides of nitrogen during anaesthesia. *Br J Anaesth* 1967; 39:388–392.

47. Greenbaum R, Bay J, Hargreaves MD, et al. Effects of higher oxides of ni-trogen on the anaesthetized dog. *Br J Anaesth* 1967;39:393–404.

48. Oda H, Kusumoto S, Nakajima T. Nitrosyl-hemoglobin formation in the blood of animals exposed to nitric oxide. *Arch Environ Health* 1975;30: 453–456.

49. Oda H, Nogami H, Kusumoto S, Nakajima T, Kurata A, Imai K. Long-term exposure to nitric oxide in mice. *J Jpn Soc Air Pollut* 1976;11:150–160.

50. Thomas HV, Mueller PK, Lyman RL. Lipid peroxydation of lung lipids in rat exposed to nitrogen dioxide. *Science* 1968;159:532–534.

51. Rasmussen TR, Kjaergaard SK, Tarp U, Pedersen OF. Delayed effects of NO$_2$ exposure on alveolar permeability and glutathione peroxidase in healthy humans. *Am Rev Respir Dis* 1992;146:654–659.

Chapter 26

Pulmonary Vascular Control Mechanisms in Sepsis and Acute Lung Injury

*Nicholas P. Curzen, PhD, MRCP and
Timothy W. Evans, BSc, MD, FRCP,PhD, EDICM*

Lung Injury, the Adult Respiratory Distress Syndrome, and "Sepsis Syndromes"

Lung injury may complicate a wide range of pulmonary and extrapulmonary pathologies (Table 1), and ranges in clinical severity from mild acute lung injury (ALI) to the acute respiratory distress syndrome (ARDS) (Table 2). Lung injury is common; in one study, 35% of a population with sepsis had mild to moderate lung injury, while 25% had severe lung injury or fully developed ARDS,[1] with an associated mortality of between 50% and 75%. Lung injury rarely occurs in isolation, and is now considered to be the pulmonary manifestation of a multisystem inflammatory vascular disorder (Figure 1).[1,2] ALI and ARDS are characterized by impaired pulmonary gas exchange and a failure of oxygen uptake in the periphery, which ultimately leads to multiple organ failure (MOF). Indeed, it is the associated clinical conditions and coexisting organ failures that appear to be the major determinants of survival.[2,3] In one study for example, respiratory failure accounted for only 16% of deaths, the majority being attributable to MOF.[4] It is therefore not surprising that sepsis occurs up to six times more commonly in patients with ARDS compared to other critically ill patients,[4,5] or that up to 25% of cases of established

N.C. is supported by a Medical Research Training Fellowship

From: Weir EK, Reeves JT (eds). *Pulmonary Edema.* Armonk, NY: Futura Publishing Company, Inc.; ©1998.

Table 1

Clinical Conditions Associated With the Development of ARDS

Respiratory	Nonrespiratory
Pneumonia (Bacterial/Viral/Fungal)	Sepsis syndrome
Aspiration of gastric contents	Major Trauma/Shock
Pulmonary contusion	Massive burns
Postpneumonectomy	DIC
Inhalation of smoke or toxins	Transfusion reactions
Near drowning	Fat embolism
Thoracic irradiation	Pregnancy-associated (eg, amniotic fluid embolism)
Oxygen toxicity	Pancreatitis
Ischemia-reperfusion	Drug/Toxin reactions (eg, paraquat, heroin)
Vasculitis (eg, Goodposture's)	Post-CP bypass
	Head injury/raised ICP
	Tumor Lysis syndrome

ARDS = acute respiratory distress syndrome; DIC = disseminated intravascular coagulopathy; CP = cardiopulmonary; ICP = intracranial pressure.

Table 2

Definitions of Acute Lung Injury (ALI) and Acute Respiratory Distress Syndrome (ARDS)

	Timing	Oxygenation	Chest Radiograph	Pulmonary Artery Occlusion Pressure
ALI criteria	Acute onset	PaO_2/FIO_2 <300 mm Hg (regardless of PEEP level)	Bilateral infiltrates seen on frontal CXR	<18 mm Hg when measured, or no clinical evidence of left atrial hypertension
ARDS criteria	Acute onset	PaO_2/FIO_2 <200 mm Hg (regardless of PEEP level)	Bilateral infiltrates seen on frontal CXR	<18 mm Hg when measured, or no clinical evidence of left atrial hypertension

PEEP = positive end-expiratory pressure; CXR = chest x-ray.

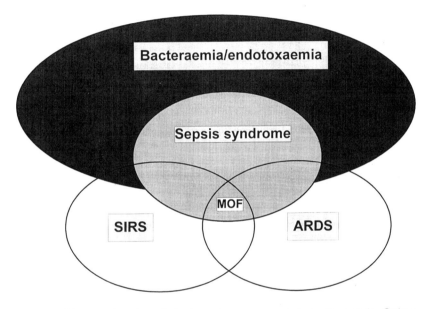

Figure 1. The overlapping clinical syndromes associated with sepsis: Only a proportion of these syndromes are associated with the identification of an infective agent. More frequently there is detectable endotoxemia, but in some, neither of these are present. SIRS = systemic inflammatory response syndrome; MOF= multiple organ failure; ARDS = acute respiratory distress syndrome. For full definitions of each syndrome, see Reference 14.

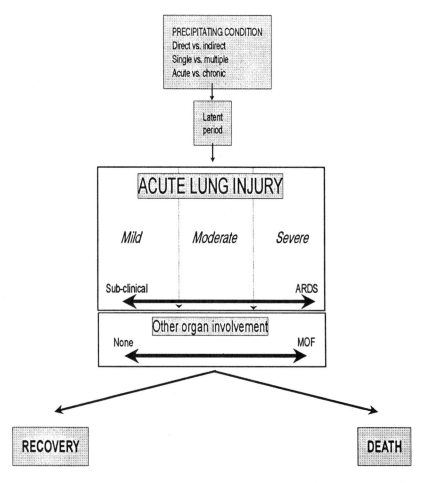

Figure 2. Acute lung injury: the spectrum of disease. Lung injury can occur in response to a wide variety of insults. The response of an individual is unpredictable, and the subsequent injury may present with characteristic clinical sequelae, the most severe form of which is full-blown ARDS, or it may be subclinical. Other organs may also be affected to a variable extent, and the most severe clinical end of this spectrum is multiple organ failure. Currently the ability to predict which patients are at high risk of developing significant lung injury (and other organ damage), as well as those with established ARDS who will survive, is seen as a research priority. MOF = multiple organ failure; ARDS = acute respiratory distress syndrome.

sepsis or systemic inflammatory response (SIRS) are complicated by ARDS. These clinical syndromes are associated with the positive identification of an infecting causative organism in less than 50% of cases. The mortality in those patients with septic shock is between 60% and 90%.

Lung injury and ARDS are thus clinically recognizable sequelae of a complex inflammatory reaction to diverse insults, so that very frequently other organs are involved in the clinical pathology (Figure 2). The vascular endothelium therefore represents the fulcrum over which this inflammatory response balances between clinical or subclinical importance.

Pathogenesis of Lung Injury

The inflammatory response to sepsis is most frequently initiated by endotoxin, a lipopolysaccharide component of the cell wall of gram-negative bacteria,[6] and the consequent generation and release of a cascade of inflammatory mediators such as tumor necrosis factor-α (TNFα), interleukins (IL)$-1,-8$, and-6, and platelet activating factor (PAF), from neutrophils, macrophages, platelets, and endothelium (Figure 3).[7] Infusion of lipopolysaccharide (LPS) or TNFα in animals reproduces some of the clinical features of sepsis, including acute lung injury.[8] Critically ill patients with sepsis have high levels of serum LPS, and those with ARDS frequently have detectable endotoxemia.[9] Further, raised levels of TNFα and IL-1 have been demonstrated in both serum and bronchoalveolar lavage fluid from patients with ARDS.[10,11] Subsequent activation of neutrophils by endotoxin or other agents is one of the earliest events in the pathogenesis of lung injury,[12] and bronchoalveolar lavage (BAL) fluid taken from patients with ARDS contains increased numbers of neutrophils, as well as excessive amounts of neutrophil-generated proteinase enzymes such as elastase and collagenase.[13]

Activation and injury of the endothelium is central to the inflammatory response to endotoxin and to the resultant functional and structural changes that occur in the pulmonary vasculature. Endotoxin, TNFα, and other cytokines are all capable of inducing endothelial cell injury,[14] thus stimulating ultrastructural changes within the cells and leading to increased permeability.[15] Endothelial cell activation also facilitates the adherence and subsequent migration from blood to tissue of activated neutrophils, mediated by adhesion molecules. Migration occurs principally in postcapillary venules, in which white cells marginate as a result of loose tethering to the underlying endothelium. Subsequently, the neutrophils become more adherent,

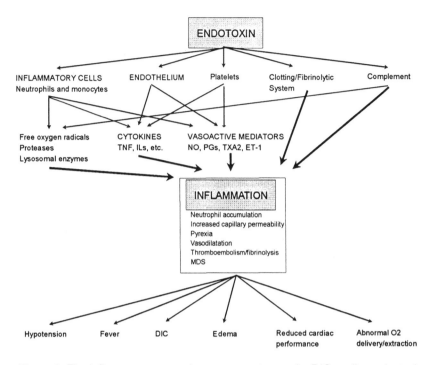

Figure 3. The inflammatory vascular response to sepsis. DIC = disseminated intravascular coagulopathy.

changing from spherical to a flatter shape. This facilitates their slow migration between endothelial cells, through the basement membrane into the interstitium. This process is now known to be mediated by interaction of specific cell adhesion molecules (CAM) on the surface of both the neutrophil and endothelial cell in a sequence known as the adhesion cascade.[16] This process is reviewed in detail elsewhere.[17]

The endothelium has other facets of its inflammatory activation, most important of which is a group of endotoxin/cytokine-inducible genes that results in the expression of mRNA coding for a range of proteins including cyclooxygenase (COX), constitutive nitric oxide synthase (cNOS), inducible nitric oxide synthase (iNOS), and endothelins (Figure 4). It is the release of these potent vasoactive and inflammatory mediators that allows the endothelium to modulate the vascular response to sepsis. When the inflammatory response is widespread and severe, intense activation of the endothelium in some areas and damage to it in others contribute to the clinical syndromes described above.

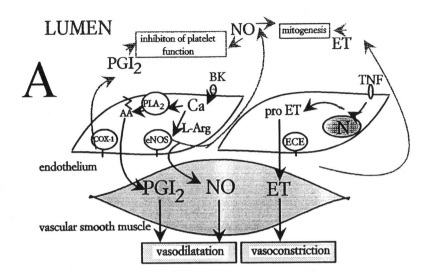

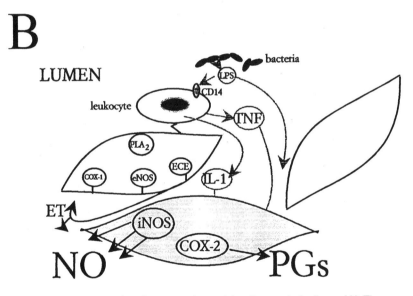

Figure 4. The vasoactive factors released by the endothelium: (A) The endothelial cell contributes to vascular tone and local anticoagulation by the tonic release of several mediators including nitric oxide (NO) via eNOS, prostacyclin (PGI_2) via COX-1, and endothelin-1 (ET-1). These are released both basally and into the vessel lumen. (B) In sepsis, the presence of endotoxin and a variety of early inflammatory cytokines results in endothelial cell activation and disruption. The activated cells produce larger quantities of NO (via iNOS), PGI_2 (via COX-2), and ET-1. At the same time, however, the underlying smooth muscle undergoes iNOS induction, resulting in the production of massive quantities of NO. It seems likely that the degree of local damage to the endothelium may determine the vascular response to the initial inflammatory insult, and that on a larger scale this may contribute to the clinical outcome.

Pathophysiology of Acute Lung Injury

Acute lung injury and ARDS are clinical diagnoses, although the criteria have only recently been standardized.[18] Pulmonary endothelial damage can lead to mild respiratory impairment or overwhelming alveolar edema, and clinical scoring systems are now commonly used to categorize patients,[19] greatly increasing the utility of such studies.[20]

Clinical studies have identified elevated pulmonary vascular resistance (PVR) as a universal finding in patients with acute respiratory failure.[21] In ARDS, PVR is increased via a combination of increased vascular tone and structural factors such as extrinsic compression by edema fluid, positive pressure ventilation, thromboemboli, or remodeling of the vessel.[22] In ARDS, pulmonary hypertension contributes to pulmonary edema formation[2] and impaired right ventricular performance and has been identified with an increased mortality.[23]

In some patients with ARDS and sepsis, an abnormal relationship between oxygen delivery (DO_2) and peripheral oxygen uptake (VO_2) has been identified.[24] Provided it is maintained above a critical level, VO_2 is normally independent of DO_2 at rest, but in ARDS, VO_2 becomes DO_2-dependent, so that the oxygen extraction ratio remains constant. Critically ill patients who manifest this pathological "supply dependency" have a higher mortality rate than those who do not.[25] This tendency, and the apparent inability of the peripheral tissues to extract oxygen, has not yet been clearly explained, but it has subsequently been shown[26] that critically ill patients in whom supraphysiological targets for cardiac output, DO_2, and VO_2 are attained have a lower incidence of MOF and mortality, although this hypothesis is the subject of some controversy. Possible pathophysiological mechanisms to account for this widespread microvascular dysfunction include: loss of microvascular control with shunting, tissue edema, compression of capillaries, and microembolization. These changes can be largely explained by the degree of endothelial injury involved in these inflammatory conditions.

Hypoxic Pulmonary Vasoconstriction and Lung Injury

Hypoxic pulmonary vasoconstriction (HPV) is a physiological response by which blood flow is diverted away from hypoxic alveoli, with the *beneficial* result that perfusion (Q) and ventilation (V) remain "matched." HPV is a homeostatic control mechanism which is disrupted in ALI/ARDS.[27] This is of significance in ARDS because alveolar edema and atelectasis can induce enormous increases in physiological dead space. Investigations using the multiple inert gas technique[28] have demonstrated that the degree of intrapulmonary shunting is large enough to account for the observed alveolar\arterial PO_2 gradient, even without invoking a reduction in diffusion capacity.

The endothelium has the capability to modulate HPV in several ways. In some species there is a requirement for an intact pulmonary vascular endothelium so that hypoxia can elicit a contractile response,[29] and hypoxia-induced contractions of pulmonary arteries are reduced by endothelial removal.[30] However, endothelial injury can enhance HPV[31] and in the longer term, structural alterations in pulmonary endothelial cells may also contribute to the development of hypoxic pulmonary hypertension.[32] The endothelium removes circulating vasoconstrictor substances[33] and, more importantly, it releases a range of vasoactive agents locally; a change in the dynamic balance of these factors can modulate the vascular tonic response.

Endothelium-Derived Factors Capable of Modifying Pulmonary Vascular Tone in Lung Injury

Nitric Oxide

In 1980, the vascular relaxation induced by acetylcholine was shown to be dependent on the presence of intact endothelium and to be mediated via the release of an endothelium-derived relaxant factor (EDRF).[34] The chemical and pharmacological properties of EDRF are shared by nitric oxide (NO). Nitric oxide is synthesized from the amino acid, L-arginine, by a group of flavin-containing oxygenase enzymes commonly termed nitric oxide synthase (NOS), a process that can be inhibited by L-arginine analogues such as N^G-monomethyl-L-arginine (L-NMMA).[35] Endothelial cells were the first mammalian cells shown to release NO, a potent vasodilator.[36] NO relaxes blood vessels by activating soluble guanylate cyclase, the resultant increase in cyclic guanine monophosphate (cGMP) causing a quenching of intracellular calcium (Figure 4, panel A).[37] It is now accepted that various cell types can release NO and that at least three distinct isoforms of NOS exist (Table 3). Endothelial NOS (eNOS) and neuronal NOS (nNOS) are constitutive and calcium-dependent enzymes. A third isoform (iNOS) is induced by LPS and inflammatory cytokines. The cDNA for all three types of NOS have now been purified, cloned, sequenced, and expressed. Although differences exist in the biochemistry of the three types of NOS, the basic pathway of metabolism of L-arginine to NO and L-citrulline is well conserved and all isoforms are inhibited by the L-arginine analogues L-NMMA and/or L-N^G nitro-L-arginine.[38-40] Such inhibitors cause a

Table 3

Vascular Isoforms of Nitric Oxide Synthase

NOS isoforms	eNOS	iNOS
Response in sepsis	Constitutive Immediate NO synthesis	Induced by LPS & cytokines Massive NO production after 2–6 hours
Location	Endothelial cell Membrane-bound	Mainly smooth muscle Cytosolic
Regulation	Estrogens, shear stress & exercise increase activity	Induction prevented by corticosteroids & inhibitors of protein synthesis
Activation	Calcium-dependent	Calcium-independent
Nonselective inhibitors	L-arginine analogues (eg, N^G-monomethyl L-arginine)	
Selective inhibitors	None known	Aminoguanidine L-canavanine

NO = Nitric oxide; NOS = Nitric oxide synthase (e = endothelial, i = inducible); LPS = Lipopolysaccharide.

rapid increase in blood pressure in animals[41]and in humans,[42] suggesting that in health, NO is required in order to maintain vascular tone.

Nitric Oxide and Sepsis (Figure 4, panel B)

Activation of the endothelium by agents such as bradykinin, PAF, and LPS causes a release of NO, following eNOS stimulation.[43] However, it has been demonstrated that both iNOS activity[44,45] and its messenger RNA expression are elevated in many organs, including the lung and pulmonary vasculature, in rats after LPS administration.[46] Furthermore, levels of NO metabolites are increased in patients with septic shock, and the administration of NOS inhibitors in those patients,[42] or in animals treated with LPS,[47] results in a recovery of blood pressure. In some models the effects of LPS are mimicked by cytokines (eg, IL-1b and TNFα) released in sepsis. Of the organs studied, the lung appears to be a major site for iNOS expression.[45,48] Indeed, iNOS messenger RNA has been demonstrated in the pulmonary artery from rats treated with LPS, where NO release seems to be responsible for the vascular hyporesponsiveness to constrictor agents observed after LPS.[49] The induction of iNOS in lung tissue[47] and in pulmonary arteries[49] is inhibited by dexamethasone. Interestingly, there seems to be a reciprocal relationship between the levels of eNOS and iNOS messenger RNA in rat tissues after LPS. Thus, preliminary data from Liu and colleagues[50] suggest that during sepsis, the well-characterized endothelial dysfunction may be compounded by a reduction in eNOS expression in any surviving cells.

Endotoxin leads to the induction of iNOS in both the endothelium and vascular smooth muscle,[51,52] as well as in the myocardium, where increased NO production has been shown to reduce contractility.[53,54] Other cytokines (TNFα, IL-1, and IL-2) also stimulate iNOS activity in vessel walls.

The time course of the increase in NO release in sepsis is the subject of considerable speculation. In a rat model of sepsis in vivo,[47] the NO-mediated hyporeactivity to noradrenaline starts within 60 minutes and may therefore be too rapid to be explained by the induction of iNOS. It seems more likely that this early increase in NO release is explained by an elevation in NO production by endothelial cNOS. However, 3 hours after the endotoxic insult, there is a massive increase in NO production as a result of iNOS activity in the endothelium and vascular smooth muscle. Furthermore, the endothelium appears to be required for maximal NO response, its removal causing a significant delay in the onset of vascular hyporesponsiveness (6 hours, compared with 4 hours) of rat aorta to LPS in vitro.

In sepsis, the induction of iNOS would be expected to reduce the degree of local HPV; however, recent evidence from pulmonary artery and aortic rings from lipopolysaccharide-treated rats investigated in vitro suggests that not only does hypoxia inhibit cNOS, but it also inhibits LPS-induced iNOS.[55]

Endothelins

In 1988 an endothelially derived vasoconstrictor was cloned and sequenced following its isolation from the culture medium of porcine aortic endothelial cells.[56] This substance, termed endothelin (ET), was found to elicit a slow sustained contraction of isolated arteries from many different species. Three ET-related genomic loci have been identified that encode for three similar but distinct 21 amino acid ET peptides (ET-1, ET-2, ET-3),[57] produced following cleavage of a prepropeptide via a propeptide. This conversion is mediated by the activity of one of a family of endothelin-converting enzymes (ECE), of which there are several types; preliminary evidence suggests that there is at least one form available on the cell membrane to handle circulating "Big ET," and two intracellular forms involved in mature ET-1 production and release.

ET-1 immunoreactivity cannot be demonstrated in homogenates of capillary endothelial cells, and release of ET from cultured endothelium can be prevented by a protein synthesis inhibitor, suggesting that ETs are not stored, but rather synthesized de novo. Factors that have been found to be capable of stimulating ET release are diverse and include vessel wall shear stress, hypoxia, endotoxin, TNFα, interferon, adrenaline, angiotensin, thrombin, activated platelets, and some prostanoids (Figure 5). Local ET release would therefore be expected during any inflammatory response. ET induces smooth muscle contraction via several secondary messenger pathways whose final common pathway is to increase free intracellular calcium (Figure 4, panel A). Phospholipase C activation with increases in inositol triphosphate and diaglycerol synthesis is thought to be the principal effector system, although protein kinase C is also involved.[58]

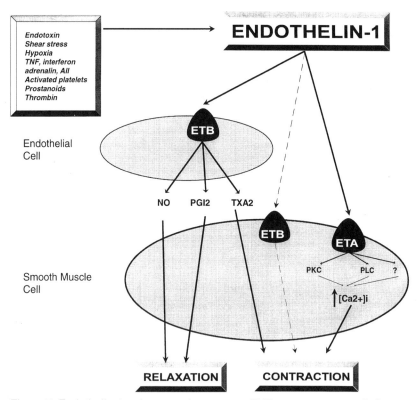

Figure 5. Endothelin-1: release and receptors. TNF = tumour necrosis factor-α; AII = angiotensin II; PKC = phosphokinase C; PLC = phospholipase C; [Ca^{2+}] = intracellular free calcium.

Two ET receptor subtypes have so far been cloned and expressed. ET_A has a higher affinity for ET-1 than ET-2 or ET-3, and has widespread expression, particularly on vascular smooth muscle, but it has not been found on endothelial cells. ET_B is nonselective, binding all three ETs equally avidly so that they are equipotent in their displacement of ^{125}ET-1. ET_B is found on vascular endothelium and also on smooth muscle in some vascular beds. At first it was thought that ET_A receptor stimulation was responsible for the direct constrictor effects of ET and that ET_B receptor stimulation resulted in the release of other vasoactive factors from those cells. ET-1 is certainly a potent vasoconstrictor in humans and animals by direct stimulation of ET_A receptors, a response which the endothelium can modulate via ET_B receptor stimulation. However, it has recently become apparent that ET_B receptors exist on some vascular smooth muscle and mediate contraction directly, and that some ET_A receptors are capable of stimulating prostanoid release.[59,61] There is now also clear evidence from both in vitro and in vivo studies that ETs release NO from the endothelium by ET_B receptor stimulation. This gives rise to the characteristic hemodynamic responses of rats (and other species) to intravenous ET-1, in which there is an initial transient fall in systemic blood pressure followed by a sustained pressor response.[56] Only the former can be attenuated by L-NMMA pretreatment[62] and only the latter can be attenuated by ET_A receptor antagonists such as BQ123.[58] There is also evidence that ET-1 can stimulate the release of prostacyclin and thromboxane from endothelial cells via ET_B receptors.

The effects of low-dose infusions of ET-1 have been studied in humans[63]; they cause a rise in systemic and pulmonary arterial vascular resistances and a small fall in cardiac output. ET-1 is largely metabolized in the pulmonary circulation, while some is eliminated by the kidneys. The plasma half-life of a bolus of radiolabeled ET-1 in anaesthetized rats was 40 seconds in one study, with 82% uptake in the lungs and 10% in the kidneys.[64]

Endothelins in Sepsis

Plasma ET-1 levels are elevated in many animal models of sepsis, as well as in patients who are critically ill with sepsis; this possibly correlates with indicators of illness severity.[65] It is probable that ET-1 effects vascular tone as a result of autocrine and paracrine activity rather than as a circulating hormone, especially since release of ET-1 from endothelial cells appears to be polarized predominantly to the basal (abluminal) direction (Figure 4, panel B).[66] The expression of ET-1 mRNA in several tissues from endotoxin-treated rats (heart, lung, aorta, pulmonary artery) is significantly increased when compared with controls, although the time course for this increase varies from tissue to tissue, and none has been seen in skeletal muscle or kidney from the same animals.[67,68] Interestingly, the marked early increases in circulating ET-1 in patients with acute lung injury seen in one study[69] appeared to be due, at least in part, to reduced pulmonary metabolism of the peptide.

Despite potent effects on vascular tone, both direct and indirect, and unequivocal increases in ET-1 production and release in sepsis, the role of these peptides in sepsis remains unclear. Isolated pulmonary arteries from endotoxemic rats demonstrate hyporesponsiveness to exogenous ET-1, and complete contraction to ET-1 in these vessels is dependent on the presence of the endothelium.[70] By contrast, the intact pulmonary circulation of septic rats is hypersensitive to ET-1, an effect exacerbated by pretreatment with L-NMMA.[71] Furthermore, administration of nonselective ET antagonists has been shown to attenuate sepsis-associated pulmonary hypertension in pigs[72] but not in rats.[73] It is tempting to speculate that, as potent vasoconstrictors, ETs contribute to the reduction of regional blood flow seen in certain organ beds such as the gut, kidney, and lung during established sepsis, but further data are required. Administration of ET_A/ET_B antagonists to rats being infused with endotoxin exacerbates the systemic hypotensive response,[74] implying that ET-1 may afford some protection against the loss of systemic vascular tone seen in sepsis.

Arachidonic Acid Metabolites

Arachidonic acid is the precursor of a variety of vasoactive and inflammatory mediators implicated in the pathogenesis of sepsis. The first step in arachidonic acid metabolism is its liberation from membrane-bound phospholipids, usually by the actions of phospholipase A_2. Once free in the cell, arachidonic acid is metabolized by various oxygenase enzymes, such as COX, to form prostaglandins (PG), thromboxanes (TX), and prostacyclin (PGI_2) or lipoxygenase (LO) to form leukotrienes (LT). COX is now known to exist in constitutive (COX-1) and inducible (COX-2) isoforms.[75] It is thought that COX-2 predominates at the site of inflammation, including in the lung of rats 6 hours after LPS challenge.[76] Thus, COX-2 may represent the main source of prostanoids released in the lung during septic shock. The identification of COX-2 as a major inflammatory enzyme has promoted attempts to develop nonsteroidal anti-inflammatory drugs (NSAIDs), which specifically inhibit this isoform.[77]

Arachidonic Acid Metabolites in Sepsis

Cytokines stimulate prostanoid release both in vivo and in vitro. During the inflammatory response, generation of prostanoids and thromboxane (TXA_2) occurs in inflammatory cells such as macrophages, as well as in the endothelium. The release of PGI_2 and TXA_2 is controlled by individual cell types. Thus, endothelial cells form mainly PGI_2, whereas platelets and to a lesser extent, eosinophils and neutrophils, are the main sources of TXB_2. COX-2 induction and accompanying increases in PGI_2 have been demonstrated in humans treated with IL-1[78] and bovine endothelial cells treated with LPS[79] in intact human vessels[37] as well as in lung homogenates and aortic smooth muscle from rats treated with LPS.[76] The increased release of PGI_2 following COX-2 induction may therefore attenuate pulmonary hypertension associated with sepsis. Thus, the balance between the local production of vasodilator (PGI_2) and vasoconstrictor (TXA_2 and endoperoxides) agents in this way undoubtedly contributes to the vascular tone in that area.[80] The induction of COX-2 occurs from about 6 hours, and at about this time PGI_2 is released from cultured endothelial cells in response to endotoxin.[79] More specifically, IL-1, known to be one of the principal mediators that amplifies the early inflammatory response in sepsis, induces PGI_2 production from human endothelial cells.[78] Both IL-1 and TNF induce COX-2 mRNA expression in human endothelial cells. TXA_2 is a vasoconstrictor, and its inhibition has been shown to diminish the early pulmonary hypertension, but not the increased vascular permeability, in an experimental model of endotoxin-induced sepsis.[81] Clinical studies of patients with ARDS have demonstrated increased serum levels of TXA_2[82] and leukotrienes in BAL.[83] The generation of COX products by the lung is suggested by the finding in endotoxemic sheep that lung lymph concentrations exceed plasma levels.[84] Several animal studies of sepsis have successfully attenuated the early changes in pulmonary hemodynamics using COX inhibitors or thromboxane receptor antagonists with a corresponding improvement in survival.[85,86] Trials of COX inhibitors in patients are currently underway in the United States.

Manipulation of Endothelium-Derived Vasoactive Factors in Lung Injury

Despite recent advances in understanding of the role of the endothelium in the modulation of the pathophysiology of lung injury, successful therapeutic intervention, as judged by a reduction in mortality reduction, remains elusive. However, this enhanced understanding has led to the development of new strategies whose potential are not yet fully realized.

Nitric Oxide Synthase Inhibitors

The theoretical attraction of inhibiting NOS in sepsis is clear: the restoration of systemic vascular tone with elevation in the systemic vascular resistance and systemic blood pressure, resulting in improved organ perfusion. Nonspecific inhibitors of NOS have been shown in small numbers of cases to improve systemic blood pressure in patients with refractory septic shock.[42] However, in one series, N-nitro-L-arginine (L-NNA) was shown to increase not only systemic vascular resistance (SVR), but also PVR.[87] This highlights the theoretical disadvantage of nonselective NOS inhibition: complete NOS inhibition, even in a patient with septic shock, may have deleterious cardiovascular side effects. In particular, the pulmonary hypertension that is characteristically seen in lung injury may be exacerbated. In addition, there is preliminary evidence that the balance between constitutive and inducible NOS isoforms is an important determinant of local vascular tone in the septic circulation,[50] and that a sweeping disruption of this balance may be disadvantageous. Laboratory-derived data suggest that certain vascular beds may require NO to maintain perfusion, even in sepsis. For example, in one study,[88] pretreatment with L-NMMA, but not with phenylephrine, increased microvascular damage in the intestine of LPS-treated rats. In the isolated perfused pulmonary circulation, rats treated with LPS exhibit hypersensitivity to constrictors including ET-1, a response exacerbated by pretreatment with L-NMMA.[71]

The theoretical disadvantages of nonselective NOS inhibition can, to a great extent, be avoided if the inhibition is either incomplete or is restricted to the inducible enzyme only. The opportunity to use a selective iNOS inhibitor has now presented itself. Aminoguanidine is approximately seven times more potent for inhibition of iNOS and 15 times less potent for inhibition of cNOS than L-NMMA.[89] In LPS-treated rats, aminoguanidine has been shown to selectively inhibit iNOS.[43,49,90] Clinical studies are now underway to investigate the therapeutic potential of NOS inhibitors in critically ill septic patients. Unfortunately, the universal application of any such agent may prove beneficial only in certain areas of the circulation while proving harmful in others.

Inhaled NO

The administration of NO by inhalation to patients with sepsis complicated by lung injury is an elegant concept by which vasodilation of blood vessels occurs only in the areas of the lung that are ventilated. The improved blood flow through the pulmonary circulation is therefore targeted to areas that can oxygenate it, hence maintaining ventilation-perfusion matching but reducing PVR, thereby also improving right ventricular ejection fraction.[91] Furthermore, NO, upon reaching the blood, is rapidly inactivated by heme, thus its potential for causing more widespread (deleterious) vasodilation is removed. Indeed, in a pig model of sepsis, inhaled NO attenuated pulmonary hypertension but did not affect SVR or cardiac output.[92] In patients with ARDS, this therapy has been shown to attenuate pulmonary hypertension and to improve the efficiency of arterial oxygenation[93] while having no effects on systemic hemodynamic parameters. Preliminary data imply that only certain subgroups of patients with lung injury are likely to benefit from inhaled NO therapy; there is inherent anxiety that some subgroups may simply not respond or may even deteriorate as a result of this therapy.[94] Large-scale randomized trials of this therapy are required to confirm its clinical utility and safety, and above all to find out which patients will have an improved outcome when exposed to it.

Cyclooxygenase Inhibitors

Experimental data derived from animal models suggest that mortality can be reduced by application of COX inhibitors in sepsis.[95] It is perhaps surprising that despite encouraging preclinical and clinical data,[1,96] this strategy has not attracted more widespread interest.

Endothelin Antagonists/Antibodies

To date there are no data to support the use of ET antagonists in sepsis or in lung injury. Further evidence is required to dissect out the precise role of ET-1 in different vascular beds before such interventions can be justified clinically. Indeed, some animal experiments suggest that nonselective antagonism of ET receptors in endotoxemia may exacerbate systemic hypotension.[97] By contrast, blood urea and creatinine levels as well as urine output were improved in a rat model of endotoxemia by the administration of an anti-ET-1 antibody.[98] It is conceivable that tailored delivery of selective ET antagonists or antibodies may attenuate the pulmonary hypertension of acute lung injury, as well as improve function of other organs, without simultaneously having deleterious effects on others.

Summary

Acute lung injury occurs in association with a variety of pulmonary and extrapulmonary pathologies. Damage to the pulmonary vascular endothelium is a fundamental step in the initiation and mediation of the inflammatory process that produces tissue injury. Clearly the endothelium and its release of NO, ET, and eicosanoids represents a dynamic fulcrum during sepsis, and the balance of these factors determine both the local pulmonary vascular tone and the extent of the inflammatory reaction. However, it is increasingly evident that other cell types, including vascular smooth muscle, can release these substances after exposure to LPS or to cytokines. Thus, during inflammatory events, the vascular smooth muscle may serve to compensate for a failing and damaged endothelium. Research is currently concerned with identifying therapeutic ways of altering the balance of these vasoactive and inflammatory mediators in a favorable way to dampen the inflammatory response and restore the usually beneficial effects of HPV, which is disrupted in lung injury.

References

1. Curzen NP, Griffiths MJD, Evans TW. Pulmonary vascular control mechanisms in lung injury. In: Morice AH (ed): *Clinical Pulmonary Hypertension.* London: Portland Press; 1995;171–202.
2. Bone RC, Balk R, Slotman G, et al. Adult respiratory distress syndrome. Sequence and importance of development of multiple organ failure. The Prostaglandin E1 Study Group. *Chest* 1992;101:320–326.
3. Fowler AA, Hamman RF, Zerbe GO, Benson KN, Hyers TM. Adult respiratory distress syndrome. Prognosis after onset. *Am Rev Respir Dis* 1985; 132:472–478.
4. Montgomery AB, Stager MA, Carrico CJ, Hudson LD. Causes of mortality in patients with the adult respiratory distress syndrome. *Am Rev Respir Dis* 1985;132:485–489.
5. Seidenfeld JJ, Pohl DF, Bell RC, Harris GD, Johanson WG Jr. Incidence, site, and outcome of infections in patients with the adult respiratory distress syndrome. *Am Rev Respir Dis* 1986;134:12–16.
6. Bone RC, Fisher CJ Jr, Clemmer TP, Slotman GJ, Metz CA, Balk RA. Sepsis syndrome: A valid clinical entity. Methylprednisolone Severe Sepsis Study Group. *Crit Care Med* 1989;17:389–393.
7. Bone RC. The pathogenesis of sepsis. *Ann Int Med* 1991;115:457–469.
8. Ferrari-Baliviera E, Mealy K, Smith RJ, Wilmore DW. Tumor necrosis factor induces adult respiratory distress syndrome in rats. *Arch Surg* 1989; 124:1400–1405.
9. Vijaykumar E, Raziuddin S, Wardle EN. Plasma endotoxin in patients with trauma, sepsis and severe haemorrhage. *Clin Int Care* 1991;2:4–9.
10. Jacobs RF, Tabor DR, Burks AW, Campbell GD. Elevated interleukin-1 release by human alveolar macrophages during the adult respiratory distress syndrome. *Am Rev Respir Dis* 1989;140:1686–1692.
11. Hyers TM, Tricomi SM, Dettenmeier PA, Fowler AA. Tumor necrosis factor levels in serum and bronchoalveolar lavage fluid of patients with the adult respiratory distress syndrome. *Am Rev Respir Dis* 1991;144:268–271.
12. Weiland JE, Davis WB, Holter JF, Mohammed JR, Dorinsky PM, Gadek JE.

Lung neutrophils in the adult respiratory distress syndrome. Clinical and pathophysiologic significance. *Am Rev Respir Dis* 1986;133:218–225.

13. Lee CT, Fein AM, Lippman M. Elastolytic activity in pulmonary lavage fluid from patients with adult respiratory distress syndrome. *N Engl J Med* 1981;304:192–194.

14. Curzen NP, Griffiths MJD, Evans TW. The role of the endothelium in modulating the vascular response to sepsis. *Clin Sci* 1994;86:359–374.

15. Phillips P, Tsan M. Cytoarchitectural aspects of endothelial barrier function in response to oxidants and inflammatory mediators. In: Johnson A, Ferro TJ (eds): *Lung Vascular Injury*. New York: Marcel Dekker; 1992.

16. Albelda SM, Smith CW, Ward PA. Adhesion molecules and inflammatory injury. *FASEB J* 1994;8:504–512.

17. Hamacher J, Schaberg T. Adhesion molecules in lung diseases. *Lung* 1994;172:189–213.

18. Macnaughton PD, Evans TW. Management of adult respiratory distress syndrome. *Lancet* 1992;339:469–472.

19. Murray JF, Matthay MA, Luce JM, Flick MR. An expanded definition of the adult respiratory distress syndrome. *Am Rev Respir Dis* 1988;138: 720–723.

20. Sloane PJ, Gee MH, Gottlieb JE, et al. A multicenter registry of patients with acute respiratory distress syndrome. Physiology and outcome. *Am Rev Respir Dis* 1992;146:419–426.

21. Zapol WM, Snider MT. Pulmonary hypertension in severe acute respiratory failure. *N Engl J Med* 1977;296:476–480.

22. Fox GA, McCormack DG. The pulmonary physician and critical care. 4. A new look at the pulmonary circulation in acute lung injury. *Thorax* 1992; 47:743–747.

23. Bernard GR, Rinaldo J, Harris T, et al. Early predictors of ARDS reversal in patients with established ARDS. *Am Rev Respir Dis* (Abstract) 1985; 131:A143.

24. Pallares LCM, Evans TW. Oxygen transport in the critically ill. *Respir Med* 1992;86:289–295.

25. Gutierrez G, Pohil RJ. Oxygen consumption is linearly related to oxygen supply in critically ill patients. *J Crit Care* 1986;1:45–53.

26. Schoemaker WC, Appel PL, Kram HB. Prospective trial of supranormal values of survivors as therapeutic goals in high risk surgical patients. *Chest* 1988;94:1176–1186.

27. Weir EK, Milczoch J, Reeves JT, Grover RF. Endotoxin and prevention of hypoxic pulmonary vasoconstriction. *J Lab Clin Med* 1976;68:975–983.

28. Dantzker DR, Brook CJ, Dehart P, Lynch JP, Weg JG. Ventilation-perfusion distributions in the adult respiratory distress syndrome. *Am Rev Respir Dis* 1979;120:1039–1052.

29. Holden WE, McCall E. Hypoxia-induced contractions of porcine pulmonary artery strips depend on intact endothelium. *Exp Lung Res* 1984; 7:101–112.

30. Rodman DM, Yamaguchi T, Hasunuma K, O'Brien RF, McMurtry IF. Effects of hypoxia on endothelium-dependent relaxation of rat pulmonary artery. *Am J Physiol* 1990;258:L207–L214.

31. Liu SF, Dewar A, Crawley DE, Barnes PJ, Evans TW. Effect of tumor necrosis factor on hypoxic pulmonary vasoconstriction. *J Appl Physiol* 1992;72:1044–1049.

32. Magee F, Wright JL, Wiggs BR, et al. Pulmonary vascular structure and

function in chronic obstructive pulmonary disease. *Thorax* 1988;43: 183–189.

33. Johnson AR, Erdos EG. Metabolism of vasoactive peptides by human endothelial cells in culture. *J Clin Invest* 1977;59:684–695.

34. Furchgott RF, Zawadzki JV. The obligatory role of endothelial cells in the relaxation of arterial smooth muscle by acetylcholine. *Nature* 1980;288: 373–376.

35. Moncada S, Higgs A. The L-arginine-nitric oxide pathway. *N Engl J Med* 1993;329:2002–2012.

36. Palmer RM, Ferrige AG, Moncada S. Nitric oxide release accounts for the biological activity of endothelium-derived relaxing factor. *Nature* 1987; 327:524–526.

37. Waldman SA, Murad F. Cyclic GMP synthesis and function. *Pharmacol Rev* (Abstract) 1987;39:163–196.

38. Bredt DS, Snyder SH. Isolation of nitric oxide synthetase, a calmodulin-requiring enzyme. *Proc Natl Acad Sci U S A* 1990;87:682–685.

39. Pollock JS, Forstermann U, Mitchell JA, et al. Purification and characterization of particulate endothelium-derived relaxant factor synthase from cultured and native bovine aortic endothelial cells. *Proc Natl Acad Sci U S A* 1991;88:10480–10484.

40. Stuehr DJ, Cho HJ, Kwon NS, Weise M, Nathan CF. Purification and characterisation of the cytokine-induced nitric oxide synthase an FAD and FMN containing protein. *Proc Natl Acad Sci U S A* 1991;88:7773–7777.

41. Rees DD, Palmer RM, Moncada S. Role of endothelium-derived nitric oxide in the regulation of blood pressure. *Proc Natl Acad Sci U S A* 1989; 86:3375–3378.

42. Petros A, Bennett D, Vallance P. Effect of nitric oxide synthase inhibitors on hypotension in patients with septic shock. *Lancet* 1991;338:1557–1558.

43. Griffiths MJD, Messent M, MacAllister RJ, Evans TW. Aminoguanidine selectively inhibits inducible nitric oxide synthase. *Br J Pharmacol* 1993; 110:963–968.

44. Salter M, Knowles RG, Moncada S. Widespread tissue distribution, species distribution and changes in activity of Ca(2+)-dependent and Ca(2+)-independent nitric oxide synthases. *FEBS Lett* 1991;291:145–149.

45. Mitchell JA, Kohlhaas KL, Sorrentino R, Warner TD, Murad F, Vane JR. Induction by endotoxin of nitric oxide synthase in the rat mesentery: Lack of effect on action of vasoconstrictors. *Br J Pharmacol* 1993;109:265–270.

46. Liu S, Adcock IM, Old RW, Barnes PJ, Evans TW. Lipopolysaccharide treatment in vivo induces widespread tissue expression of inducible nitric oxide synthase mRNA. *Biochem Biophys Res Commun* 1993;196:1208–1213.

47. Szabo C, Mitchell JA, Thiemermann C, Vane JR. Nitric oxide-mediated hyporeactivity to noradrenaline precedes the induction of nitric oxide synthase in endotoxin shock. *Br J Pharmacol* 1993;108:786–792.

48. Martin JF, Booth RF, Moncada S. Arterial wall hypoxia following thrombosis of the vasa vasorum is an initial lesion in atherosclerosis. *Eur J Clin Invest* 1991;21:355–359.

49. Griffiths MJD, Liu S, Curzen N, Messent M, Evans TW. In vivo treatment with endotoxin induces nitric oxide synthase in rat main pulmonary artery. *Am J Physiol* 1995;268:L509–L518.

50. Liu S, Adcock IM, Barnes PJ, Evans TW. Differential regulation of the constitutive and inducible NO synthase mRNA by endotoxin in vivo in the rat. *Am J Respir Crit Care Med* (Abstract) 1995;151:A15.

51. Busse R, Mulsch A, Fleming I, Hecker M. Mechanisms of nitric oxide release from the vascular endothelium. *Circulation* 1993;87:V18–V25.
52. Fleming I, Gray GA, Schott C, Stoclet JC. Inducible but not constitutive production of nitric oxide by vascular smooth muscle cells. *Eur J Pharmacol* 1991;200:375–376.
53. Brady AJ, Poole-Wilson PA, Harding SE, Warren JB. Nitric oxide production within cardiac myocytes reduces their contractility in endotoxemia. *Am J Physiol* 1992;263:H1963–H1966.
54. Brady AJB, Warren JB, Poole-Wilson PA, Williams TJ, Harding SE. Nitric oxide attenuates cardiac myocyte contraction. *Am J Physiol* 1993;265: H176–H182.
55. Zelenkov P, McLoughlin T, Johns RA. Endotoxin enhances hypoxic constriction of rat aorta and pulmonary artery through induction of EDRF/ NO synthase. *Am J Physiol* 1993;9:346–354.
56. Yanagisawa M, Kurihara H, Kimura S, et al. A novel potent vasoconstrictor peptide produced by vascular endothelial cells *Nature* 1988;332:411–415.
57. Haynes WG, Webb DJ. The endothelin family of peptides: Local hormones with diverse roles in health and disease? *Clin Sci* 1993;84:485–500.
58. Rubanyi GM, Polokoff MA. Endothelins: Molecular biology, biochemistry, pharmacology, physiology, and pathophysiology. *Pharmacol Rev* 1994;46:325–415.
59. Bax WA, Saxena PR. The current endothelin receptor classification: time for reconsideration? *Trends Pharmacol Sci* 1994;15:379–386.
60. Reynolds EE, Mok LLS. Role of thromboxane A2/prostaglandin H2 receptor in the vasoconstrictor response of rat aorta to endothelin. *J Pharmacol Exp Ther* 1989;252:915–921.
61. de Nucci G, Thomas R, D'Orleans-Juste P, et al. Pressor effects of circulating endothelin are limited by its removal in the pulmonary circulation and by the release of prostacyclin and EDRF. *Proc Natl Acad Sci U S A* 1988;85:9797–9800.
62. Gardiner SM, Compton AM, Kemp PA, Bennett T. Regional and cardiac haemodynamic effects of NG-nitro-L-arginine methyl ester in conscious, Long Evans rats. *Br J Pharmacol* 1990;101:625–631.
63. Weitzberg E. Circulatory responses to endothelin-1 and nitric oxide. *Acta Physiol Scand* 1993;148:S611–S672.
64. Sirvio ML, Metsarinne K, Fyhrquist F. Tissue distribution and half-life of ^{125}I-endothelin in the rat: Importance of pulmonary clearance. *Biochem Biophys Res Commun* 1990;167:1191–1195.
65. Pittet JF, Morel DR, Hemsen A, et al. Elevated plasma endothelin-1 concentrations are associated with the severity of illness in patients with sepsis. *Ann Surg* 1991;213:261–264.
66. Wagner OF, Christ G, Wojta J, et al. Polar secretion of endothelin-1 by cultured endothelial cells. *J Biol Chem* 1992;267:16066–16068.
67. Kaddoura S, Curzen N, Firth J, Sugden PH, Poole-Wilson PA, Evans TW. Tissue expression of endothelin-1 mRNA in endotoxaemia. *Clin Sci* 1995; 88:12P.
68. Curzen NP, Kaddoura S, Sugden PH, Poole-Wilson PA, Evans TW. Vascular expression of endothelin-1 mRNA increases in sepsis. *Br Heart J* (Abstract) 1995;73:P46.
69. Langleben D, De Marchie M, Laporta D, Spanier AH, Schlesinger RD, Stewart DJ. Endothelin-1 in acute lung injury and the adult respiratory distress syndrome. *Am Rev Respir Dis* 1993;148:1646–1650.

70. Curzen NP, Griffiths MJD, Evans TW. Contraction to endothelin-1 in pulmonary arteries from endotoxin-treated rats is modulated by endothelium. *Am J Physiol* 1995;37:H2260–H2266.
71. Curzen NP, Griffiths MJD, Evans TW. Is the pulmonary circulation hypersensitive to endothelin-1 in sepsis? *Heart* (Abstract) 1996;75:P9.
72. Lundberg JM, Weitzberg E, Rudehill A, Hemsen A, Modin A. The endothelin receptor antagonist bosentan reduces pulmonary hypertension in endotoxin shock. *Am J Respir Crit Care Med* 1995;151:A317.
73. Curzen NP, Griffiths MJD, Evans TW. Bosentan does not reduce systemic or pulmonary artery pressures in rat endotoxaemia. *Thorax* (Abstract) 1995.
74. Gardiner SM, Kemp PA, March JE, Bennett T. Effects of the non-peptide, non-selective endothelin antagonist, bosentan, on regional haemodynamic responses to N^G-mono-methyl-L-arginine in conscious rats. *Br J Pharmacol* 1996;118:352–354.
75. Mitchell JA, Larkin S, Williams TJ. Cyclooxygenase-2: Regulation and relevance in inflammation. *Biochem Pharmacol* 1995;50:1535–1542.
76. Swierkosz TA, Mitchell JA, Warner TD, Botting RM, Vane JR. Co-induction of nitric oxide synthase and cyclooxygenase: Interactions between nitric oxide and prostanoids. *Br J Pharmacol* 1995;114:1335–1342.
77. Masferrer JL, Zweifel BS, Manning PT, et al. Selective inhibition of inducible cyclooxygenase 2 in vivo is anti-inflammatory and non-ulcerogenic. *Proc Natl Acad Sci U S A* 1994;91:3228–3232.
78. Hla T, Neilson K. Human cyclooxygenase-2 cDNA. *Proc Natl Acad Sci U S A* 1992;89:7384–7388.
79. Akarasereenont P, Mitchell JA, Appleton I, Thiemermann C, Vane JR. Involvement of protein tyrosine phosphorylation in the induction of cyclooxygenase and nitric oxide synthase by endotoxin in cultured cells. *Br J Pharmacol* (Abstract) 1994;113:1522–1528.
80. Petrak RA, Balk RA, Bone RC. Prostaglandins, cyclo-oxygenase inhibitors, and thromboxane synthetase inhibitors in the pathogenesis of multiple systems organ failure. *Crit Care Clin* 1989;5:303–314.
81. Winn R, Harlan J, Nadir B, et al. Thromboxane A2 mediates vasoconstriction but not permeability after endotoxin. *J Clin Invest* 1983;72:911–918.
82. Leeman M, Boeynaems JM, Degaute JP, Vincent JL, Kahn RJ. Administration of dazoxiben, a selective thromboxane synthetase inhibitor, in the adult respiratory distress syndrome. *Chest* 1985;87:726–730.
83. Matthay MA, Eschenbacher WL, Goetzel EJ. Elevated concentrations of leukotriene D4 in pulmonary oedema fluid of patients with the adult respiratory distress syndrome. *J Clin Immunol* 1984;4:479–483.
84. Ogletree ML, Begley CJ, King GA, Brigham KL. Influence of steroidal and nonsteroidal anti-inflammatory agents on the accumulation of arachidonic acid metabolites in plasma and lung lymph after endotoxemia in awake sheep. Measurements of prostacyclin and thromboxane metabolites and 12-HETE. *Am Rev Respir Dis* 1986;133:55–61.
85. Ahmed T, Wasserman MA, Muccitelli R, Tucker S, Gazeroglu H, Marchette B. Endotoxin-induced changes in pulmonary hemodynamics and respiratory mechanics: Role of lipoxygenase and cyclooxygenase products. *Am Rev Respir Dis* 1986;134:1149–1157.
86. Harlan RWJ, Harker BNL, Hilderbrandt J. Thromboxane A2 mediates lung vasoconstriction but not permeability after endotoxin. *J Clin Invest* 1983;72:911–918.

87. Lorente JA, Landin L, de Pablo R, Renes E, Liste D. L-arginine pathway in the sepsis syndrome. *Crit Care Med* 1993;21:1287–1295.
88. Hutcheson IR, Whittle BJ, Boughton-Smith NK. Role of nitric oxide in maintaining vascular integrity in endotoxin-induced acute intestinal damage in the rat. *Br J Pharmacol* 1990;101:815–820.
89. Tilton RG, Chang C, Hasan KS, et al. Prevention of diabetic vascular dysfunction by guanidines: Inhibition of nitric oxide synthase versus advanced glycation end-product formation. *Diabetes* 1993;42:221–232.
90. Misko TP, Moore WM, Kasten TP, et al. Selective inhibition of the inducible nitric oxide synthase by aminoguanidine. *Eur J Pharmacol* 1993; 233:119–125.
91. Rossaint R, Slama K, Steudel W, et al. Effects of inhaled nitric oxide on right ventricular function in severe acute respiratory distress syndrome. *Intensive Care Med* 1995;21:197–203.
92. Weitzberg E, Rudehill A, Lundberg JM. Nitric oxide inhalation attenuates pulmonary hypertension and improves gas exchange in endotoxin shock. *Eur J Pharmacol* 1993;233:85–94.
93. Rossaint R, Falke KJ, Lopez F, Slama K, Pison U, Zapol WM. Inhaled nitric oxide for the adult respiratory distress syndrome. *N Engl J Med* 1993;328:399–405.
94. Krafft P, Fridrich P, Fitzgerald RD, Koc D, Steltzer H. Effectiveness of nitric oxide inhalation in septic ARDS. *Chest* 1996;109:486–493.
95. Metz C, Sibbald WJ. Anti-inflammatory therapy for acute lung injury. A review of animal and clinical studies. *Chest* 1991;100:1110–1119.
96. Bernard GR, Reines HD, Metz CA, et al. Effects of a short course of ibuprofen in patients with severe sepsis. *Am Rev Respir Dis* (Abstract) 1988; 137:A138.
97. Gardiner SM, Kemp PA, March JE, Bennett T. Enhancement of the hypotensive and vasodilator effects of endotoxaemia in conscious rats by the endothelin antagonist, SB 209670. *Br J Pharmacol* 1995;116:1718–1719.
98. Morise Z, Ueda M, Aiura K, Endo M, Kitajima M. Pathophysiologic role of endothelin-1 in renal function in rats with endotoxin shock. *Surgery* 1994;115:199–204.

Index